Interventional and Device Therapy in Heart Failure

Editors

DEEPAK L. BHATT
MICHAEL R. GOLD

HEART FAILURE CLINICS

www.heartfailure.theclinics.com

Consulting Editors
MANDEEP R. MEHRA
JAVED BUTLER

April 2015 • Volume 11 • Number 2

ELSEVIER

1600 John F. Kennedy Boulevard • Suite 1800 • Philadelphia, Pennsylvania, 19103-2899

http://www.theclinics.com

HEART FAILURE CLINICS Volume 11, Number 2
April 2015 ISSN 1551-7136, ISBN-13: 978-0-323-35975-7

Editor: Adrianne Brigido
Developmental Editor: Susan Showalter

Heart Failure Clinics (ISSN 1551-7136) is published quarterly by Elsevier Inc., 360 Park Avenue South, New York, NY 10010-1710. Months of publication are January, April, July, and October. Business and editorial offices: 1600 John F. Kennedy Boulevard, Suite 1800, Philadelphia, PA 19103-2899. Periodicals postage paid at New York, NY, and additional mailing offices. Subscription prices are USD 235.00 per year for US individuals, USD 382.00 per year for US institutions, USD 80.00 per year for US students and residents, USD 280.00 per year for Canadian individuals, USD 442.00 per year for Canadian institutions, USD 300.00 per year for international individuals, USD 442.00 per year for international institutions, and USD 100.00 per year for Canadian and foreign students/residents. To receive student and resident rate, orders must be accompanied by name of affiliated institution, date of term, and the *signature* of program/residency coordinator on institution letterhead. Orders will be billed at individual rate until proof of status is received. Foreign air speed delivery is included in all *Clinics* subscription prices. All prices are subject to change without notice. **POSTMASTER:** Send address changes to *Heart Failure Clinics*, Elsevier Health Sciences Division, Subscription Customer Service, 3251 Riverport Lane, Maryland Heights, MO 63043. **Customer Service: 1-800-654-2452 (US and Canada). From outside of the US and Canada, call 314-447-8871. Fax: 314-447-8029. For print support, E-mail: JournalsCustomerService-usa@elsevier.com. For online support, E-mail: JournalsOnlineSupport-usa@elsevier.com.**

Reprints. For copies of 100 or more of articles in this publication, please contact the Commercial Reprints Department, Elsevier Inc., 360 Park Avenue South, New York, NY 10010-1710. Tel.: 212-633-3874; Fax: 212-633-3820; E-mail: reprints@elsevier.com.

Heart Failure Clinics is covered in *MEDLINE/PubMed (Index Medicus).*

Contributors

CONSULTING EDITORS

MANDEEP R. MEHRA, MD
Professor of Medicine, Harvard Medical
School; Medical Director, BWH Heart and
Vascular Center, Brigham and Women's
Hospital, Boston, Massachusetts

JAVED BUTLER, MD, MPH
Division Chief, Cardiology and Co-Director,
Stony Brook University Heart Institute
Professor, Department of Internal Medicine,
Stony Brook School of Medicine, Stony Brook
University Medical Center, Stony Brook,
New York

EDITORS

DEEPAK L. BHATT, MD, MPH, FACC, FAHA, FSCAI, FESC
Executive Director of Interventional
Cardiovascular Programs, Brigham and
Women's Hospital Heart & Vascular Center;
Professor of Medicine, Harvard Medical
School, Boston, Massachusetts

MICHAEL R. GOLD, MD, PhD, FACC, FHRS
Michael E. Assey Professor of Medicine;
Chief of Cardiology, Medical University of
South Carolina, Charleston, South Carolina

AUTHORS

PHILIP AAGAARD, MD, PhD
Albert Einstein College of Medicine, Montefiore
Hospital, Bronx, New York

WILLIAM T. ABRAHAM, MD, FACP, FACC, FAHA, FESC, FRCP
Professor of Internal Medicine, Physiology, and
Cell Biology, Chair of Excellence in
Cardiovascular Medicine, Director, Division of
Cardiovascular Medicine, The Ohio State
University, Columbus, Ohio

SADEER G. AL-KINDI, MD
Advanced Heart Failure and Transplant Center,
Harrington Heart & Vascular Institute,
University Hospitals Case Medical Center,
Department of Medicine; Case Western
Reserve University, Cleveland, Ohio

GUILHERME ATTIZZANI, MD
Advanced Heart Failure and Transplant Center,
Harrington Heart & Vascular Institute,
University Hospitals Case Medical Center,
Department of Medicine; Case Western
Reserve University, Cleveland, Ohio

JOHN P. BOEHMER, MD
Professor of Medicine; Director, Heart Failure
Program, Division of Cardiology, Penn State
Hershey Medical Center, Hershey,
Pennsylvania

NEAL A. CHATTERJEE, MD
Cardiology Division, Department of
Medicine, Massachusetts General Hospital,
Harvard Medical School, Boston,
Massachusetts

WILLIAM W.B. CHIK, MBBS, MD, PhD
Division of Cardiovascular Medicine,
Department of Cardiac Electrophysiology,
Hospital of the University of Pennsylvania,
Philadelphia, Pennsylvania

MARCO COSTA, MD
Advanced Heart Failure and Transplant
Center, Harrington Heart & Vascular
Institute, University Hospitals Case
Medical Center, Department of Medicine;
Case Western Reserve University,
Cleveland, Ohio

LUIGI DI BIASE, MD, PhD, FACC, FHRS
Albert Einstein College of Medicine, Montefiore Hospital, Bronx, New York; Texas Cardiac Arrhythmia Institute, St David's Medical Center, Austin, Texas; Department of Cardiology, University of Foggia, Foggia, Italy

STEPHEN G. ELLIS, MD
Section Head of Invasive/Interventional Cardiology, Department of Cardiovascular Medicine, The Cleveland Clinic Foundation, Cleveland, Ohio

MICHELE ESPOSITO, MD
The Cardiovascular Center, Tufts Medical Center, Boston, Massachusetts

TED FELDMAN, MD, FESC, FACC, MSCAI
NorthShore University HealthSystem, Evanston, Illinois

DOMINIQUE HIMBERT, MD
Director of the Structural Program, Department of Cardiology, Bichat-Claude Bernard Hospital, Assistance Publique Hôpitaux de Paris, Paris, France

MOBOLAJI IGE, MD
Advanced Heart Failure and Transplant Center, Harrington Heart & Vascular Institute, University Hospitals Case Medical Center, Department of Medicine; Case Western Reserve University, Cleveland, Ohio

NAVIN K. KAPUR, MD
The Cardiovascular Center, Tufts Medical Center, Boston, Massachusetts

FRANCIS E. MARCHLINSKI, MD
Professor of Medicine, Division of Cardiovascular Medicine, Director, Department of Cardiac Electrophysiology, Hospital of the University of Pennsylvania, Philadelphia, Pennsylvania

ANDREA NATALE, MD, FACC, FHRS, FESC
Texas Cardiac Arrhythmia Institute, St David's Medical Center, Austin, Texas; Department of Biomedical Engineering, University of Texas, Austin, Texas; Division of Cardiology, Stanford University, Stanford, California; Case Western Reserve University, Cleveland, Ohio; EP Services, California Pacific Medical Center, San Francisco, California; Interventional Electrophysiology, Scripps Clinic, San Diego, California

GUILHERME H. OLIVEIRA, MD
Associate Professor of Medicine, Director, Advanced Heart Failure and Transplant Center, Harrington Heart & Vascular Institute, University Hospitals Case Medical Center, Department of Medicine; Case Western Reserve University, Cleveland, Ohio

AMIT N. PATEL, MD, MS
University of Utah School of Medicine, Salt Lake City, Utah; Director of Cardiovascular Regenerative Medicine, Director of the Optimist Program, Associate Professor of Surgery (Tenured), University of Utah, Salt Lake City, Utah

HARSH C. PATEL, MD
Fellow, Department of Cardiovascular Medicine, The Cleveland Clinic Foundation, Cleveland, Ohio

MOHAMMAD SARRAF, MD
NorthShore University HealthSystem, Evanston, Illinois

MARK J. SHEN, MD
Krannert Institute of Cardiology, Department of Medicine, Indiana University School of Medicine, Indianapolis, Indiana

FRANCISCO SILVA, MS
University of Utah School of Medicine, Salt Lake City, Utah

JAGMEET P. SINGH, MD, DPhil
Associate Professor of Medicine, Harvard Medical School, Cardiology Division, Electrophysiology Laboratory, Cardiac Arrhythmia Service, Department of Medicine, Massachusetts General Hospital, Boston, Massachusetts

ALEC VAHANIAN, MD
Professor, Head of the Cardiology Department, Department of Cardiology, Bichat-Claude Bernard Hospital, Assistance Publique Hôpitaux de Paris, Paris, France

AMALIA A. WINTERS, BSc
University of Utah School of Medicine, Salt Lake City, Utah

DOUGLAS P. ZIPES, MD
Krannert Institute of Cardiology, Department of Medicine, Indiana University School of Medicine, Indianapolis, Indiana

Contents

and human testing, with proved feasibility and safety, and is currently being studied in a pivotal randomized clinical trial. This article discusses ventricular remodeling and therapies attempted in the past, details the components of the ventricular partitioning device, describes the implanting technique, and reviews the most current experience of this device in humans.

implantable cardiac defibrillators (ICD). Although ICDs are highly effective in reducing sudden cardiac death by termination of VA, they do not prevent arrhythmia recurrences. Recurrent shocks are not only associated with poor quality of life but also progressive HF and increased mortality and morbidity. Radiofrequency catheter ablation has emerged as an important therapeutic option for patients with drug-refractory ventricular tachycardia to reduce or prevent ICD shocks.

Heart failure is an increasingly prevalent disease with high mortality and public health burden. It is associated with autonomic imbalance characterized by sympathetic hyperactivity and parasympathetic hypoactivity. Evolving novel interventional and device-based therapies have sought to restore autonomic balance by neuro-modulation. Results of preclinical animal studies and early clinical trials have demon-strated the safety and efficacy of these therapies in heart failure. This article discusses specific neuromodulatory treatment modalities individually—spinal cord stimulation, vagus nerve stimulation, baroreceptor activation therapy, and renal sympathetic nerve denervation.

HEART FAILURE CLINICS

NOW AVAILABLE FOR YOUR iPhone and iPad

Foreword

The Hi-Tech Age of Heart Failure Management

 CrossMark

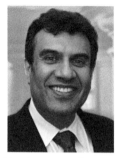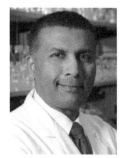

Mandeep R. Mehra, MD   Javed Butler, MD, MPH

Consulting Editors

It is hard to believe the progress of medicine in our lifetime. Up until the 1970s, there was practically no therapy available for the management of patients with heart failure barring the use of diuretics for symptom and congestion improvement, and an experience-based use of digoxin without any definitive evidence for either its safety or its efficacy.

This paradigm shifted in the 1980s with better understanding of cardiovascular hemodynamics. Subsequent studies tested the effects of both oral and intravenous vasodilators for the management of patients with heart failure. With evidence that hemodynamic modulation with vasodilators can improve cardiac output and patient symptoms acutely, longer-term trials initially with the combination of hydralazine and isosorbide dinitrate, and later with angiotensin-converting enzyme inhibitors, were conducted. These studies showed that vasodilator therapy improves patient symptoms, stops the adverse cardiac remodeling process, and decreases the risk of hospitalization and mortality among outpatients with heart failure and reduced ejection fraction.

The hemodynamic paradigm of heart failure management was augmented in the 1990s with the use of neurohormonal modulation. This evolution was aided by studies showing that angiotensin-converting enzyme inhibitors improve outcomes better than direct vasodilators without an incremental added hemodynamic benefit to explain the clinical outcome improvement. This led to further studies with neurohormonal modula-

tors targeting the sympathetic nervous system as well as aldosterone. While the pharmacologic advances were moving ahead, so was device-based therapy for the management of patients with heart failure and reduced ejection fraction with implanted defibrillators and with cardiac resynchronization therapy.

While these advances targeting the vast majority of *routine* heart failure patients with reduced ejection fraction in the outpatient setting in the 1990s were being successfully conducted, there was a growing appreciation of the need for treatment options for the two extremes of heart failure: one for prevention of worsening heart failure episodes and the other for options for patients with more advanced disease, including those with structural heart disease. These gaps were the focus of innovation and research in the 2000s and have led now to many hi-tech options for the management of these patients.

Under the erudite editorship of Drs Deepak L. Bhatt and Michael R. Gold, we are very proud to present this issue of the *Heart Failure Clinics* focusing on interventional and device-based therapy for heart failure. The expert commentaries included in this issue are both varied and extremely important. They include the use of hemodynamic and nonhemodynamic data from an implanted device that can be captured remotely and may affect early detection and treatment of worsening heart failure episodes, preventing unnecessary hospitalization. Also discussed is the fast growing field of percutaneous procedural options for patients with

Heart Failure Clin 11 (2015) xi–xii
http://dx.doi.org/10.1016/j.hfc.2015.01.002
1551-7136/15/$ – see front matter © 2015 Published by Elsevier Inc.

heartfailure.theclinics.com

aortic or mitral valve disease, remodeled ventricles, advanced coronary disease, or those requiring hemodynamic support. Management of both atrial and ventricular arrhythmias continues to evolve, and the latest advances are presented. Other topics include the promising but not yet ready for clinical use application of autonomic modulation as well as stem cell therapies.

We hope that these hi-tech advances for the management of heart failure patients will continue to evolve and improve the longevity and quality of lives for our patients. We also hope that with ongoing research and innovation, soon we will look back at these *hi-tech* advances as not-so-hi-tech. But, in the meantime, this issue of *Heart Failure Clinics* will be an invaluable resource for both clinicians and researchers alike.

Mandeep R. Mehra, MD
Harvard Medical School
BWH Heart and Vascular Center
Brigham and Women's Hospital
75 Francis Street
A Building, 3rd Floor, Room AB324
Boston, MA 02115, USA

Javed Butler, MD, MPH
Stony Brook University Heart Institute
Department of Internal Medicine
Stony Brook School of Medicine
Stony Brook University Medical Center
101 Nicolls Rd, Stony Brook, NY 11794, USA

E-mail addresses:
mmehra@partners.org (M.R. Mehra)
javed.butler@emory.edu (J. Butler)

Preface

Expanding the Boundaries of Heart Failure Care with Interventional and Device Therapy

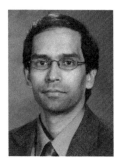   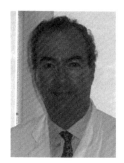

Deepak L. Bhatt, MD, MPH, FACC, FAHA, FSCAI, FESC   Michael R. Gold, MD, PhD, FACC, FHRS

Editors

Pharmacologic therapy has been the mainstay of treatment of heart failure for decades. More recently, interventional and device therapies have revolutionized the management of patients with heart failure. Advances in these areas of cardiology have improved the prognosis of patients with left ventricular dysfunction in both the acute and the chronic stages of the disease process. In this issue of *Heart Failure Clinics*, we have been fortunate to assemble the foremost electrophysiologists, heart failure specialists, and interventionalists to provide their expertise in these evolving, multidisciplinary areas. Notably, these leaders bring both academic knowledge and clinical acumen to their writing.

The timing of this issue could not have been better, as multiple lines of investigation are converging to benefit patients with heart failure. Advances in diagnosis, such as with implantable hemodynamic monitoring, are completely changing our paradigm for managing heart failure—both with reduced ejection fraction and with preserved ejection fraction. Revascularization with coronary artery bypass surgery and, increasingly, via percutaneous techniques provides effective therapy for many patients with ischemic heart failure. Exciting developments in percutaneous hemodynamic support and transcatheter therapies for aortic and mitral disease are redefining the limits of care. Percutaneous left ventricular remodeling and percutaneous delivery of stem cells are being actively studied in several trials. Ablation of atrial and ventricular arrhythmia as well as cardiac resynchronization therapy provides hope for many patients with heart failure. Device therapy to achieve autonomic modulation is being explored as a new approach to treat heart failure and should provide insight into underlying mechanisms of disease.

The evidence base in these areas is growing rapidly, and the authors have synthesized the relevant issues quite nicely. We hope our readers find this collection of topics interesting, informative, and useful in their daily care of patients with heart failure.

Deepak L. Bhatt, MD, MPH, FACC, FAHA, FSCAI, FESC
Brigham and Women's Hospital Heart & Vascular Center
Harvard Medical School
Boston, MA 02115, USA

Michael R. Gold, MD, PhD, FACC, FHRS
Medical University of South Carolina
Charleston, SC 29425, USA

E-mail addresses:
dlbhattmd@post.harvard.edu (D.L. Bhatt)
goldmr@musc.edu (M.R. Gold)

Heart Failure Clin 11 (2015) xiii
http://dx.doi.org/10.1016/j.hfc.2015.01.001
1551-7136/15/$ – see front matter © 2015 Published by Elsevier Inc.

The Role of Implantable Hemodynamic Monitors to Manage Heart Failure

William T. Abraham, MD, FACP, FACC, FAHA, FESC, FRCP

KEYWORDS

- Disease management • Heart failure • Hemodynamics • Hospitalization • Left atrial pressure
- Pulmonary artery pressure • Quality of life

KEY POINTS

- Heart failure is associated with high rates of hospitalization and rehospitalization.
- Current approaches to monitoring heart failure have done little to reduce these high rates of hospitalization and rehospitalization.
- Implantable hemodynamic monitors provide direct measurements of intracardiac and pulmonary artery pressures in ambulatory patients with heart failure.
- Heart failure care guided by implantable hemodynamic monitors reduces the risk of heart failure hospitalization and improves quality of life.

INTRODUCTION

Heart failure represents a major and growing public health concern, associated with high rates of hospitalization and rehospitalization. Heart failure is the primary diagnosis in more than 1 million hospitalizations annually in the United States.[1] It is associated with the highest rate of hospital readmission compared with all other medical or surgical causes of hospitalization.[2] Approximately 25% of discharged patients are readmitted within 30 days and about 67% are readmitted within 1 year, following the index hospitalization.[2–4] Lack of improvement in health-related quality of life after discharge from the hospital is a powerful predictor of rehospitalization and mortality.[5]

Hospitalization for heart failure results in a substantial economic burden. In 2012, the US total economic burden from heart failure was estimated at $31 billion.[1] The direct costs of heart failure in the United States are estimated at $21 billion annually; of this amount, 80% of costs are from hospitalizations.[6] Without improvements in current clinical outcomes, the US total economic burden from heart failure is expected to rise to $70 billion annually by the year 2030.[1,6] Consequently, a major goal in heart failure management is to keep patients well and out of the hospital and to reduce these costs.

Unfortunately, current approaches to monitoring patients with heart failure have generally focused on insensitive noninvasive markers of heart failure clinical status and failed to improve quality of life or to reduce hospitalization rates. Worsening heart failure symptoms, changes in vital signs, and weight gain are late and unreliable markers of worsening heart failure. Implantable hemodynamic monitors, which remotely provide direct measurement of intracardiac and pulmonary artery pressures (PAP) in ambulatory patients with heart

Disclosures: Dr W.T. Abraham has received consulting fees from CardioMEMS for his role as Co-Principal Investigator of the CHAMPION trial and from St. Jude Medical for his role as Principal Investigator of the HOMEOSTASIS and LAPTOP-HF trials.
Division of Cardiovascular Medicine, The Ohio State University, 473 West 12th Avenue, Room 110P, Columbus, OH 43210–1252, USA
E-mail address: William.Abraham@osumc.edu

Heart Failure Clin 11 (2015) 183–189
http://dx.doi.org/10.1016/j.hfc.2014.12.011
1551-7136/15/$ – see front matter © 2015 Elsevier Inc. All rights reserved.

failure, enable a proactive approach that shifts the focus from crisis management to stability management in patients with heart failure. This article reviews current knowledge on the role of implantable hemodynamic monitors in heart failure management.

LIMITATIONS OF CURRENT STANDARD OF CARE MONITORING IN HEART FAILURE

Noninvasive remote monitoring of patients with heart failure generally involves regularly scheduled structured telephone contact between patients and health care providers and/or the electronic transfer of physiologic data using remote access technology via electronic devices. This approach allows for the assessment of symptoms, vital signs, and daily weights, and other noninvasive parameters of interest. The efficacy of such noninvasive monitoring methods remains uncertain, although a growing body of evidence suggests that its value is limited.

Two recent large meta-analyses of randomized controlled trials and observational cohort studies suggest that remote monitoring of symptoms, vital signs, and daily weights may be beneficial for reducing death, hospitalizations, and rehospitalizations for heart failure.[7,8] In contrast, two recent large prospective randomized controlled trials challenge these findings.

In a study sponsored by the National Institutes of Health called TELE-HF, 1653 patients recently hospitalized for heart failure were randomized to undergo either remote monitoring or usual care.[9] Remote monitoring was accomplished by means of a telephone-based interactive voice-response system that collected daily information about symptoms and weight that was reviewed by clinicians, providing the opportunity for outpatient intervention to avoid hospitalization. There was no significant difference between groups in the primary end point of readmissions or death for any cause at 180 days. Hospitalizations for heart failure, the number of days in hospital, and the total number of hospitalizations were not significantly reduced by use of the remote monitoring system.

Similarly, the European randomized controlled TIM-HF trial assigned patients with heart failure with reduced left ventricular ejection fractions (LVEF) to daily remote monitoring, including an electrocardiogram, blood pressure measurement, and assessment of body weight, coupled with medical telephone support or to usual care directed by the patient's local physician.[10] After 2 years of follow-up, there was no significant difference in the primary end point of all-cause mortality or in the composite of cardiovascular death or heart failure hospitalization between the two groups.

One reason for the failure of noninvasive remote monitoring to consistently improve clinical outcomes may be the relatively low sensitivity of changes in symptoms, vital signs, and daily weights to predict heart failure hospitalizations. For example, the sensitivity of weight change in predicting worsening heart failure events is on the order of only 10% to 20%.[11,12] In addition, weight gain and symptoms of clinical congestion (eg, worsening shortness of breath) are late manifestations of worsening heart failure. Thus, when these changes occur, the opportunity to prevent heart failure hospitalization may already be lost. Earlier markers of worsening heart failure may include autonomic adaptation and changes in intrathoracic impedance reflective of increasing lung water.[12–16] However, because clinical congestion, weight change, autonomic adaptation, and changes in intrathoracic impedance are all preceded for many days or weeks by increases in intracardiac pressure and PAP (or hemodynamic congestion), targeting pressure changes in the monitoring and management of heart failure may provide the earliest opportunity for intervention and avoidance of heart failure hospitalizations (**Fig. 1**). This is the premise supporting the use of implantable hemodynamic monitors in the management of heart failure.

IMPLANTABLE HEMODYNAMIC MONITORING

A variety of approaches to remote ambulatory monitoring of intracardiac pressure and PAP have been developed over the years. Devices targeting measurement of right ventricular pressure, PAP, and left atrial pressure (LAP) have been studied. Recently, one system for PAP monitoring received regulatory approval in the United States, ushering in a new era of implantable hemodynamic monitoring for the management of patients with heart failure.

Right Ventricular Pressure Monitors

The ability to estimate pulmonary artery end-diastolic pressure (ePAD) from the right ventricle (RV) was described in 1995.[17] Based on the observation that RV pressure at the time of pulmonary valve opening is equal to pulmonary artery diastolic pressure, RV pressure at the time of RV maximum change in pressure over time (dP/dt) was considered the ePAD and this correlated with directly measured pulmonary artery diastolic pressures at baseline, during isometric work, and during the Valsalva maneuver. This observation

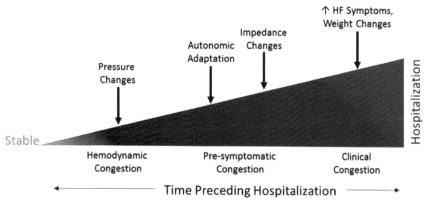

Fig. 1. Progression from stable compensated to decompensated heart failure. The earliest manifestations of worsening heart failure leading to hospitalization are increase in intracardiac pressure and PAP that occur several days to weeks before worsening symptoms and weight gain. Intermediate markers of worsening heart failure may include autonomic adaptation and changes in intrathoracic impedance reflective of increasing lung water. Changes in symptoms and daily weights occur late in this progression. HF, heart failure.

was incorporated into an implantable leaded RV pressure monitoring system, which looked similar to a single-lead permanent pacemaker, to continuously measure RV systolic and diastolic pressures, ePAD, RV dP/dt, heart rate, patient activity level, and temperature. In 32 New York Heart Association (NYHA) class II and class III patients with heart failure evaluated in an observational study of this device, RV pressures and the ePAD were shown to increase several days before worsening symptoms and heart failure hospitalization.[18] This pilot study led to the first randomized controlled trial of implantable hemodynamic monitoring for heart failure.

That study was called the Chronicle Offers Management to Patients with Advanced Signs and Symptoms of Heart Failure (COMPASS-HF) trial. COMPASS-HF randomized 274 NYHA class III and ambulatory class IV patients with heart failure to usual care alone versus usual care plus care guided by knowledge from the RV sensor system.[19] The study demonstrated a nonsignificant 21% reduction in the RV sensor group compared with the control group in the primary efficacy end point of heart failure events (hospitalizations, emergency or urgent care visits requiring intravenous therapy). COMPASS-HF was underpowered for its primary end point, and clinicians generally failed to adequately lower ePAD without target values or an algorithm to guide therapy. Thus, the hypothesis that lower pressures result in reduced rates of heart failure events was not adequately tested in this study.

However, COMPASS-HF did confirm the association of elevated PAP with increased risk of worsening heart failure events.[20] It also defined a range of pressures associated with a reduced

risk of heart failure events. Based on the 24-hour mean ePAD, pressures between 10 and 24 mm Hg were associated with a significantly lower risk of heart failure events compared with pressures of 25 mm Hg or higher. These observations suggest that lowering pressures into the normal or near normal range, even in the absence of heart failure symptoms, might reduce the risk of heart failure hospitalizations. This hypothesis was carried forward to subsequent studies of implantable hemodynamic monitors in heart failure.

Pulmonary Artery Pressure Monitors

A novel wireless PAP measurement system was recently evaluated in the CardioMEMS Heart Sensor Allows Monitoring of Pressure to Improve Outcomes in NYHA Class III Heart Failure Patients (CHAMPION) trial.[21,22] This system was previously shown to be safe and accurate in a pilot study.[23] The PAP sensor is comprised of a coil and a pressure-sensitive capacitor encased in a capsule (**Fig. 2**A). It has no battery, so there is nothing to run out or to be replaced. It is implanted into a branch of the pulmonary artery during right heart catheterization, using a specialized delivery system. Pressure applied to the sensor causes deflections of the pressure-sensitive surface, resulting in a characteristic shift in the resonant frequency. Electromagnetic coupling is achieved by an external antenna, which is held against the patient's body or embedded in a pillow (see **Fig. 2**B). The antenna provides power to the device, continuously measuring its resonant frequency, which is then converted to a pressure waveform. Pressure data are then transmitted wirelessly to a secure Web site, where clinicians

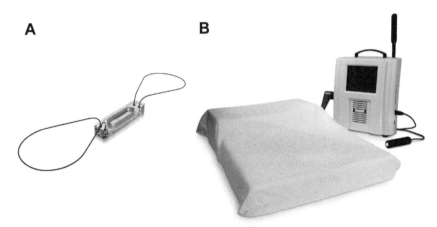

Fig. 2. PAP measurement system. (*A*) The PAP MEMS-based sensor. (*B*) An antenna embedded in a pillow simultaneously powers and interrogates the sensor using radiofrequency. (*Courtesy of* St. Jude Medical, St Paul, MN; with permission.)

can inspect discrete data or pressure trends graphed longitudinally over time.

The CHAMPION trial randomized 550 NYHA class III patients with heart failure, regardless of LVEF, to a treatment group (N = 270) where clinicians had access to daily PAP measurements and used them, in addition to standard of care heart failure monitoring, to manage patients versus a control group (N = 280) where clinicians had no access to daily PAP measurements and managed patients using standard of care heart failure monitoring alone. The CHAMPION trial differed from prior studies of implantable hemodynamic monitors in that specific pressure targets and treatment algorithms were mandated by protocol to ensure adequate testing of the hypothesis. Protocol-specified pressure goals were pulmonary artery systolic pressure 15 to 35 mm Hg, pulmonary artery diastolic pressure 8 to 20 mm Hg, and pulmonary artery mean pressure 10 to 25 mm Hg. Patients were consider hypervolemic and at-risk for heart failure hospitalization if their pressures were higher than these ranges. The goal in these patients was to lower PAP to within the target ranges, unless limited by an untoward clinical effect of PAP lowering (eg, symptomatic hypotension, clinically meaningful worsening of renal function). Protocol-guided responses to hypervolemia included initiation or intensification of diuretics, initiation or intensification of long-acting nitrates, and initiation or intensification of education regarding dietary salt and fluid restrictions. An example of PAP-guided heart failure therapy in a hypervolemic patient is shown in **Fig. 3**.

The primary end point of the CHAMPION trial was the rate of heart failure hospitalizations over 6 months. However, all patients were kept in their randomized, single-blind study assignment until

the last patient reached 6 months of follow-up, so that the long-term effectiveness of the approach could be evaluated.

There were few device-related or system-related complications and no pressure sensor failures in the CHAMPION trial. Freedom from device-related or system-related complications was 98.6%, and overall freedom from pressure-sensor failures was 100%. During the first 6 months following randomization, significantly fewer heart failure hospitalizations occurred in the treatment group (83 hospitalizations) compared with the control group (120 hospitalizations), yielding a relative risk reduction of 28% (*P*<.00002). During the entire single-blinded follow-up period averaging more than 15 months, the treatment group demonstrated a 37% relative risk reduction in heart failure hospitalizations compared with the control group. Most pressure-based medication changes involved diuretics and long-acting nitrates. Heart failure management guided by daily PAP measurement also resulted in significant PAP reduction, a decrease in the proportion of patients hospitalized for heart failure, an increase in the number of days alive and out of the hospital for heart failure, and an improvement in quality of life score. This first positive randomized controlled trial of implantable hemodynamic monitoring in patients with heart failure led to the regulatory approval of the PAP measurement system on May 28, 2014 (http://www.fda.gov/NewsEvents/Newsroom/PressAnnouncements/ucm399024.htm).

An important prespecified subgroup analysis of the CHAMPION trial evaluated the efficacy of PAP-guided heart failure therapy in patients with a preserved LVEF.[22,24] Heart failure hospitalizations were analyzed in subgroups by baseline LVEF less than 40% and 40% or greater.[22] In an

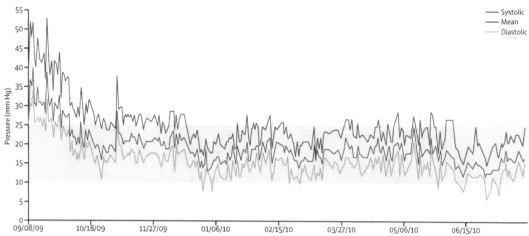

Fig. 3. Example of PAP-guided heart failure therapy from the CHAMPION trial. Pressure data uploaded to a secure Web site are used to guide pressure-based medication changes, with the goal of reducing PAP into the target range depicted by the shaded area for PA mean pressure. In this patient example, increased diuretic dosing was used to lower the initially elevated pressures into the target range and to keep it there, to reduce the risk of heart failure rehospitalization. This patient was not rehospitalized during CHAMPION trial follow-up. (*Courtesy of* St. Jude Medical, St Paul, MN; with permission.)

additional analysis, the subgroup of patients with LVEF of 50% or greater was also analyzed.[24] Patients in the treatment group had a significant reduction in the rate of heart failure hospitalizations compared with those in the control group for preserved and reduced LVEF during 6 months (**Table 1**). Thus, PAP-guided heart failure management represents the first approach to demonstrate improved clinical outcomes in patients with heart failure with a preserved LVEF.

Another key subgroup analysis of CHAMPION trial data evaluated the utility of PAP-guided therapy in patients with heart failure with World Health Organization group II pulmonary hypertension.[25] This retrospective analysis demonstrated the following significant findings: patients with heart failure without pulmonary hypertension were at significantly lower risk for mortality than those with pulmonary hypertension; and in patients with and without pulmonary hypertension, ongoing knowledge of PAP data resulted in a reduction in heart failure hospitalizations.

Left Atrial Pressure Monitors

An implantable system for the direct measurement of LAP has been developed[26,27] and is under ongoing investigation. The system consists of an implantable sensor lead coupled to a subcutaneous antenna coil, a patient advisory module, and remote clinician access via a secure computer-based data management system. Using a transvenous approach and transseptal crossing of the interatrial septum, the tip of the sensor system lead is oriented to the left atrium, providing measurement of LAP, temperature, and an intracardiac electrogram. The implant is powered and interrogated through the skin by wireless transmissions from the patient advisory module, and high-fidelity

Table 1
Heart failure hospitalization rates at 6 months by baseline LVEF in the CHAMPION trial

Ejection Fraction	Randomization Group	6 Mo Rates of Hospitalization for Heart Failure	Incidence Rate Ratio (95% Confidence Interval) [P Value]
≥40%	Treatment group (N = 62)	0.18	0.54 (0.38–0.70) [P<.0001]
	Control group (N = 57)	0.33	
≥50%	Treatment group (N = 35)	0.18	0.50 (0.29–0.86) [P = .0129]
	Control group (N = 31)	0.35	
<40%	Treatment group (N = 208)	0.36	0.76 (0.61–0.91) [P = .0085]
	Control group (N = 222)	0.47	

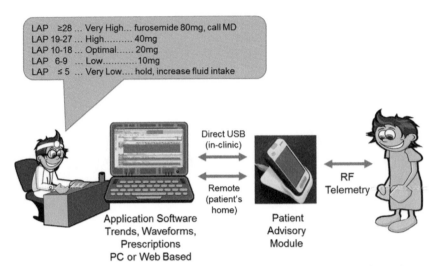

Fig. 4. Physician-directed, patient self-management of intracardiac pressure or PAP. Within physician-prescribed guidelines, patients with heart failure may one day manage their own intracardiac pressure or PAP like the approach shown. This approach is similar to how patients with diabetes use glucometers to self-manage their diabetes medications. The example shown uses LAP to monitor and manage heart failure.

LAP waveforms are captured and stored in the patient advisory module.

Using the physician-directed, patient self-management approach depicted in **Fig. 4**, a prospective, observational, first-in-human study of this LAP monitoring system provided preliminary evidence of efficacy.[28] In this study, LAP monitoring improved hemodynamics, symptoms, and outcomes in NYHA class III and class IV patients with heart failure. Following a 3-month blinding period, LAP and individualized therapy instructions guided by these pressures were disclosed to the patient. The mean daily LAP decreased from 17.6 mm Hg in the first 3 months to 14.8 mm Hg ($P<.003$) during pressure-guided therapy. The frequency of readings greater than 25 mm Hg was reduced by 67% ($P<.001$). LVEF and NYHA class improved. Compared with the year before LAP monitor implantation and with the 3-month period of observation postimplantation, the annualized rate of heart failure hospitalization was significantly reduced following initiation of the physician-directed, patient self-management approach. These findings are being evaluated further in a large prospective randomized controlled outcomes study.

SUMMARY

An implantable PAP measurement system was recently approved for the management of NYHA class III patients with heart failure with a history of heart failure hospitalization in the past 12 months. Therapy guided by knowledge of PAP significantly reduces the risk of heart failure hospitalization and improves quality of life in systolic and diastolic patients with heart failure. This ushers in a new era of heart failure management based on information derived from implantable hemodynamic monitoring systems. Other implantable hemodynamic monitoring systems are under investigation, as is the approach of physician-directed, patient self-management based on direct measurement of intracardiac pressure or PAP.

REFERENCES

1. Go AS, Mozaffarian D, Roger VL, et al. Heart disease and stroke statistics: 2014 update. A report from the American Heart Association. Circulation 2014;129:e27–292.
2. Jencks SF, Williams MV, Coleman EA. Rehospitalizations among patients in the Medicare fee-for-service program. N Engl J Med 2009;360:1418–28.
3. Ross JS, Chen J, Lin Z, et al. Recent national trends in readmission rates after heart failure hospitalization. Circ Heart Fail 2010;3:97–103.
4. Kociol RD, Hammill BG, Fonarow GC, et al. Generalizability and longitudinal outcomes of a national heart failure clinical registry: comparison of Acute Decompensated Heart Failure National Registry (ADHERE) and non-ADHERE Medicare beneficiaries. Am Heart J 2010;160:885–92.
5. Moser DK, Yamokoski L, Sun JL, et al. Improvement in health-related quality of life after hospitalization predicts event-free survival in patients with advanced heart failure. J Card Fail 2009;15:763–9.
6. Heidenreich PA. Forecasting the impact of heart failure in the United States: a policy statement from the American Heart Association. Circ Heart Fail 2013;6: 606–19.

7. Klersy C, De Silvestri A, Gabutti G, et al. A meta-analysis of remote monitoring of heart failure patients. J Am Coll Cardiol 2009;54:1683–94.

8. Inglis SC, Clark RA, McAlister FA, et al. Structured telephone support or telemonitoring programmes for patients with chronic heart failure. Cochrane Database Syst Rev 2010;(8):CD007228.

9. Chaudhry SI, Mattera JA, Curtis JP, et al. Telemonitoring in patients with heart failure. N Engl J Med 2010;363:2301–9.

10. Koehler F, Winkler S, Schieber M, et al. Impact of remote telemedical management on mortality and hospitalizations in ambulatory patients with chronic heart failure: the Telemedical Interventional Monitoring in Heart Failure study. Circulation 2011;123:1873–80.

11. Lewin J, Ledwidge M, O'Loughlin C, et al. Clinical deterioration in established heart failure: what is the value of BNP and weight gain in aiding diagnosis? Eur J Heart Fail 2005;7:953–7.

12. Abraham WT, Compton S, Haas G, et al. Intrathoracic impedance vs daily weight monitoring for predicting worsening heart failure events: results of the Fluid Accumulation Status Trial (FAST). Congest Heart Fail 2011;17:51–5.

13. Yu CM, Wang L, Chau E, et al. Intrathoracic impedance monitoring in patients with heart failure: correlation with fluid status and feasibility of early warning preceding hospitalization. Circulation 2005;112:841–8.

14. Ypenburg C, Bax JJ, van der Wall EE, et al. Intrathoracic impedance monitoring to predict decompensated heart failure. Am J Cardiol 2007;99:554–7.

15. Adamson PB, Smith AL, Abraham WT, et al. Continuous autonomic assessment in patients with symptomatic heart failure: prognostic value of heart rate variability measured by an implanted cardiac resynchronization device. Circulation 2004;110:2389–94.

16. Whellan DJ, Ousdigian KT, Al-Khatib SM, et al. Combined heart failure device diagnostics identify patients at higher risk of subsequent heart failure hospitalizations: results from PARTNERS HF (Program to Access and Review Trending Information and Evaluate Correlation to Symptoms in Patients With Heart Failure) study. J Am Coll Cardiol 2010;55:1803–10.

17. Reynolds DW, Bartelt N, Taepke R, et al. Measurement of pulmonary artery diastolic pressure from the right ventricle. J Am Coll Cardiol 1995;25:1176–82.

18. Adamson PB, Magalski A, Braunschweig F, et al. Ongoing right ventricular hemodynamics in heart failure: clinical value of measurements derived from an implantable monitoring system. J Am Coll Cardiol 2003;41:565–71.

19. Bourge RC, Abraham WT, Adamson PB, et al. Randomized controlled trial of an implantable continuous hemodynamic monitor in patients with advanced heart failure: the COMPASS-HF study. J Am Coll Cardiol 2008;51:1073–9.

20. Stevenson LW, Zile M, Bennett TD, et al. Chronic ambulatory intracardiac pressures and future heart failure events. Circ Heart Fail 2010;3:580–7.

21. Adamson PB, Abraham WT, Aaron M, et al. CHAMPION trial rationale and design: the long-term safety and clinical efficacy of a wireless pulmonary artery pressure monitoring system. J Card Fail 2011;17:3–10.

22. Abraham WT, Adamson PB, Bourge RC, et al. Wireless pulmonary artery haemodynamic monitoring in chronic heart failure: a randomised controlled trial. Lancet 2011;377:658–66.

23. Abraham WT, Adamson PB, Hasan A, et al. Safety and accuracy of a wireless pulmonary artery pressure monitoring system in patients with heart failure. Am Heart J 2011;161:558–66.

24. Adamson PB, Abraham WT, Bourge RC, et al. Wireless pulmonary artery pressure monitoring guides management to reduce decompensation in heart failure with preserved ejection fraction. Circ Heart Fail 2014;7:935–44.

25. Benza RL, Raina A, Abraham WT, et al. Pulmonary hypertension related to left heart disease: insight from a wireless implantable hemodynamic monitor. J Heart Lung Transpl 2014. [Epub ahead of print].

26. Ritzema J, Melton IC, Richards AM, et al. Direct left atrial pressure monitoring in ambulatory heart failure patients: initial experience with a new permanent implantable device. Circulation 2007;116:2952–9.

27. Troughton RW, Ritzema J, Eigler NL, et al. Direct left atrial pressure monitoring in severe heart failure: long-term sensor performance. J Cardiovasc Transl Res 2011;4:3–13.

28. Ritzema J, Troughton R, Melton I, et al. Physician-directed patient self-management of left atrial pressure in advanced chronic heart failure. Circulation 2010;121:1086–95.

Nonhemodynamic Parameters from Implantable Devices for Heart Failure Risk Stratification

John P. Boehmer, MD

KEYWORDS

- Heart failure • Remote monitoring • Implantable defibrillator • Vital signs • Thoracic impedance

KEY POINTS

- Vital signs are ubiquitously monitored by the physician because they provide important information about the condition of a patient.
- In the setting of heart failure, heart rate and blood pressure carry important prognostic information, whereas respiration may provide important information about the short-term risk of acute heart failure events.
- Implantable cardioverter defibrillators (ICDs) can monitor several parameters that contain important prognostic information or provide a risk assessment of acute heart failure events.
- The occurrence of atrial and ventricular arrhythmias, heart rate variability (HRV), and activity level may be used to assess long-term prognosis. Thoracic impedance can provide a short-term risk assessment of acute heart failure events.
- Although no single parameter precisely defines long-term prognosis for survival or short-term risk of acute heart failure events, combining such parameters may provide a means to a more accurate risk assessment.

Chronic heart failure is common, and there are more than 1 million hospital admissions annually in the United States for acute decompensated heart failure.[1] Much of the medical expense and morbidity associated with heart failure is derived from these hospitalizations.[2] Further, heart failure hospitalizations are associated with an increased risk of subsequent mortality.[3] Accordingly, there is a continuing search for methods for the early detection of worsening heart failure. There are several parameters that are monitored by implantable electronic devices currently in practice or that could easily be obtained clinically, which provide important prognostic information and may be useful in remote patient monitoring. However, several of these parameters have been limited by their

sensitivity and specificity in assessing the condition of a given patient. Despite these limitations, the data provided can be useful clinically and may be even more useful when incorporated into the entirety of the clinical information available regarding a patient.

INFORMATION GATHERED FROM REMOTE MONITORING VITAL SIGNS
Blood Pressure

Blood pressure is a ubiquitously monitored parameter, obtained in every clinic and hospital visit. However, the importance of blood pressure as a prognostic indicator is often overlooked. In patients with acute heart failure, there is a U-shaped

Division of Cardiology, Penn State Hershey Medical Center, Mail Code H047, 500 University Drive, Hershey, PA 17033, USA
E-mail addresses: jboehmer@psu.edu; jboehmer@hmc.psu.edu

Heart Failure Clin 11 (2015) 191–201
http://dx.doi.org/10.1016/j.hfc.2014.12.001
1551-7136/15/$ – see front matter © 2015 Elsevier Inc. All rights reserved.

curve describing risk of death for patients hospitalized with acute heart failure (**Fig. 1**).[4] The mortality seems to nadir in the range of 140 to 150 mm Hg systolic, whereas the nadir is in the range of 70 to 80 mm Hg diastolic. The reasons for this are not entirely clear, but part of it seems to be related to the association of low blood pressure with poor systolic function; this is made clearer when grouping patients into those with heart failure with preserved ejection fraction and heart failure with reduced ejection fraction (**Fig. 2**).[5] The greatest risk of death is in patients with reduced ejection fraction and low blood pressure. Further, higher blood pressures in the preserved ejection fraction group are not associated with an increase in the risk of mortality, whereas the typical U-shaped curve is present for patients with heart failure with reduced ejection fraction.

The utility of blood pressure monitoring in the management of patients with heart failure lies with the impact on prognosis. There may be further utility in using the data to titrate standard heart failure therapy, including beta-blockers, angiotensin converting enzyme inhibitors, and angiotensin receptor blockers, but there are no compelling data to demonstrate that this strategy is superior to the use of symptoms and clinic-measured blood pressures. The data may also be used to assist in the management of hypertension. Most patients with heart failure have a history of hypertension, and many patients, particularly those with heart failure with preserved ejection fraction, have ongoing issues with high blood pressure. Remotely monitored blood pressure measurements may be useful in the management of these patients.[6]

Heart Rate

Heart rate is another vital sign that is monitored in all patients. Historically, heart rate was used as a prognostic indicator in patients with heart failure and provided solid predictive value.[7] However, with the common use of β-blockers and some antiarrhythmic drugs that lower heart rates, the ability to use heart rate as a prognostic metric has diminished. Despite this, there is still predictive value in heart rates, best seen with the use of implantable pacemakers and ICDs, which monitor heart rates continuously. In doing so, they are well positioned to measure heart rates under several conditions, including at rest as detected by the accelerometer inside the device, at night, or averages during the day. Even considering the ability of such devices to continuously monitor heart rate, the predictive value for either mortality or heart failure events is modest.

Measurements of HRV have been evaluated for several decades in patients with heart failure.[8] Even in the presence of β-blockers and other medications that affect heart rate, HRV has shown solid prognostic value in patients with heart failure, although the predictive value may be diminished.[9] The measurement has been made in several ways

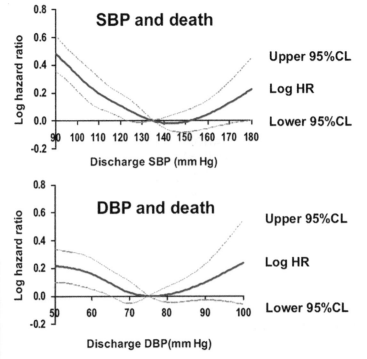

Fig. 1. Spline curves relating discharge systolic blood pressures (SBP) and diastolic blood pressures (DBP) with mortality in patients who were admitted with heart failure, adjusted for covariates and medications. CL, confidence limit; HR, hazard ratio. (*From* Lee DS, Ghosh N, Floras JS, et al. Association of blood pressure at hospital discharge with mortality in patients diagnosed with heart failure. Circ Heart Fail 2009;2(6):618; with permission.)

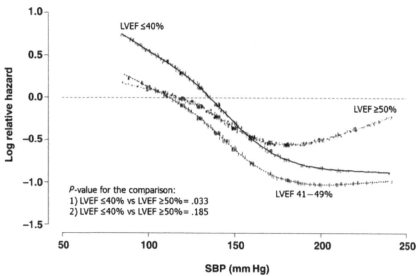

Fig. 2. Spline curves of systolic blood pressure (SBP) stratified by left ventricular ejection fraction (LVEF) status. The risk of all-cause mortality decreased as SBP increased in patients with LVEF less than 40%, and the pattern was similar in patients with mild left-ventricular systolic dysfunction (LVEF 41%–49%). Conversely, in the presence of preserved systolic function, the relationship between SBP and all-cause mortality was nonlinear, showing a U- or J-curve pattern. (*From* Nunez J, Nunez E, Fonarow GC, et al. Differential prognostic effect of systolic blood pressure on mortality according to left-ventricular function in patients with acute heart failure. Eur J Heart Fail 2010;12(1):42; with permission.)

but most commonly involves the measurement of the standard deviation of beat-to-beat intervals, typically measured from one P wave to the next and abbreviated as SDANN.[10] Fourier transformation, which changes the measurement of this variability from the time domain to the frequency domain, demonstrates a low-frequency peak, generally in the range of the respiratory frequency.

The amplitude of this peak is proportional to the beat-to-beat variability in heart rate. The measurement of HRV is limited by arrhythmias such as atrial fibrillation or when the atria are paced electronically, which eliminates beat-to-beat variability. In patients with implantable devices, HRV as measured by the implanted device has been shown to be predictive of outcome (**Fig. 3**).[11–13]

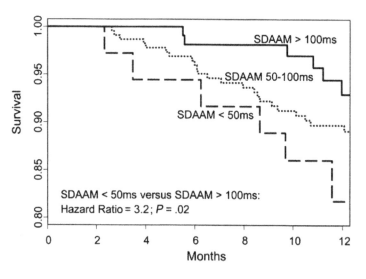

Fig. 3. Kaplan-Meier survival curve for all-cause mortality based on the standard deviation of a 5-minute median atrial-atrial sensed interval (SDAAM that is similar to SDANN) measured as a 4-week average between weeks 5 and 8 after implantation. There were 36 patients in the SDAAM less than 50 ms group, 227 in the 50 to 100 ms group, and 167 in the greater than 100 ms group. The SDAAM less than 50 ms group was associated with increased mortality risk compared with the SDAAM greater than 100 ms group (hazard ratio, 3.20; P = .02). (*From* Adamson PB, Smith AL, Abraham WT, et al. Continuous autonomic assessment in patients with symptomatic heart failure: prognostic value of heart rate variability measured by an implanted cardiac resynchronization device. Circulation 2004;110 (16):2391; with permission.)

Respiratory Changes

Acute heart failure is often manifested by acute tachypnea and the sensation of dyspnea. In the Acute Decompensated Heart Failure National Registry (ADHERE), 89% of patients admitted for acute decompensated heart failure presented with dyspnea at the time of admission.[14] Respiratory rate is another commonly measured vital sign that would seem to be a natural metric to monitor in patients at risk for an acute heart failure event. However, until recently, the ability to chronically monitor respirations in patients with heart failure has not been possible. Several years ago, changes in minute ventilation as estimated by an implanted pacemaker were used to guide rate-responsive pacing[15]; this provided a new metric to guide rate-adaptive pacing in addition to the typical motion detected by an accelerometer, which is still used to guide rate-responsive pacing.[16] However, this technology was not applied to the monitoring and management of patients with heart failure. There have been several observational studies in which respiration is monitored in patients with chronic heart failure. As heart failure worsens, several changes occur in respiration. The respiratory rate increases, and at the same time, the tidal volume drops as the lungs become wet and heavy. Minute ventilation increases as dead space breathing increases with the smaller and more frequent respirations but only modestly so until heart failure becomes symptomatic. This pattern of rapid shallow breathing may be a more useful signal to monitor during the development of acute heart failure.

A study is underway which utilizes investigational software applied to an approved ICD in order to measure respiratory rate and provide a relative measure of tidal volume. It uses the signal from thoracic impedance, but rather than measuring the average impedance, it uses the impedance to monitor the change in air between the intracardiac lead and the ICD generator. As air enters the lungs, the impedance increases because air is a poor conductor. As air leave the lungs, the impedance drops. The more the air that enters the lungs, the larger the change in impedance. Accordingly, impedance is used as a relative measure of tidal volume, whereas respiratory rate is measured from the curve directly. Studies are underway to determine the usefulness of this type of measurement.

ARRHYTHMIAS

Many arrhythmias are common in patients with heart failure. For example, atrial fibrillation typically occurs in 15% to 20% of patients with chronic heart failure. However, the incidence of atrial fibrillation increases as the severity of heart failure increases. Maisel and Stevenson[17] took data available from several heart failure clinical trials and demonstrated that in trials of mild heart failure, such as the Studies of Left Ventricular Dysfunction (SOLVD) prevention trial, the incidence of heart failure was low at 4.2% and increased with the severity of heart failure, worsening to an incidence of 49.8% in the Cooperative North Scandinavian Enalapril Survival Study (CONSENSUS) (**Fig. 4**).

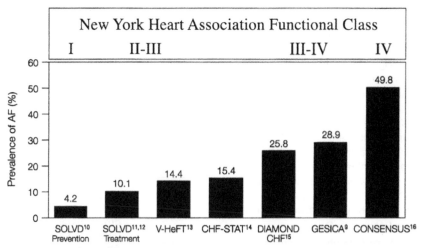

Fig. 4. Prevalence of atrial fibrillation (AF) in several major heart failure trials arranged from lowest to highest heart failure severity and mortality. CHF-STAT, Congestive Heart Failure Survival Trial of Antiarrhythmic Therapy; CONSENSUS, Cooperative North Scandinavian Enalapril Survival Study; DIAMOND CHF, Danish Investigations of Arrhythmia and Mortality on Dofetilide Congestive Heart Failure study; GESICA, Grupo de Estudio de la Sobrevida en la Insuficiencia Cardiaca en Argentina; SOLVD, Studies of Left Ventricular Dysfunction; V-HeFT, Vasodilator in Heart Failure Trial. (*From* Maisel WH, Stevenson LW. Atrial fibrillation in heart failure: epidemiology, pathophysiology, and rationale for therapy. Am J Cardiol 2003;91(6A):3D; with permission.)

Accordingly, the severity of heart failure in a population may be estimated by measuring the incidence of atrial fibrillation within the population. However, this is not useful in patient management, as predictions need to be made for the individual patient and many patients with atrial fibrillation do well. Indeed, after correcting for other risk factors, a patient with atrial fibrillation has nearly equal survival to similar patients without atrial fibrillation.[18]

Atrial arrhythmias are, however, predictors of acute heart failure events. In the Framingham Study of patients who had either atrial fibrillation or a diagnosis of heart failure, both conditions were present in 26% of patients, and of those patients, both conditions occurred together on the same day in 21%.[19] Patients who are diagnosed with atrial fibrillation have a rising incidence of a diagnosis of heart failure over the ensuing years. The risk is attributed to several hemodynamic changes that occur in the setting of atrial fibrillation, including poor filling of the left ventricle, reduced stroke volume, higher left atrial pressures, the irregular rhythm, and the adverse effects of sustained tachycardia.

Implantable devices are capable of detecting atrial arrhythmias, particularly in devices that incorporate an atrial lead. Several assessments of the risk of an acute heart failure event following the onset of atrial arrhythmias have been made using implantable devices. This method has been particularly useful in assessing stroke risk in patients with heart failure and ICDs.[20] The early detection of atrial arrhythmias, particularly when associated with a rapid ventricular response, may provide an opportunity for treatment before worsening heart failure associated with the atrial arrhythmia is manifest.[21] In addition, in patients with atrial fibrillation who have cardiac resynchronization devices, the arrhythmia may limit the ability of the device to pace the ventricles, which may in turn have an adverse effect on patient outcomes.[22]

Ventricular arrhythmias are also common in patients with heart failure and are associated with a poor prognosis. The initial observation of the risk of death from progressive heart failure following ventricular arrhythmias came from the Comparison of Medical Therapy, Pacing, and Defibrillation in Heart Failure (COMPANION) trial, in which patients receiving an ICD shock also had a high risk of death due to progressive heart failure.[23] This study demonstrated that patients who received an ICD shock were at high risk of sudden death, and this risk was primarily related to the risk of death due to progressive heart failure. This observation was confirmed in the Sudden Cardiac Death Heart Failure Trial, SCD-HeFT.[24] Finally, data from a large registry in which the electrograms before ICD shocks were adjudicated by an expert panel of electrophysiologists demonstrated that the risk is associated with arrhythmias, both rapid atrial and ventricular arrhythmias, but not related to ICD shocks due to artifact.[25] It is recommended that ventricular arrhythmias prompt an assessment of a patient's heart failure condition in addition to further management of arrhythmia. Therefore, the occurrence of arrhythmias provides important prognostic and patient management information.

THORACIC IMPEDANCE

The presence of implantable electronic devices has led to a search for parameters that could be monitored to assess the heart failure condition. One such parameter is the measurement of thoracic impedance. Impedance cardiography has been used for many decades to assess heart function by measuring stroke volume and cardiac output by the changes in thoracic impedance that occur during the cardiac cycle.[26] Although it is accurate in skilled hands and can be used to study populations as an investigational tool, the utility of impedance cardiography in the management of patients with heart failure has not been demonstrated to date.

The use of thoracic impedance to assess lung water content has gained a great deal of interest. Most admissions for heart failure are necessary for the management of volume overload, and in most instances, it is shortness of breath that prompts the visit to the hospital. Subclinical pulmonary edema may occur for several weeks before patients notice overt symptoms. As a result, a window of opportunity to identify increasing lung water is present before the need for hospitalization.

Most studies of thoracic impedance in patients with heart failure have been made by ICDs. Although ICDs are well suited for the measurement of impedance, the leads of the device are oriented to deliver an ICD shock rather than to monitor lung water content. There is only a modest amount of lung present between the intracardiac leads and ICD pulse generator. Despite this, a signal that takes into account lung water content can be measured. Several studies have evaluated the utility of thoracic impedance measured this way to detect worsening heart failure before an acute heart failure event. The first significant study evaluating the performance of this type of monitoring was published by Yu and colleagues.[27] The reduction in impedance predated symptoms by an average of 15 days; this is important, because it provides a window of opportunity for corrective action to be taken before presentation to the hospital with symptoms of acute heart failure. The impedance measurements correlated well with pulmonary capillary wedge pressures measured while in hospital, as well as fluid balance measured while in hospital (**Fig. 5**). As the patient diuresed, the thoracic impedance increased, whereas the pulmonary capillary wedge pressure dropped. This observational study estimated that the measurement had a 77% sensitivity to detect a heart failure event before its occurrence, although presenting about 1.5 false-positive alerts per patient-year of monitoring. It is the occurrence of false-positive alerts that has slowed the adoption of this technology in practice. Although the sensitivity is reasonable and the lead time is good for the detection of worsening heart failure, the number of false-positive alerts outnumber the true-positive alerts in a low-risk population. Another challenge in analyzing these types of data is the lack of a true gold standard for assessing worsening heart failure. Typically, a heart failure hospitalization is taken as an objective end point. However, the need for urgent care, parenteral therapy, and adjustment of oral therapy have all been suggested as meaningful end points that indicate worsening heart failure. Further, patients may experience worsening heart failure that could be associated with increase in lung water content and is able to manage the event by reducing their dietary sodium intake or adjusting their oral diuretic therapy on their own. Many of the alerts that are designated as false positive may be associated with meaningful true changes in the patient but did not rise to the level to require hospitalization for heart failure. As a result of these challenges, the use of thoracic impedance as an isolated measurement seems to serve as a measure of short-term risk in a high-risk patient population, such as those with a recent hospitalization for acute heart failure.[28]

COMBINING MEASUREMENTS FOR REMOTE PHYSIOLOGIC MONITORING

To be useful, sensors for the detection of worsening heart failure must provide warning in the weeks leading up to an acute heart failure event to allow sufficient time for patient evaluation and the administration of new therapy to prevent an event. Further, the metric must supply reasonable specificity to the heart failure condition to avoid adverse effects of heart failure therapy in circumstances in which it may not be needed. In clinical practice, no one sign, symptom, or laboratory finding is interpreted in isolation but rather in the context of all available clinical data. The clinical criteria for identifying heart failure are multifaceted and do not rely on any single parameter.[29] Attempts to combine different means of assessing the heart failure condition may be helpful to better ensure both the sensitivity and specificity of the detection of worsening heart failure.

Implantable electronic devices monitor several parameters that may provide insight into the heart failure condition of a patient as described earlier. Some studies have suggested an overall benefit for remote monitoring of ICD parameters monitoring rhythm and other physiologic parameters, which led to a reduction in the number of emergency department or urgent in-office visits for episodes of worsening heart failure.[30]

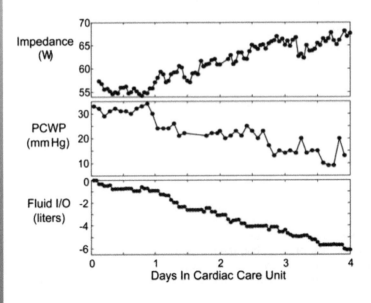

Fig. 5. Example from a single patient demonstrating the relationship between intrathoracic impedance, pulmonary capillary wedge pressure (PCWP), and net fluid loss (Fluid I/O) during 4 days of intensive diuresis.

However, other studies have been less convincing.[31] There have been several attempts to combine these metrics to provide a more meaningful evaluation of these data. One example combined data from mean heart rate over 24 hours, heart rate at rest, patient activity, impedance measured between the right ventricular lead and the pulse generator, and the number of ventricular extrasystoles.[32] HRV and impedance from the shock electrode to the pulse generator were added. Combining the metrics led to an improved assessment over any individual measurement. The algorithm had a 65% sensitivity to predict a heart failure event. But because of a low event rate, the positive predictive value of an alert was only 7.8%, with the remainder being false-positive alerts that did not precede a worsening heart failure event. However, there was a robust negative predictive value of 99.96% for those who did not have an alert, which is clinically important, as most patients did not have an alert, and the algorithm could provide solid assurance that the risk of an event was very low.

An attempt at combining such metrics, along with adding new metrics, is under investigation. In the Multisensor Chronic Evaluations in Ambulatory Heart Failure Patients (MultiSENSE) study, in addition to heart rate and thoracic impedance data, respiration, posture, and heart sounds are assessed, along with the change in heart rate and respirations with activity. In this study, a market release device is converted to an investigational device with the use of research software uploaded to the device. The device then dedicates more resources to the collection of these parameters.

Respiration is evaluated as described earlier using the impedance signal between the right ventricular lead and the pulse generator. The periodic changes in impedance during the respiratory cycle can be used to measure respiratory rate, the amplitude of the impedance changes can be used as a relative measure of tidal volume, and the product of respiratory rate and relative tidal volume can be used as a relative measure of minute ventilation (**Fig. 6**). In addition, the impedance respiration sensor can also be used to detect sleep disordered breathing. Sleep apnea, and particularly central sleep apnea, is common in patients with heart failure. Further, the incidence of sleep disordered breathing increases with worsening heart failure. Sleep disordered breathing is a known risk factor for adverse outcomes in patients with heart failure. It is unknown whether changes in sleep disordered breathing correlate with the short-term risk of a heart failure event, but this can be investigated by long-term implantation of a device that measures this parameter daily.

Heart sounds can be detected using the accelerometer present in a typical ICD if the signal from the device is processed to detect frequencies in the audible, or just infrasonic, range (**Fig. 7**). The third heart sound is widely known to be one of the

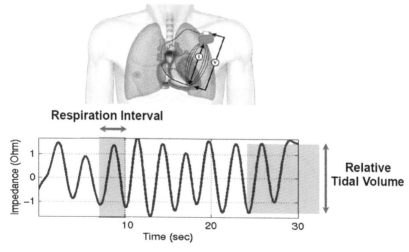

Minute Ventilation = 60/Respiration Interval x Tidal Volume

Fig. 6. Measurement of impedance by placing a small voltage between an intracardiac lead and the pulse generator. The graph demonstrates how the impedance varies with the respiratory cycle, increasing as more air enters the lungs and decreasing as the air exits. The respiratory rate can be measured using the respiratory interval; a relative measure of tidal volume in ohms can be measured, and the product of both is a relative measure of minute ventilation. (*Courtesy of* Boston Scientific Corporation, Marlborough, MA; with permission.)

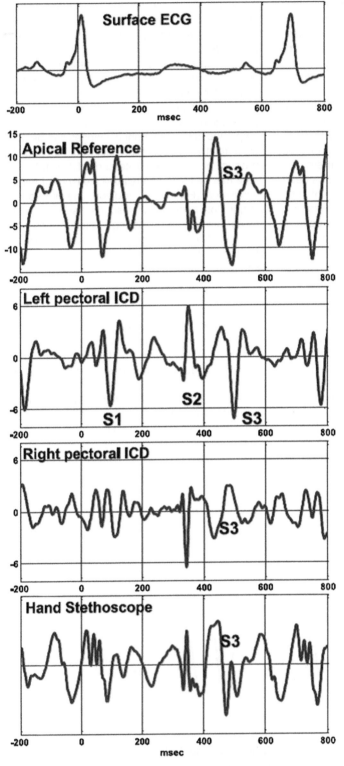

Fig. 7. The panels depict simultaneous ensemble averages recorded using an accelerometer at the cardiac apex or left or right pectoral areas compared with an apically placed hand stethoscope. The band used for the recording is extended to the subaudibal range (20 Hz is used as the typical lower limit of the audible range). The recordings are from a heart failure patient who had a loud audible S3 on clinical examination. The electrocardiogram R-wave reference was placed at t = 0 ms in this example. (*From* Siejko KZ, et al. Feasibility of heart sounds measurements from an accelerometer within an ICD pulse generator. Pacing Clin. Electrophysiol. Mar 2013;36(3):338; with permission.)

**Extended band (6-70Hz)
Ensemble Averages**

most specific clinical signs of heart failure. The S3 originates from left ventricular mechanical vibrations resulting from the rapid deceleration of blood during early diastolic filling. These vibrations propagate as waves throughout the torso and can be heard with a stethoscope, provided they are of sufficient energy and have components in the audible frequency range. Electronic vibration sensors such as accelerometers or microphones can more reliably detect S3 vibrations than a stethoscope.[33] The ability of such sensors to detect S3 sounds has been demonstrated in canine models of heart failure and in human studies.[34,35]

Posture can be measured with a multidimensional accelerometer. Although the study described earlier using a market release device contains a 1-dimensional accelerometer, a stand-alone device is used in a subset of patients worn on the chest wall to evaluate the potential of this sensor. Orthopnea is a common symptom in patients with heart failure.[36,37] A posture sensor in the thorax would be capable of detecting the recumbent angle of a patient. In addition, other parameters could be evaluated, including the percentage of time patients are upright or the number of times a patient gets up during the night, which could be a measure of the frequency of nocturia or simply patient restlessness.

Finally, the change in heart rate and respiration during activity can be evaluated. The accelerometer in the ICD has a long history of being used to evaluate activity and is used to drive rate-adaptive pacing. Conversely, this same metric can be used to evaluate the patient's heart rate response to exercise as well as their respiratory response. During activity, patients with heart failure exhibit increased ventilation for a given level of metabolic demand and do not require maximal effort testing. In cardiopulmonary exercise tests, the ratio of the minute ventilation to carbon dioxide excretion (a measure of metabolic demand) is a powerful prognostic indicator, similar or possibly superior to peak oxygen consumption.[38,39] This measurement does not require maximal effort. Patients with heart failure also exhibit a rapid shallow breathing pattern compared with normal subjects,[40,41] and this pattern is accentuated with exertion. Heart rate responses to activity are also different in patients with heart failure. These patients exhibit an increased heart rate for a given level of activity.[42] As heart failure progresses, chronotropic insufficiency becomes more common.[43–45] The presence of chronotropic insufficiency has been shown to be nearly as valuable in predicting morbidity and mortality as peak oxygen consumption or the ventilatory response to exercise.[45–47]

SUMMARY

Clinicians use vital signs every day as a means to evaluate a patient's condition. For patients with heart failure, the vital signs contain important information regarding prognosis and change in their condition. Additional metrics have been evaluated with the advent of implantable electronic devices. Information in the history of a patient, such as the presence of orthopnea, and the patient's activity level may be correlated to implantable sensors that measure posture and activity. Heart sounds have long been used clinically, and an S3 is considered a specific clinical sign for heart failure. An implantable device can detect heart sounds in the audible range and may be useful in assessing prognosis or predicting worsening heart failure. Thoracic impedance has shown promise in the detection of worsening heart failure, but the specificity of changes in impedance to correlate with clinical worsening heart failure has limited its application. Combining these measures to make an assessment, much as a clinician combines symptoms, clinical signs, and laboratory data, may lead to improved means of detecting worsening heart failure.

REFERENCES

1. Rosamond W, Flegal K, Furie K, et al. Heart disease and stroke statistics–2008 update: a report from the American Heart Association Statistics Committee and Stroke Statistics Subcommittee. Circulation 2008;117(4):e25–146.
2. Heart Failure Society Of America. HFSA 2006 Comprehensive Heart Failure Practice Guideline. J Card Fail 2006;12(1):e1–2.
3. Dickstein K, Cohen-Solal A, Filippatos G, et al. ESC Guidelines for the diagnosis and treatment of acute and chronic heart failure 2008: the Task Force for the Diagnosis and Treatment of Acute and Chronic Heart Failure 2008 of the European Society of Cardiology. Developed in collaboration with the Heart Failure Association of the ESC (HFA) and endorsed by the European Society of Intensive Care Medicine (ESICM). Eur Heart J 2008;29(19):2388–442.
4. Lee DS, Ghosh N, Floras JS, et al. Association of blood pressure at hospital discharge with mortality in patients diagnosed with heart failure. Circ Heart Fail 2009;2(6):616–23.
5. Nunez J, Nunez E, Fonarow GC, et al. Differential prognostic effect of systolic blood pressure on mortality according to left-ventricular function in patients with acute heart failure. Eur J Heart Fail 2010;12(1):38–44.
6. Verberk WJ, Kessels AG, Thien T. Telecare is a valuable tool for hypertension management, a

systematic review and meta-analysis. Blood Press Monit 2011;16(3):149–55.

7. Ho KK, Anderson KM, Kannel WB, et al. Survival after the onset of congestive heart failure in Framingham Heart Study subjects. Circulation 1993;88(1):107–15.

8. Bilchick KC, Fetics B, Djoukeng R, et al. Prognostic value of heart rate variability in chronic congestive heart failure (Veterans Affairs' Survival Trial of Antiarrhythmic Therapy in Congestive Heart Failure). Am J Cardiol 2002;90(1):24–8.

9. Huikuri HV, Tapanainen JM, Lindgren K, et al. Prediction of sudden cardiac death after myocardial infarction in the beta-blocking era. J Am Coll Cardiol 2003;42(4):652–8.

10. Bilchick KC, Berger RD. Heart rate variability. J Cardiovasc Electrophysiol 2006;17(6):691–4.

11. Tereshchenko LG, Henrikson CA, Berger RD. Strong coherence between heart rate variability and intracardiac repolarization lability during biventricular pacing is associated with reverse electrical remodeling of the native conduction and improved outcome. J Electrocardiol 2011;44(6):713–7.

12. Molon G, Solimene F, Melissano D, et al. Baseline heart rate variability predicts clinical events in heart failure patients implanted with cardiac resynchronization therapy: validation by means of related complexity index. Ann Noninvasive Electrocardiol 2010;15(4):301–7.

13. Adamson PB, Smith AL, Abraham WT, et al. Continuous autonomic assessment in patients with symptomatic heart failure: prognostic value of heart rate variability measured by an implanted cardiac resynchronization device. Circulation 2004;110(16):2389–94.

14. Fonarow GC. The Acute Decompensated Heart Failure National Registry (ADHERE): opportunities to improve care of patients hospitalized with acute decompensated heart failure. Rev Cardiovasc Med 2003;4(Suppl 7):S21–30.

15. Kappenberger LJ, Herpers L. Rate responsive dual chamber pacing. Pacing Clin Electrophysiol 1986;9(6 Pt 2):987–91.

16. Coman J, Freedman R, Koplan BA, et al. A blended sensor restores chronotropic response more favorably than an accelerometer alone in pacemaker patients: the LIFE study results. Pacing Clin Electrophysiol 2008;31(11):1433–42.

17. Maisel WH, Stevenson LW. Atrial fibrillation in heart failure: epidemiology, pathophysiology, and rationale for therapy. Am J Cardiol 2003;91(6A):2D–8D.

18. Deedwania PC, Lardizabal JA. Atrial fibrillation in heart failure: a comprehensive review. Am J Med 2010;123(3):198–204.

19. Wang TJ, Larson MG, Levy D, et al. Temporal relations of atrial fibrillation and congestive heart failure and their joint influence on mortality: the Framingham Heart Study. Circulation 2003;107(23):2920–5.

20. Shanmugam N, Boerdlein A, Proff J, et al. Detection of atrial high-rate events by continuous home monitoring: clinical significance in the heart failure - cardiac resynchronization therapy population. Europace 2012;14(2):230–7.

21. Varma N, Stambler B, Chun S. Detection of atrial fibrillation by implanted devices with wireless data transmission capability. Pacing Clin Electrophysiol 2005;28(Suppl 1):S133–6.

22. Hayes DL, Boehmer JP, Day JD, et al. Cardiac resynchronization therapy and the relationship of percent biventricular pacing to symptoms and survival. Heart Rhythm 2011;8(9):1469–75.

23. Saxon LA, Bristow MR, Boehmer J, et al. Predictors of sudden cardiac death and appropriate shock in the Comparison of Medical Therapy, Pacing, and Defibrillation in Heart Failure (COMPANION) Trial. Circulation 2006;114(25):2766–72.

24. Poole JE, Johnson GW, Hellkamp AS, et al. Prognostic importance of defibrillator shocks in patients with heart failure. N Engl J Med 2008;359(10):1009–17.

25. Saxon LA, Hayes DL, Gilliam FR, et al. Long-term outcome after ICD and CRT implantation and influence of remote device follow-up: the ALTITUDE survival study. Circulation 2010;122(23):2359–67.

26. Kubicek WG, Karnegis JN, Patterson RP, et al. Development and evaluation of an impedance cardiac output system. Aerosp Med 1966;37(12):1208–12.

27. Yu CM, Wang L, Chau E, et al. Intrathoracic impedance monitoring in patients with heart failure: correlation with fluid status and feasibility of early warning preceding hospitalization. Circulation 2005;112(6):841–8.

28. Packer M, Abraham WT, Mehra MR, et al. Utility of impedance cardiography for the identification of short-term risk of clinical decompensation in stable patients with chronic heart failure. J Am Coll Cardiol 2006;47(11):2245–52.

29. Levy D, Larson MG, Vasan RS, et al. The progression from hypertension to congestive heart failure. JAMA 1996;275(20):1557–62.

30. Landolina M, Perego GB, Lunati M, et al. Remote monitoring reduces healthcare use and improves quality of care in heart failure patients with implantable defibrillators: the evolution of management strategies of heart failure patients with implantable defibrillators (EVOLVO) study. Circulation 2012;125(24):2985–92.

31. Daubert JC, Saxon L, Adamson PB, et al. 2012 EHRA/HRS expert consensus statement on cardiac resynchronization therapy in heart failure: implant and follow-up recommendations and management. Heart Rhythm 2012;9(9):1524–76.

32. Sack S, Wende CM, Nagele H, et al. Potential value of automated daily screening of cardiac resynchronization therapy defibrillator diagnostics for prediction of major cardiovascular events: results from Home-CARE (Home Monitoring in Cardiac Resynchronization Therapy) study. Eur J Heart Fail 2011; 13(9):1019–27.

33. Marcus GM, Gerber IL, McKeown BH, et al. Association between phonocardiographic third and fourth heart sounds and objective measures of left ventricular function. JAMA 2005;293(18):2238–44.

34. Ozawa Y, Smith D, Craige E. Origin of the third heart sound. II. Studies in human subjects. Circulation 1983;67(2):399–404.

35. Ozawa Y, Smith D, Craige E. Origin of the third heart sound. I. Studies in dogs. Circulation 1983;67(2): 393–8.

36. Stevenson LW, Perloff JK. The limited reliability of physical signs for estimating hemodynamics in chronic heart failure. JAMA 1989;261(6):884–8.

37. Duguet A, Tantucci C, Lozinguez O, et al. Expiratory flow limitation as a determinant of orthopnea in acute left heart failure. J Am Coll Cardiol 2000; 35(3):690–700.

38. Agostoni P, Pellegrino R, Conca C, et al. Exercise hyperpnea in chronic heart failure: relationships to lung stiffness and expiratory flow limitation. J Appl Physiol (1985) 2002;92(4):1409–16.

39. Johnson BD, Beck KC, Olson LJ, et al. Ventilatory constraints during exercise in patients with chronic heart failure. Chest 2000;117(2):321–32.

40. Sullivan MJ, Higginbotham MB, Cobb FR. Increased exercise ventilation in patients with chronic heart failure: intact ventilatory control despite hemodynamic and pulmonary abnormalities. Circulation 1988;77(3):552–9.

41. Dimopoulou I, Tsintzas OK, Alivizatos PA, et al. Pattern of breathing during progressive exercise in chronic heart failure. Int J Cardiol 2001;81(2–3): 117–21 [discussion: 121–2].

42. McElroy PA, Janicki JS, Weber KT. Physiologic correlates of the heart rate response to upright isotonic exercise: relevance to rate-responsive pacemakers. J Am Coll Cardiol 1988;11(1):94–9.

43. Huang PH, Leu HB, Chen JW, et al. Comparison of endothelial vasodilator function, inflammatory markers, and N-terminal pro-brain natriuretic peptide in patients with or without chronotropic incompetence to exercise test. Heart 2006;92(5): 609–14.

44. Khan MN, Pothier CE, Lauer MS. Chronotropic incompetence as a predictor of death among patients with normal electrograms taking beta blockers (metoprolol or atenolol). Am J Cardiol 2005;96(9): 1328–33.

45. Witte KK, Cleland JG, Clark AL. Chronic heart failure, chronotropic incompetence, and the effects of beta blockade. Heart 2006;92(4):481–6.

46. Arena R, Myers J, Abella J, et al. The prognostic value of the heart rate response during exercise and recovery in patients with heart failure: influence of beta-blockade. Int J Cardiol 2010;138(2):166–73.

47. Robbins M, Francis G, Pashkow FJ, et al. Ventilatory and heart rate responses to exercise: better predictors of heart failure mortality than peak oxygen consumption. Circulation 1999;100(24):2411–7.

Role of Revascularization to Improve Left Ventricular Function

Harsh C. Patel, MD, Stephen G. Ellis, MD*

KEYWORDS

- Revascularization • LV function • Viability • Ischemic cardiomyopathy
- Percutaneous coronary intervention • Coronary artery bypass grafting

KEY POINTS

- Coronary revascularization to improve left ventricular (LV) function and improve mortality in patients with ischemic cardiomyopathy remains controversial, especially in the absence of angina or ischemia.
- A large body of observational evidence suggests that patients with dysfunctional but viable myocardium may experience improvement in mortality and LV function after revascularization.
- Results of randomized trials conducted in the last decade dispute the value of viability testing or coronary revascularization in improving outcomes of patients with ischemic cardiomyopathy.
- Clinical equipoise persists regarding the role of coronary revascularization in certain patients.
- Surgical revascularization has been preferred over percutaneous revascularization in patients with LV dysfunction based on observational data, but high-quality randomized comparative effectiveness data are lacking.

INTRODUCTION

Mortality from coronary artery disease (CAD) has decreased in developed countries over the past several decades.[1] As a result, however, the prevalence of ischemic cardiomyopathy is increasing and presently it is the most common cause of heart failure in developed countries. In the large ADHERE registry of patients hospitalized for heart failure in the United States, almost 60% had a history of CAD.[2] Despite improvement in medical therapy and increased utilization of implantable cardioverter defibrillators and cardiac resynchronization therapies, mortality from ischemic cardiomyopathy remains high.

Left ventricular (LV) function has generally been considered to be one of the strongest prognostic factors in patients with CAD.[3] The role of coronary revascularization to improve LV function and reduce mortality has been investigated in several studies over the past few decades. Most of these studies, which have largely been retrospective and nonrandomized and containing small sample sizes, have demonstrated a benefit from revascularization, especially in those patients with a significant amount of viable myocardium. More recently, however, 3 prospective randomized studies, the Surgical Treatment for Ischemic Heart Disease (STICH) trial,[4] the Heart Failure Revascularization (HEART) trial,[5] and the PET And Recovery following Revascularization (PARR-2) trial,[6] have contested the value of revascularization or viability testing in patients with ischemic cardiomyopathy. Unfortunately, all of these studies had several

Conflict of Interest: None.
Disclosures: None.
Department of Cardiovascular Medicine, The Cleveland Clinic Foundation, 9500 Euclid Avenue, Cleveland, OH 44195, USA
* Corresponding author. Cleveland Clinic Main Campus, 9500 Euclid Avenue, Desk J2-3, Cleveland, OH 44195.
E-mail address: elliss@ccf.org

Heart Failure Clin 11 (2015) 203–214
http://dx.doi.org/10.1016/j.hfc.2014.12.002

major limitations, thus tempering their impact on clinical practice. Furthermore, most of these studies focused primarily on surgical revascularization, making it even more difficult to draw conclusions regarding the role of percutaneous revascularization.

The objectives of this article are to provide a brief overview of the concepts of myocardial hibernation and stunning, compare the various methods of viability testing, and review the current literature including analysis of the recent trials on the role of coronary revascularization in ischemic cardiomyopathy. Recent guideline recommendations from various societies are reviewed and factors affecting the choice of surgical versus percutaneous revascularization are discussed.

THEORETIC BASIS OF FUNCTIONAL IMPROVEMENT WITH REVASCULARIZATION IN ISCHEMIC CARDIOMYOPATHY

The proposed mechanism by which LV function improves following revascularization in ischemic cardiomyopathy is the revitalization of previously dysfunctional but still viable myocardial tissue. The concept of stunning was originally described more than 30 years ago[7] to explain the observation that myocardium that is transiently ischemic displays contractile dysfunction, which ultimately recovers early after restoration of normal resting blood flow. Studies with serial assessment of ventricular function showed that approximately two-thirds of stunned segments display early recovery of contractility by 3 months and only 10% show delayed recovery at 14 months after revascularization.[8] Although stunned myocardium has normal resting blood flow with blunted coronary flow reserve, hibernating myocardium has severely reduced resting blood flow, yet remains viable by adaptively reducing contractility and cellular activity to decrease basal metabolic demand. In contrast to stunned myocardium, hibernating myocardium generally shows delayed recovery after revascularization, with approximately two-thirds of hibernating segments recovering after 14 months in one study.[8] This time dependence of recovery has important implications because early evaluation after revascularization may underestimate the degree of true functional recovery.[9]

According to the current paradigm, stunning and hibernation exist along a continuum of chronic myocardial dysfunction. Repeated episodes of transient ischemia over time lead to progression from stunned to hibernating myocardium and ultimately to necrosis and scar. Several animal and human studies with histologic evaluation have shown that these processes often coexist in the same myocardial segments with hibernating myocytes showing more severe ultrastructural changes than stunned myocytes.[9,10] Clinically, the distinction between stunned and hibernating myocardium may be more difficult to discern and less relevant because they both constitute viable myocardium. Studies have shown that up to 60% of patients with ischemic LV dysfunction may have viable myocardium that may recover with revascularization.[11,12] However, not all viable myocardium recovers after revascularization and the probability of recovery and reverse remodeling is affected by several factors including the timeliness,[13,14] completeness,[15] and long-term patency of revascularization. Prolonged myocardial hibernation may progress to necrosis, limiting functional recovery after revascularization. Extent of viability is also important and several studies have shown that at least 25% to 30% of dysfunctional myocardium needs to be viable for improvement in LV ejection fraction (EF) after revascularization.[16,17] However, extensively remodeled ventricles with severe dilation may not recover after revascularization even in the presence of viability.[18]

ASSESSMENT OF MYOCARDIAL VIABILITY AND ISCHEMIA

The role of viability testing has been at the center of the discussion regarding the value of revascularization in patients with ischemic LV dysfunction. Many studies, including the recent randomized trials (STICH[4] and HEART[5]), have not distinguished between patients evaluated using different viability testing methods. However, there are important fundamental differences between the tests that must be emphasized. The various imaging modalities can be broadly divided into those that assess cellular integrity (such as single-photon emission computed tomography or SPECT, PET, and late gadolinium enhancement cardiac magnetic resonance or CMR) and those that assess contractile reserve (such as dobutamine echo or dobutamine CMR).

Among the tests of cellular integrity, SPECT is by far the most commonly used because of the ready availability of the nuclear isotopes thallium-201 and technetium-99m. However, SPECT has the lowest spatial resolution (10–14 mm) of any test of cellular integrity, which can affect diagnostic accuracy.[19,20] Furthermore, technetium-99m agents sestamibi and tetrofosmin do not undergo significant redistribution following initial myocyte uptake, which is proportional to myocardial blood flow. Thallium-201, by contrast, is a potassium analogue that is actively transported into myocytes and redistributes extensively into viable myocardium over time. Thus, the true extent of hibernating myocardium may be underestimated by technetium-99m compared with thallium-201 SPECT.[21] Despite this theoretic difference, studies have found technetium-99m and thallium-201 SPECT to have equivalent accuracy in predicting functional recovery after revascularization.[22] Overall use of thallium-201 has declined significantly because of relatively higher absorbed dose and poorer image quality in comparison to technetium-99m.

PET is clearly the most advanced nuclear imaging test of cellular integrity. It has superior spatial resolution (5–7 mm) in comparison to SPECT because of the higher energy of photons and in-built attenuation correction technology. Furthermore, it is the only nuclear test that can also evaluate metabolic activity using radiolabeled fluorodeoxyglucose (FDG) detecting residual myocardial viability in areas of severe hypoperfusion. Thus, PET is likely to be more sensitive than technetium-99m or thallium-201 SPECT in identifying hibernating myocardium.[23,24] However, extensive use of PET is limited by equipment costs and restricted availability of radiotracers.

CMR is used most commonly for the evaluation of cellular integrity through the assessment of late gadolinium enhancement. Gadolinium-III is a paramagnetic ion that distributes into myocardial tissue in proportion to the amount of extracellular space and therefore accumulates in areas of fibrosis.[25] Nonviable myocardial segments have a visually estimated transmural extent of late gadolinium enhancement above a predefined threshold percentage (usually >50%) of the myocardial thickness. Not surprisingly, the sensitivity, specificity, and value of this test in predicting functional recovery after revascularization are significantly dependent on the threshold value of the transmural extent of late gadolinium enhancement used to define viability.[26] Extensive use of late gadolinium CMR is also limited by cost, presence of implanted hardware such as pacemakers or defibrillators, patient intolerance due to claustrophobia, and the presence of advanced renal insufficiency preventing the use of gadolinium contrast agents.

CMR can also be used to test viability by evaluating contractile reserve in response to dobutamine, often in conjunction with late gadolinium enhancement technique. When the transmural extent of late gadolinium exceeds 75%, the likelihood of functional recovery is very low.[26] However, in segments wherein the transmural extent of late gadolinium enhancement is less than 75%, demonstration of contractile reserve through dobutamine CMR provides incremental value in predicting functional recovery.[27] Dobutamine CMR protocols, however, lead to tachycardia, which can degrade image quality and significantly prolong image acquisition time, which can exacerbate patient claustrophobia.

Dobutamine echocardiography, however, is the most commonly used test of contractile reserve. Low-dose dobutamine is generally used to augment contractility and thereby demonstrate viability in myocardial segments with baseline contractile dysfunction. With higher doses of dobutamine, the hibernating or stunned myocardium may become ischemic as metabolic demand exceeds oxygen delivery and once again display contractile dysfunction. Some studies have suggested that this "biphasic response" indicating both viability and ischemia may be an excellent predictor of functional recovery following revascularization.[28,29]

The sensitivities and specificities of the various viability testing modalities for detecting viable myocardium calculated from a pooled analysis of the available literature are presented in **Table 1**.[30,31] In general, tests of cellular integrity may be considered to have higher sensitivity than tests of contractile reserve, which may have higher specificity and predictive accuracy for functional recovery.[32] A greater amount of viable myocardial mass is needed to demonstrate contractile reserve and subsequent functional recovery than to simply achieve radiotracer uptake.[33,34] Unfortunately, there are very limited contemporary studies comparing the effectiveness of the various viability tests in improving outcomes after revascularization and therefore no testing modality can currently be considered to be the gold standard.

EFFECT OF REVASCULARIZATION IN PATIENTS WITH ISCHEMIC CARDIOMYOPATHY—THE OBSERVATIONAL EVIDENCE

Over the past several decades, a large number of observational studies have attempted to evaluate the impact of revascularization in patients with LV dysfunction because of obstructive CAD.[27,35–46] Most of these studies showed that in the presence of viable myocardium, revascularization of patients with ischemic cardiomyopathy leads to improvement in mortality as well as LV systolic function in comparison to medical therapy alone. In addition to demonstration of viability by imaging, the presence of angina, which can be considered a clinical marker of extensive viability, was required for inclusion of patients in many of

Table 1
Comparison of the various imaging techniques for detecting hibernating myocardium: pooled analysis of available literature

Technique	No. of Studies	No. of Patients	Mean EF (%)	Sensitivity (%)	Specificity (%)
Dobutamine echocardiography, total	41	1421	25–48	80	78
Low-dose dobutamine echo	33	1121	25–48	79	78
High-dose dobutamine echo	8	290	29–38	83	79
Thallium scintigraphy, total	40	1119	23–45	87	54
Thallium rest-redistribution	28	776	23–45	87	56
Thallium reinjection	12	343	31–49	87	50
Technetium scintigraphy, total	25	721	23–54	83	65
Without nitrates protocol	17	516	23–52	83	57
With nitrates protocol	8	205	35–54	81	69
PET, total	24	756	23–53	92	63
CMR, total	14	450	24–53	80	70
Low-dose dobutamine protocol	9	272	24–53	74	82
Late gadolinium-enhancement protocol	5	178	32–52	84	63

Adapted from Shah BN, Khattar RS, Senior R. The hibernating myocardium: current concepts, diagnostic dilemmas, and clinical challenges in the post-STICH era. Eur Heart J 2013;34:1323–34; with permission.

these studies. Other studies, in fact, showed that in patients with ischemic LV dysfunction without angina, revascularization provided no benefit in mortality or improvement in ventricular function.[47,48] However, O'Connor and colleagues[49] reported a large single-center experience that showed that revascularization improved outcomes in patients with ischemic cardiomyopathy even in the absence of angina.

In 2002, Allman and colleagues[50] reported a meta-analysis of 24 observational studies (comprising 3088 patients with mean LV EF of 32%) that demonstrated an 80% lower long-term mortality in patients with viable myocardium who underwent revascularization compared with medical therapy alone (3.2% vs 16%, respectively). By contrast, in patients without viability, there was no mortality benefit with revascularization. A subsequent large single-center study of outcomes in ischemic cardiomyopathy patients who underwent PET viability testing showed a significantly lower mortality with early revascularization regardless of the presence or extent of viability.[51] Another review of 29 studies including 758 patients with severe ischemic systolic dysfunction showed that revascularization in the presence of viable myocardium led to an average improvement in EF of 8% compared with no improvement in the absence of viability.[12]

Despite this extensive body of observational data in support of revascularization in patients with ischemic cardiomyopathy, multiple concerns

remained. The studies were highly variable in terms of methodology and likely to be affected by several biases including selection and publication bias. Furthermore, most of the studies were conducted before extensive use of current evidence-based medical and device therapies, thereby raising uncertainty regarding the role of revascularization in contemporary management of patients with ischemic cardiomyopathy.

EFFECT OF REVASCULARIZATION IN PATIENTS WITH ISCHEMIC CARDIOMYOPATHY—SUMMARY AND ANALYSIS OF RECENT RANDOMIZED TRIALS

Three prospective randomized trials (summarized in **Table 2**) were conducted in the last decade to address the continuing uncertainty regarding the value of revascularization in ischemic cardiomyopathy. The PARR-2 trial randomized 430 patients with average EF of 27% to either management based on results of PET viability testing or standard care.[6] In the PET group, revascularization (coronary artery bypass grafting [CABG] or coronary artery bypass grafting [PCI]) was recommended in patients with demonstrated viability. The study reported no significant difference in primary composite endpoint of cardiac death, myocardial infarction, or rehospitalization between the 2 groups. However, a major drawback of the study was that 25% of patients in the PET group did not undergo recommended revascularization despite moderate and even large amounts of ischemia. In fact, in the subgroup of patients with viability on PET that actually underwent revascularization, there was a significant decrease in mortality compared with the standard care group.[52]

The HEART trial, conducted at multiple centers in the United Kingdom, aimed to randomize 800 patients with ischemic cardiomyopathy, EF less than 35%, without angina but with evidence of viable myocardium to either revascularization (CABG or PCI) with medical therapy or medical therapy alone.[5] However, only 138 of the intended 800 patients were enrolled because of slow recruitment and withdrawal of funding. In this severely underpowered trial, no difference in mortality was detected between the 2 groups.

After the inconclusive results of the PARR-2 and HEART trials, the outcome of the landmark STICH trial was highly anticipated. It was an international multicenter trial that randomized 1212 patients with ischemic cardiomyopathy and EF less than 35% to surgical revascularization with medical therapy or medical therapy alone.[4] After a mean 56 months of follow-up, intention-to-treat analysis of the results showed no significant difference in all-cause mortality between the 2 groups. There was, however, a significant reduction in secondary outcomes of cardiovascular mortality or rehospitalization in the surgical revascularization group.

Despite being the largest randomized trial of its kind, STICH generated a significant amount of controversy due to its notable limitations. First, patient recruitment for the study was quite slow, with average enrollment rate being only 2 patients per site per year, suggesting a strong component of selection bias. Many eligible patients were not enrolled in the study by providers with a priori assumptions about the most beneficial treatment plan. Furthermore, patients with significant left main disease were not enrolled in the study due to the previously demonstrated mortality benefit in such patients with revascularization compared with medical therapy alone.[53] Given that there was a trend toward reduction in all-cause mortality in the surgical revascularization group, inclusion of left main stenosis patients in the study might have allowed the results to reach statistical significance. There was also a suggestion that a longer duration of follow-up may have allowed the results to reach statistical significance, and the study is currently being continued to provide 10-year follow-up. Finally, there was a significant amount of crossover between the 2 groups in the study. Among the patients randomized to medical therapy, 17% crossed over to CABG and an additional 6% underwent PCI. Furthermore, 9% of those randomized to CABG did not have surgery. In fact, after accounting for the crossover, the as-treated analysis *did* show a significant mortality reduction in patients who underwent revascularization compared with medical therapy alone.

Following the main STICH trial, the investigators published a subgroup analysis of outcomes in 601 patients (of 1212 enrolled in the main trial) that had undergone viability testing (SPECT or dobutamine echo).[54] They reported no difference in all-cause mortality in those with or without evidence of viability, after adjustment for other baseline variables. Furthermore, viability testing did not seem to identify patients with increased mortality benefit from CABG. This study, however, also had several major limitations. First, the decision to pursue viability testing was optional and left to the discretion of the recruiting investigator. Thus, the study was not truly randomized and it is likely that many patients with evidence of viability were not even enrolled in the study. In fact, the presence of selection bias is evident by the fact that patients who underwent viability testing had more significant LV remodeling and were therefore less likely to derive a functional benefit from revascularization.[55] Finally, the study used 2 fundamentally different types of viability tests (SPECT and dobutamine echo) with variable definitions of viability. Viability by SPECT was defined as radiotracer uptake in greater than 11 segments, whereas by dobutamine echo, it was defined as contractile reserve in greater than 5 segments. It is also important to note that the presence of radiotracer uptake specifically in dysfunctional segments was not necessary for demonstration of viability by SPECT. Moreover, most patients with SPECT imaging did not undergo evaluation for ischemia, which has been shown to add incremental value in predicting functional recovery, especially in patients with less severe CAD.[56]

Thus, despite the negative results of the STICH trial and the viability substudy, uncertainty persists regarding the role of revascularization as well as viability testing in ischemic cardiomyopathy as reflected in the guidelines discussed later.

COMPARATIVE EFFECTIVENESS OF PERCUTANEOUS VERSUS SURGICAL REVASCULARIZATION IN PATIENTS WITH SYSTOLIC DYSFUNCTION

Several large observational studies have suggested better outcomes with CABG compared with PCI in the setting of LV dysfunction. A propensity analysis of long-term survival in 6033 patients who underwent CABG or PCI (with 70% stents) in late 1990s showed a trend toward reduction in

Table 2
Summary of randomized trials of revascularization in patients with severe ischemic cardiomyopathy

	PARR-2	HEART	STICH, Main Trial	STICH, Viability Substudy
Number of patients	430	138	1212	601
Number of enrollment sites	9	13	99	99
Study question	Does FDG-PET-assisted management in patients with severe LV dysfunction and suspected CAD improve outcomes?	Does revascularization compared with OMT alone improve outcomes in patients with LV dysfunction and viable myocardium?	Does CABG compared with OMT alone improve outcomes in patients with LV dysfunction with or without viable myocardium?	Does presence of viability improve survival in patients with ischemic LV dysfunction? Does viability testing identify patients with differential survival benefit from CABG compared with OMT alone?
Primary endpoint	Composite of cardiac death, MI, or recurrent hospitalization for cardiac cause	All-cause mortality	All-cause mortality	All-cause mortality
Secondary endpoints	Time to occurrence of the composite event and time to cardiac death	n/a	Cardiovascular mortality and composite of all-cause mortality and hospitalization for any cause	Cardiovascular mortality and composite of all-cause mortality and hospitalization for any cause
Median duration of follow-up (mo)	12	59	56	56

Viability testing modality	PET	SPECT, PET, or dobutamine echo	SPECT or dobutamine echo	SPECT or dobutamine echo
Revascularization strategy	CABG or PCI vs OMT alone	CABG or PCI vs OMT alone	CABG or OMT alone	CABG or OMT alone
Results/conclusion	No difference in primary outcome with FDG-PET-assisted management compared with standard care (HR 0.78; 95% CI 0.58 to 1.1; $P = .15$)	No difference in primary outcome with revascularization compared with OMT alone	• No difference in primary outcome (HR with CABG 0.86; 95% CI 0.72 to 1.04; $P = .12$) • Reduction in cardiovascular mortality (HR with CABG 0.81; 95% CI 0.66 to 1.00, $P = .05$) • Reduction in all-cause mortality + cardiac hospitalization (HR with CABG 0.74; 95% CI, 0.64 to 0.85; $P<.001$)	• Reduced mortality in patients with viable myocardium compared with without viable myocardium (HR 0.64; 95% CI 0.48 to 0.86; $P = .003$). However, results not significant ($P = .21$) after adjustment for other baseline variables • No mortality difference with respect to treatment assignment in patients with or without viability
Major limitations	25% of patients in PET group did not undergo recommended revascularization despite moderate or large amounts of ischemia	Severely underpowered; only 138 of planned 800 patients enrolled due to lack of funding	• Very slow recruitment raising concern for selection bias • Significant crossover between groups; significant difference in primary outcome in as-treated patients • Exclusion of left main patients	• Not truly a randomized study • Decision to pursue viability testing was optional and at discretion of recruiting investigator • Used fundamentally different viability tests with variable definitions of viability

Abbreviations: CI, confidence interval; HR, hazard ratio; MI, myocardial infarction; n/a, none; OMT, optimal medical therapy.

5-year mortality with CABG over PCI (28% vs 37%) in patients with EF less than 30%.[57] Another large nonrandomized study of 59,314 patients from the New York registry who underwent CABG or PCI with bare-metal stenting between 1997 and 2000 reported higher risk-adjusted survival rates with CABG in patients with EF less than 40% and 3-vessel CAD or 2-vessel CAD with involvement of the proximal LAD.[58] A similar New York registry study of patients who underwent PCI with DES or CABG between 2003 and 2004 also reported improved survival with CABG.[59]

Unfortunately, high-quality comparative effectiveness data of PCI versus CABG in patients with chronic systolic dysfunction are scant. The vast majority of randomized trials of PCI versus CABG excluded patients with reduced LV function. Only the BARI[60] and AWESOME[61] trials reported comparative outcomes based on LV function. The BARI trial, which randomized 1829 patients with multivessel CAD and severe angina or ischemia to either percutaneous transluminal coronary angioplasty or CABG, showed no significant difference in 5-year mortality with either revascularization strategy in nondiabetic patients with reduced LV function. In diabetic patients, the recent FREEDOM[62] trial showed that CABG compared with PCI was associated with a significant reduction in mortality and myocardial infarction, but the study did not include a meaningful number of patients with reduced LV function. The AWESOME trial, which randomized 454 high-risk patients with CAD and medically refractory unstable angina to CABG or PCI with or without stents, showed no significant difference in 3-year mortality in the subgroup of patients with LV EF less than 35%.

A limitation of most randomized trials of PCI versus CABG is that they excluded a significant portion of "real world" patients, for example, enrolling only those that can feasibly undergo both PCI and CABG based on anatomy. Unfortunately, even the relatively recent SYNTAX[63] trial comparing PCI with Taxus DES versus CABG did not include many patients with reduced LV function despite having an "all-comer" design with respect to anatomy. On the other hand, although large observational studies are more inclusive and provide the power to detect a difference in mortality that may remain hidden in smaller randomized trials, they are also prone to several biases that are often not eliminated by statistical techniques such as propensity matching.[64] For example, PCI is generally preferred over CABG in patients with life-limiting noncardiac illnesses, and such confounders are seldom ascertained

from observational databases. Furthermore, there has been significant evolution in both technologies (CABG and PCI) as well as medical management of CAD in the last 15 years, limiting the conclusions that can be drawn from older studies. Thus, even though CABG currently appears to be favored over PCI in patients with severe systolic dysfunction, the evidence base for their comparative effectiveness in this high-risk subgroup remains weak.

CURRENT GUIDELINES AND OPINION STATEMENTS REGARDING REVASCULARIZATION IN PATIENTS WITH REDUCED LEFT VENTRICULAR FUNCTION

According to the 2013 American College of Cardiology Foundation/American Heart Association (ACCF/AHA) Heart Failure Guidelines,[65] revascularization with either CABG or PCI is given a class I recommendation in heart failure patients with angina in the presence of suitable anatomy, especially left main or left main equivalent stenosis. In patients with mild to moderate LV systolic dysfunction without angina, CABG is given a class IIA recommendation to improve survival, when viable myocardium is present. In those with severe systolic dysfunction (EF <30%) with heart failure but without angina, either CABG or medical therapy is given a class IIA recommendation to improve morbidity and mortality. Notably, no recommendations are given regarding the role of PCI in patients with systolic dysfunction without angina. By contrast, the 2012 ESC Heart Failure Guidelines[66] give a class IIB recommendation for PCI as an alternative to CABG in patients considered unsuitable for surgery.

Although CABG may be considered the standard of care in patients with LV dysfunction, PCI has been used with increasing frequency in certain situations. In the absence of high-quality data to guide choice of revascularization strategy based on LV function alone, other factors may be important. Completeness of revascularization, which is generally higher with CABG, has been shown to be an important predictor of outcomes in patients with ischemic LV dysfunction.[15] The SYNTAX trial concluded that in patients with multivessel or left-main CAD, CABG is associated with a higher rate of complete revascularization and lower rates of major adverse cardiovascular events (MACE) compared with PCI with Taxus DES.[62] Of note, the difference in MACE rates between the 2 groups was driven primarily by rate of repeat revascularization, which, not surprisingly, was significantly higher in the patients undergoing PCI. However, subgroup analysis showed that patients with less complex multivessel disease (SYNTAX score <22) have equivalent rates of complete revascularization and MACE with PCI or CABG. Furthermore, residual SYNTAX score of 0 in patients who were randomized to PCI in the trial was shown to be a powerful indicator of survival at 5 years.[67] Thus, in patients with LV dysfunction due to multivessel CAD and high operative risk, the authors think that PCI may be a reasonable alternative to CABG if complete percutaneous revascularization is feasible based on anatomy.

Left main CAD is another situation in which PCI may be comparable with CABG in selected patients. The PRECOMBAT trial, which randomized 600 patients with unprotected left main disease to CABG or PCI with sirolimus-eluting stents, showed that at 2 years, MACE rates were not significantly different between the 2 groups.[68] In the subgroup analysis, patients with isolated left main or left main with single-vessel disease had trended toward superior outcomes with PCI, whereas patients with multivessel disease had trended toward superior outcomes with CABG. Similar analysis was also reported in the left main subset of patients in the SYNTAX trial.[61] Unfortunately, patients with significant LV dysfunction were not enrolled in either study. However, the authors think that in patients with LV dysfunction and isolated left main or left main with single-vessel disease and high operative risk, PCI may be considered a reasonable alternative to CABG.

SUMMARY

Coronary revascularization to improve LV function and improve mortality in patients with ischemic cardiomyopathy remains controversial, especially in the absence of angina or ischemia. A large body of observational evidence suggests that patients with dysfunctional but viable myocardium may experience improvement in mortality and LV function after revascularization. However, results of randomized trials conducted in the last decade dispute the value of viability testing or coronary revascularization in improving outcomes of patients with ischemic cardiomyopathy. However, because of the numerous methodological limitations of these studies, clinical equipoise persists regarding the role of coronary revascularization in certain patients; this is reflected in the 2013 ACCF/AHA Heart Failure Guidelines, which continue to give a class I or class IIA recommendation to revascularization in ischemic cardiomyopathy patients with or without angina but with evidence of viability, respectively. Surgical revascularization has been preferred over percutaneous

revascularization in patients with LV dysfunction based on observational data, but high-quality randomized comparative effectiveness data are lacking. Based on results of randomized studies of PCI versus CABG in patients with normal LV function, PCI may be considered as an alternative to CABG in patients in whom complete revascularization is feasible based on anatomy—such as less complex 3-vessel CAD (SYNTAX score <22), isolated left main, or isolated left main plus one-vessel CAD.

REFERENCES

1. Rogers WJ, Canto JG, Lambrew CT, et al. Temporal trends in the treatment of over 1.5 million patients with myocardial infarction in the US from 1990 through 1999: the National Registry of Myocardial Infarction 1, 2 and 3. J Am Coll Cardiol 2000;36: 2056–63.
2. Adams KF Jr, Fonarow GC, Emerman CL, et al. Characteristics and outcomes of patients hospitalized for heart failure in the United States: rationale, design, and preliminary observations from the first 100,000 cases in the Acute Decompensated Heart Failure National Registry (ADHERE). Am Heart J 2005;149:209–16.
3. Curtis JP, Sokol SI, Wang Y, et al. The association of left ventricular ejection fraction, mortality, and cause of death in stable outpatients with heart failure. J Am Coll Cardiol 2003;42:736–42.
4. Velazquez EJ, Lee KL, Deja MA, et al. Coronary-artery bypass surgery in patients with left ventricular dysfunction. N Engl J Med 2011;364:1607–16.
5. Cleland JG, Calvert M, Freemantle N, et al. The heart failure revascularisation trial (HEART). Eur J Heart Fail 2011;13:227–33.
6. Beanlands RS, Nichol G, Huszti E, et al. F-18-fluorodeoxyglucose positron emission tomography imaging-assisted management of patients with severe left ventricular dysfunction and suspected coronary disease: a randomized, controlled trial (PARR-2). J Am Coll Cardiol 2007;50:2002–12.
7. Braunwald E, Kloner RA. The stunned myocardium: prolonged, postischemic ventricular dysfunction. Circulation 1982;66:1146–9.
8. Bax JJ, Visser FC, Poldermans D, et al. Time course of functional recovery of stunned and hibernating segments after surgical revascularization. Circulation 2001;104(Suppl 1):I314–8.
9. Haas F, Jennen L, Heinzmann U, et al. Ischemically compromised myocardium displays different time-courses of functional recovery: correlation with morphological alterations? Eur J Cardiothorac Surg 2001;20:290–8.
10. Firoozan S, Wei K, Linka A, et al. A canine model of chronic ischemic cardiomyopathy: characterization

of regional flow-function relations. Am J Phys 1999; 276:H446–55.

11. Auerbach MA, Schöder H, Hoh C, et al. Prevalence of myocardial viability as detected by positron emission tomography in patients with ischemic cardiomyopathy. Circulation 1999;99(22):2921.

12. Bax JJ, van der Wall EE, Harbinson M. Radionuclide techniques for the assessment of myocardial viability and hibernation. Heart 2004;90(Suppl 5): v26–33.

13. Bax JJ, Schinkel AF, Boersma E, et al. Early versus delayed revascularization in patients with ischemic cardiomyopathy and substantial viability: impact on outcome. Circulation 2003;108:II39–42.

14. Beanlands RS, Hendry PJ, Masters RG, et al. Delay in revascularization is associated with increased mortality rate in patients with severe left ventricular dysfunction and viable myocardium on fluorine 18-fluorodeoxyglucose positron emission tomography imaging. Circulation 1998;98:II51–6.

15. Bell MR, Gersh BJ, Schaff HV, et al. Effect of completeness of revascularization on long-term outcome of patients with three-vessel disease undergoing coronary artery bypass surgery. A report from the Coronary Artery Surgery Study (CASS) Registry. Circulation 1992;86:446–57.

16. Bax JJ, Maddahi J, Poldermans D, et al. Sequential (201) Tl imaging and dobutamine echocardiography to enhance accuracy of predicting improved left ventricular ejection fraction after revascularization. J Nucl Med 2002;43:795–802.

17. Pagano D, Bonser RS, Townend JN, et al. Predictive value of dobutamine echocardiography and positron emission tomography in identifying hibernating myocardium in patients with postischaemic heart failure. Heart 1998;79:281–8.

18. Bax JJ, Poldermans D, Elhendy A, et al. Assessment of myocardial viability by nuclear imaging techniques. Curr Cardiol Rep 2005;7:124–9.

19. Wagner A, Mahrholdt H, Holly TA, et al. Contrast-enhanced MRI and routine single photon emission computed tomography (SPECT) perfusion imaging for detection of subendocardial myocardial infarcts: an imaging study. Lancet 2003;361:374–9.

20. Di Carli MF. Assessment of myocardial viability after myocardial infarction. J Nucl Cardiol 2002;9:229–35.

21. Dilsizian V, Arrighi JA, Diodati JG, et al. Myocardial viability in patients with chronic coronary artery disease. Comparison of 99Tc-sestamibi with thallium reinjection and 18F-fluorodeoxyglucose. Circulation 1994;89:578–87.

22. Udelson JE, Coleman PS, Metherall J, et al. Predicting recovery of severe regional ventricular dysfunction. Comparison of resting scintigraphy with 201Tl and 99mTc-sestamibi. Circulation 1994;89:2552–61.

23. Sawada S, Allman K, Muzik O, et al. Positron emission tomography detects evidence of viability in rest technetium-99m sestamibi defects. J Am Coll Cardiol 1994;23:92–8.

24. Alexanderson E, Ricalde A, Romero-Ibarra JL, et al. Comparison of 18FDG PET with thallium SPECT in the assessment of myocardial viability. A segmental model analysis. Arch Cardiol Mex 2006;76(1):9–15.

25. Abraham JL, Higgins CB, Newell JD. Uptake of iodinated contrast material in ischemic myocardium as an indicator of loss of cellular membrane integrity. Am J Pathol 1980;101:319–30.

26. Kim RJ, Wu E, Rafael A, et al. The use of contrast-enhanced magnetic resonance imaging to identify reversible myocardial dysfunction. N Engl J Med 2000;343:1445–53.

27. Wellnhofer E, Olariu A, Klein C, et al. Magnetic resonance low-dose dobutamine test is superior to SCAR quantification for the prediction of functional recovery. Circulation 2004;109(18):2172–4.

28. Afridi I, Kleiman NS, Raizner AE, et al. Dobutamine echocardiography in myocardial hibernation. Optimal dose and accuracy in predicting recovery of ventricular function after coronary angioplasty. Circulation 1995;91:663–70.

29. Afridi I, Grayburn PA, Panza JA, et al. Myocardial viability during dobutamine echocardiography predicts survival in patients with coronary artery disease and severe left ventricular systolic dysfunction. J Am Coll Cardiol 1998;32:921–6.

30. Shah BN, Khattar RS, Senior R. The hibernating myocardium: current concepts, diagnostic dilemmas, and clinical challenges in the post-STICH era. Eur Heart J 2013;34:1323–34.

31. Schinkel AF, Bax JJ, Poldermans D, et al. Hibernating myocardium: diagnosis and patient outcomes. Curr Probl Cardiol 2007;32:375–410.

32. Bax JJ, Wijns W, Cornel JH, et al. Accuracy of currently available techniques for prediction of functional recovery after revascularization in patients with left ventricular dysfunction due to chronic coronary artery disease: comparison of pooled data. J Am Coll Cardiol 1997;30:1451–60.

33. Gunning MG, Kaprielian RR, Pepper J, et al. The histology of viable and hibernating myocardium in relation to imaging characteristics. J Am Coll Cardiol 2002;39:428–35.

34. Baumgartner H, Porenta G, Lau YK, et al. Assessment of myocardial viability by dobutamine echocardiography, positron emission tomography and thallium-201 SPECT: correlation with histopathology in explanted hearts. J Am Coll Cardiol 1998;32: 1701–8.

35. Brundage BH, Massie BM, Botvinick EH. Improved regional ventricular function after successful surgical revascularization. J Am Coll Cardiol 1984;3(4):902.

36. Tillisch J, Brunken R, Marshall R, et al. Reversibility of cardiac wall-motion abnormalities predicted by positron tomography. N Engl J Med 1986;314(14):884.

37. Eitzman D, al-Aouar Z, Kanter HL, et al. Clinical outcome of patients with advanced coronary artery disease after viability studies with positron emission tomography. J Am Coll Cardiol 1992;20(3):559.

38. Elefteriades JA, Tolis G Jr, Levi E, et al. Coronary artery bypass grafting in severe left ventricular dysfunction: excellent survival with improved ejection fraction and functional state. J Am Coll Cardiol 1993;22(5):1411.

39. Ragosta M, Beller GA, Watson DD, et al. Quantitative planar rest-redistribution 201Tl imaging in detection of myocardial viability and prediction of improvement in left ventricular function after coronary bypass surgery in patients with severely depressed left ventricular function. Circulation 1993;87(5):1630.

40. Lee KS, Marwick TH, Cook SA, et al. Prognosis of patients with left ventricular dysfunction, with and without viable myocardium after myocardial infarction. Relative efficacy of medical therapy and revascularization. Circulation 1994;90(6):2687.

41. Pagley PR, Beller GA, Watson DD, et al. Improved outcome after coronary bypass surgery in patients with ischemic cardiomyopathy and residual myocardial viability. Circulation 1997;96(3):793.

42. Baer FM, Theissen P, Schneider CA, et al. Dobutamine magnetic resonance imaging predicts contractile recovery of chronically dysfunctional myocardium after successful revascularization. J Am Coll Cardiol 1998;31(5):1040.

43. Bax JJ, Poldermans D, Elhendy A, et al. Improvement of left ventricular ejection fraction, heart failure symptoms and prognosis after revascularization in patients with chronic coronary artery disease and viable myocardium detected by dobutamine stress echocardiography. J Am Coll Cardiol 1999;34(1):163.

44. Samady H, Elefteriades JA, Abbott BG, et al. Failure to improve left ventricular function after coronary revascularization for ischemic cardiomyopathy is not associated with worse outcome. Circulation 1999;100(12):1298.

45. Chareonthaitawee P, Gersh BJ, Araoz PA, et al. Revascularization in severe left ventricular dysfunction: the role of viability testing. J Am Coll Cardiol 2005;46(4):567.

46. Gerber BL, Rousseau MF, Ahn SA, et al. Prognostic value of myocardial viability by delayed-enhanced magnetic resonance in patients with coronary artery disease and low ejection fraction: impact of revascularization therapy. J Am Coll Cardiol 2012;59(9):825.

47. Alderman EL, Fisher LD, Litwin P, et al. Results of coronary artery surgery in patients with poor left ventricular function (CASS). Circulation 1983;68:785–95.

48. Baker DW, Jones R, Hodges J, et al. Management of heart failure, III: the role of revascularization in the treatment of patients with moderate or severe left ventricular systolic dysfunction. JAMA 1994;272:1528–34.

49. O'Connor CM, Velazquez EJ, Gardner LH, et al. Comparison of coronary artery bypass grafting versus medical therapy on long-term outcome in patients with ischemic cardiomyopathy (a 25-year experience from the Duke Cardiovascular Disease Databank). Am J Cardiol 2002;90:101–7.

50. Allman KC, Shaw LJ, Hachamovitch R, et al. Myocardial viability testing and impact of revascularization on prognosis in patients with coronary artery disease and left ventricular dysfunction: a meta-analysis. J Am Coll Cardiol 2002;39:1151–8.

51. Tarakji KG, Brunken R, McCarthy PM, et al. Myocardial viability testing and the effect of early intervention in patients with advanced left ventricular systolic dysfunction. Circulation 2006;113:230–7.

52. Abraham A, Nichol G, Williams KA, et al. 18F-FDG PET imaging of myocardial viability in an experienced center with access to 18-FDG and integration with clinical management teams: the Ottawa-FIVE substudy of the PARR 2 Trial. J Nucl Med 2010;51:567–74.

53. Eagle KA, Guyton RA, Davidoff R, et al. ACC/AHA 2004 guideline update for coronary artery bypass graft surgery: a report of the American College of Cardiology/American Heart Association Task Force on Practice Guidelines. Circulation 2004;110(14):e340.

54. Bonow RO, Maurer G, Lee KL, et al. Myocardial viability and survival in ischemic left ventricular dysfunction. N Engl J Med 2011;364:1617–25.

55. Schinkel AF, Poldermans D, Rizzello V, et al. Why do patients with ischemic cardiomyopathy and a substantial amount of viable myocardium not always recover in function after revascularization? J Thorac Cardiovasc Surg 2004;127:385–90.

56. Kitsiou AN, Srinivasan G, Quyyumi AA, et al. Stress-induced reversible and mild-to-moderate irreversible thallium defects: are they equally accurate for predicting recovery of regional left ventricular function after revascularization? Circulation 1998;98:501–8.

57. Brener SJ, Lytle BW, Casserly IP, et al. Propensity analysis of long-term survival after surgical or percutaneous revascularization in patients with multivessel coronary artery disease and high-risk features. Circulation 2004;109:2290–5.

58. Hannan EL, Racz MJ, Walford G, et al. Long-term outcomes of coronary-artery bypass grafting versus stent implantation. N Engl J Med 2005;352:2174–83.

59. Hannan EL, Wu C, Walford G, et al. Drug eluting stents vs. coronary artery bypass grafting in multivessel coronary disease. N Engl J Med 2008;358:331–41.

60. Chaitman BR, Rosen AD, Williams DO, et al. Myocardial infarction and cardiac mortality in the Bypass

Angioplasty Revascularization Investigation (BARI) randomized trial. Circulation 1997;96(7):2162–70.

61. Morrison DA, Sethi G, Sacks J, et al. Percutaneous coronary intervention versus coronary artery bypass graft surgery for patients with medically refractory myocardial ischemia and risk factors for adverse outcomes with bypass: a multicenter, randomized trial. J Am Coll Cardiol 2001;38(1):143–9.

62. Farkouh ME, Domanski M, Sleeper LA, et al. Strategies for multivessel revascularization in patients with diabetes. N Engl J Med 2012;367: 2375–84.

63. Serruys PW, Morice MC, Kappetein AP, et al. Percutaneous coronary intervention versus coronary-artery bypass grafting for severe coronary artery disease. N Engl J Med 2009;360:916–72.

64. Casserly IP. The optimal revascularization strategy for multivessel coronary artery disease: the debate continues. Cleve Clin J Med 2006;73:317–28.

65. Yancy CW, Jessup M, Bozkurt B, et al. 2013 ACCF/ AHA guideline for the management of heart failure: executive summary. J Am Coll Cardiol 2013;62: 1495–539.

66. McMurray JJ, Adamopoulos S, Anker SD, et al. ESC guidelines for the diagnosis and treatment of acute and chronic heart failure 2012: the task force for the diagnosis and treatment of acute and chronic heart failure 2012 of the European Society of Cardiology. Developed in collaboration with the Heart Failure Association (HFA) of the ESC. Eur Heart J 2012;33:1787–847.

67. Farooq V, Serruys PW, Bourantas CV, et al. Quantification of incomplete revascularization and its association with five-year mortality in the surgery between percutaneous coronary intervention with Taxus and cardiac surgery (SYNTAX) trial validation of residual SYNTAX score. Circulation 2013;128: 141–51.

68. Park SJ, Kim YH, Park DW, et al. Randomized trial of stents versus bypass surgery for left main coronary artery disease. N Engl J Med 2011;364(18): 1718.

Hemodynamic Support with Percutaneous Devices in Patients with Heart Failure

CrossMark

Navin K. Kapur, MD*, Michele Esposito, MD

KEYWORDS

- Percutaneous mechanical support • Impella • TandemHeart • ECMO • Cardiogenic shock
- Refractory heart failure • Decompensated heart failure • Assist device

KEY POINTS

- The use of surgically implanted durable mechanical circulatory support (MCS) in high-risk patients with heart failure is declining and short-term, nondurable MCS device use is growing.
- Percutaneously delivered MCS options for advanced heart failure include the intra-aortic balloon pump, Impella axial flow catheter, TandemHeart (TH) centrifugal pump, and venoarterial extracorporeal membrane oxygenation.
- Each nondurable MCS device has unique implantation characteristics and hemodynamic effects on left ventricular function.
- Algorithms and guidelines for optimal nondurable MCS device selection do not exist.
- Emerging technologies and applications will address the need for improved left ventricular unloading using lower-profile devices, longer-term ambulatory support, and the potential for myocardial recovery.

 Videos of TandemHeart Pump and Impella RP (Investigational) Pump implantation accompany this article at http://www.heartfailure.theclinics.com

ADVANCED HEART FAILURE AND CARDIOGENIC SHOCK

An estimated 2.6% of the American population and nearly 11% of the elderly population more than 80 years of age experiences heart failure, which is defined as a syndrome caused by cardiac dysfunction, generally resulting from myocardial muscle dysfunction or loss and characterized by either left ventricular dilatation or hypertrophy or both.[1] By 2030, more than 8 million people in the United States (1 in every 33) will be diagnosed with heart failure.[2] The clinical spectrum of heart failure often begins with an initial event such as acute myocardial infarction (AMI), progressive valvular heart disease, myocarditis, or onset of a primary dilated cardiomyopathy. With initial medical stabilization, these patients often survive to develop chronic heart failure, which is characterized by neurohormonal activation, increased sympathetic tone, and maladaptive cardiac remodeling, and, despite optimal medical therapy,

Disclosures: Dr N.K. Kapur receives speaker/consultant honoraria from Abiomed Inc, CardiacAssist Inc, Thoratec Inc, Heartware Inc, and Maquet Inc. Dr M. Esposito has no disclosures.
The Cardiovascular Center, Tufts Medical Center, 800 Washington Street, BOX 80, Boston, MA 02111, USA
* Corresponding author.
E-mail address: nkapur@tuftsmedicalcenter.org

Heart Failure Clin 11 (2015) 215–230
http://dx.doi.org/10.1016/j.hfc.2014.12.012
1551-7136/15/$ – see front matter © 2015 Elsevier Inc. All rights reserved.

ultimate leads to recurrent hospitalizations for acute-on-chronic heart failure and death. At both ends of this clinical spectrum, low cardiac output and multiorgan hypoperfusion are primary indications for the use of advanced therapies, including durable mechanical circulatory support (MCS) devices, which include surgically implanted left, right, or biventricular assist devices, or cardiac transplantation.

In the United States, cardiac transplant volumes have remained stable at approximately 2000 to 2500 per year. In contrast, based on supportive data from the HeartMate-II and Heartware bridge to transplant (BTT) trials and the HeartMate-II destination therapy trial, left ventricular assist device (LVAD) use increased to more than 2500 implants in 2013 in the United States alone.[3] Prospective registry data from the Interagency for Mechanically Assisted Circulatory Support (INTERMACS) reports an increase in the use of LVADs for so-called destination therapy and a reduction in their use as part of a bridge to recovery or rescue strategy (Fig. 1). This shift in LVAD use away from unstable, high-risk INTERMACS profiles (1 and 2) toward more stable candidates (profiles 3 and 4) is partly driven by data showing increased mortality after LVAD implantation for INTERMACS profiles 1 and 2 after the age of 65 years and the increasing availability of nondurable MCS devices, which include short-term, percutaneously inserted devices without the need for cardiac surgery (see Fig. 1). Potential indications for nondurable MCS in patients with advanced heart failure

being considered for durable MCS are listed in Box 1.

Consistent with this observation, a recent analysis of the Nationwide Inpatient Sample from the Healthcare Cost and Utilization Project identified a 1511% increase in the use of nondurable MCS devices, including the TandemHeart (Cardiac Assist Inc) and Impella (Abiomed Inc), and no significant change in intra-aortic balloon pump (IABP) use from 2007 to 2011 compared with 2004 to 2007 (Fig. 2).[4] Use of the TandemHeart and Impella devices was associated with a reduced length of stay and cost for patients admitted with a diagnosis of congestive heart failure, but no change in inhospital mortality. Primary predictors of mortality included advanced age, coagulopathy, metabolic dyscrasia, a diagnosis of cardiogenic shock, and IABP use or cardiopulmonary resuscitation before application of the TandemHeart or Impella devices. This article provides a fundamental understanding of the nondurable MCS device options, hemodynamic effects, candidate selection, and supportive clinical trials in patients with advanced heart failure.

CLASSIFICATION AND INDICATIONS FOR NONDURABLE MECHANICAL CIRCULATORY SUPPORT IN HEART FAILURE

The primary goals of nondurable MCS devices are to (1) increase vital organ perfusion, (2) augment coronary perfusion, and (3) reduce ventricular volume and filling pressures, thereby reducing wall stress, stroke work, and myocardial oxygen consumption. Clinical scenarios in

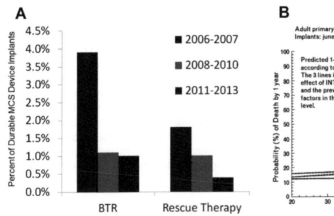

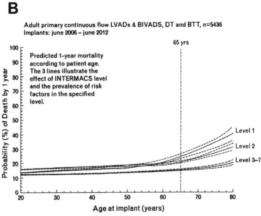

Fig. 1. Trends in the use of durable MCS. (A) Since 2006, use of surgically implanted durable MCS as a bridge to recovery (BTR) or as rescue therapy is declining, caused in part by (B) higher 1-year predicted mortality in patients more than 65 years of age who present with INTERMACS level 1 or 2 advanced heart failure. BIVADS, biventricular assist devices; DT, destination therapy. (From Kirklin JK, Naftel DC, Kormos RL, et al. Fifth INTERMACS annual report: risk factor analysis from more than 6,000 mechanical circulatory support patients. J Heart Lung Transplant 2013;32:144, 147; with permission.)

Box 1
Indications for nondurable MCS in patients with advanced heart failure being considered for durable MCS

- Cardiogenic shock refractory to maximal medical therapy
- Irreversible end-organ damage
- Neurologic status unknown
- Severe hemodynamic instability
- Major coagulopathy
- Prolonged mechanical ventilation
- Sepsis or active infection
- Right ventricular failure
- Noncompliant

which these devices are commonly used include advanced heart failure, cardiogenic shock, mechanical complications after AMI, high-risk coronary and noncoronary intervention, and high-risk electrophysiologic ablations. **Box 2** summarizes current guideline recommendations for nondurable MCS in patients with advanced heart failure.

COUNTERPULSATION PUMPS: INTRA-AORTIC BALLOON PUMPS

The IABP is the most widely used nondurable MCS device, with more than 50,000 implants per year in the United States alone.[5–9] The IABP is a catheter-mounted balloon that augments pulsatile blood flow by inflating during diastole, which displaces blood volume in the descending aorta and

increases mean aortic pressure, thereby potentially augmenting coronary perfusion. On deflation, during systole, the IABP generates a pressure sink, which is filled by ejecting blood from the heart. Optimal IABP function increases diastolic aortic pressure, reduces aortic and left ventricular systolic pressure, increases systemic mean arterial pressure, reduces left ventricular diastolic volume and pressure, and increases coronary perfusion pressure. The hemodynamic effect of an IABP can be directly measured using tracings obtained from the IABP console to determine the magnitude of systolic unloading and diastolic augmentation (**Fig. 3**).

The pioneering work of Kantrowitz, Weber, Janicki, Sarnoff, Schreuder, Kern, and many others have established that the hemodynamic impact of balloon counterpulsation is primarily determined by 4 factors: (1) the magnitude of diastolic pressure augmentation, (2) the magnitude of reduced systolic pressure, (3) the magnitude of volume displacement, and (4) the timing of balloon inflation and deflation.[7,8,10–15] IABP balloon capacity ranges from 34 to 50 cm³. Larger capacity IABPs potentially offer better hemodynamic support than standard 40-cm³ IABPs.[16] We recently reported that larger capacity, 50-cm³ IABPs, provide greater diastolic augmentation and systolic unloading compared with the 40-cm³ IABP in a retrospective analysis of IABP tracings from 52 consecutive patients (**Fig. 4**).[17] We further showed that the magnitude of systolic unloading correlates directly with the magnitude of diastolic augmentation and inversely with pulmonary artery occlusion pressure. In addition to balloon capacity, the hemodynamic effects of IABP are determined by frequency and timing of IABP inflation and deflation, its position in the descending aorta, shape and

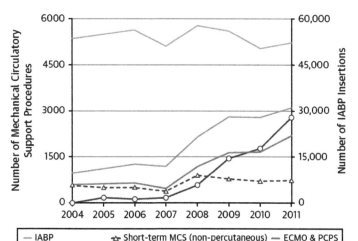

Fig. 2. Trends in the use of nondurable MCS. Coincident with the growth in use of durable or permanent MCS, the use of short-term percutaneous MCS, ECMO, and percutaneous cardiopulmonary support options has been steadily increasing because 2007. ECMO, extracorporeal membrane oxygenation. (*From* Stretch R, Sauer CM, Yuh DD, et al. National trends in the utilization of short-term mechanical circulatory support: Incidence, outcomes, and cost analysis. J Am Coll Cardiol 2014;64:1407–15; with permission.)

Box 2
Current guideline recommendations for nondurable MCS in patients with heart failure

ISHLT Mechanical Circulatory Support Guidelines 2012:

- Class 1: nondurable MCS indicated for acute decompensated heart failure failing maximal medical therapy, multiorgan failure, sepsis, or ventilator-dependent patients to optimize hemodynamics and evaluate neurologic status.
- Class 1: right ventricular assist device is indicated for postoperative right ventricular failure refractory to maximal medical therapy after LV assist device implantation

AHA Heart Failure Guidelines 2013:

- Class 2A (level of evidence, B): nondurable MCS is reasonable as a bridge to recovery or decision for carefully selected patients with heart failure and acute profound disease

HFSA Heart Failure Guidelines 2010:

- Urgent MCS is indicated for bridge to decision in unstable heart failure refractory to maximal medical therapy complicated by multiorgan dysfunction and with a relative contraindication to transplant or durable MCS

---

occlusivity, as well as biological factors including heart rate, blood pressure, and aortic compliance.[18–21] These observations suggest that future clinical trials employing the 50-cm^3 IABPs may show better clinical outcomes than studies predominantly using the 40-cm^3 IABP. Because these devices are designed to unload the heart of excess volume congestion and pressure overload, measuring hemodynamic variables before device deployment may help identify optimal candidates for IABP therapy versus a nondurable MCS option.

IABP advantages include its cost compared with other assist devices, ease of insertion, and widespread familiarity with its insertion technique. Major complications, including acute limb ischemia, severe bleeding, IABP failure or leak, or death directly related to IABP insertion, occurred at a frequency of 2.6% in 16,909 patients in case records in the Benchmark Registry.[22] Clinician expertise, sheathless insertion, and smaller IABPs are associated with decreased incidence of vascular complications.[23,24]

Registry data have historically supported the use of IABPs,[6,25,26] but recent studies attempting to identify optimal candidates for IABP support in high-risk percutaneous coronary intervention (HR-

PCI), AMI, or cardiogenic shock have shown no significant benefit associated with elective IABP insertion. The Counterpulsation Reduces Infarct Size Acute Myocardial Infarction (CRISP-AMI) trial showed that IABP implantation immediately before revascularization for an anterior ST-elevation myocardial infarction (MI) did not reduce infarct size or improve short-term survival.[27] The IABP-SHOCK II (Should We Emergently Revascularize Occluded Coronaries for Cardiogenic Shock) study suggested that not all patients presenting with an acute coronary syndromes (ACS) with marginal blood pressures and clinical evidence of hypoperfusion benefit from IABP activation.[28] In patients with HR-PCI, the PROTECT II (Prospective Multicenter Randomized Trial Comparing IMPELLA to IABP in High Risk PCI) study showed no difference in major adverse cardiovascular events between IABP and the Impella 2.5 axial flow catheter.[29] The Balloon Pump Assisted Coronary Intervention Study (BCIS)-1 also showed no reduction in short-term mortality with IABP insertion before HR-PCI; however, follow-up data suggested a possible long-term benefit up to 5 years after percutaneous coronary intervention (PCI).[30,31] Recent analysis of trends for acute MCS use have reported an increase in the cost of hospital stays associated with IABP use.[4] No clinical studies have rigorously examined the clinical utility of IABP therapy in advanced heart failure.

THE IMPELLA FAMILY OF AXIAL FLOW CATHETERS

The Impella devices are catheter-mounted axial flow pumps that are placed into the left ventricle (LV) in retrograde fashion across the aortic valve (**Fig. 5**). The pumps transfer kinetic energy from a circulating impeller to the blood stream, which generates continuous blood flow from the LV to ascending aorta (**Fig. 6**). The Impella 2.5 left percutaneous (LP) and cardiac power (CP) devices can be deployed without the need for surgery, whereas the Impella 5.0 device requires surgical vascular access through a conduit graft. Unlike left ventricular apical cannulation for durable MCS, transaortic delivery may initially increase left ventricular stroke work (LVSW) until the Impella pump is activated by inducing transient aortic regurgitation.[32] Remmelink and colleagues[33] reported decreased left ventricular end-diastolic pressure, but no change in LVSW, left ventricular volumes, or cardiac output with maximal activation of the Impella 2.5 LP device in 11 patients presenting for high-risk coronary intervention. In 2007, Sauren and colleagues[34] reported a 50% reduction in LVSW with a larger Impella prototype device that generated 3.8 L/min of

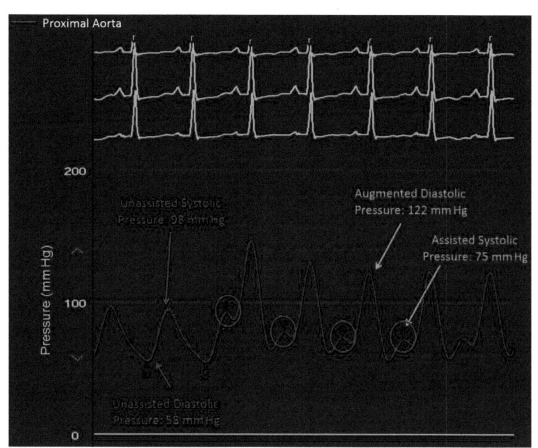

Fig. 3. Optimal effects of IABP counterpulsation. A hemodynamic tracing of proximal aortic pressure at the time of IABP activation shows a reduction in systolic pressure and augmented diastolic pressure. Reduced aortic systolic pressure is an indicator of mechanical unloading of left ventricular pressure.

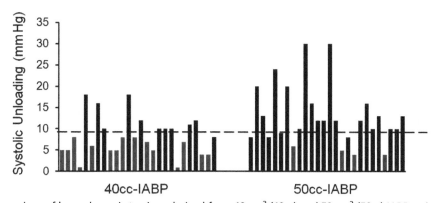

Fig. 4. Comparison of hemodynamic tracings derived from 40-cm^3 (40cc) and 50-cm^3 (50cc) IABP recipients. More patients failed to show a reduction in aortic systolic pressure greater than 10 mm Hg (*red bars*) after receiving a 40-cm^3 IABP compared with patients receiving a 50-cm^3 IABP. (*From* Kapur NK, Paruchuri V, Majithia A, et al. Hemodynamic effects of standard versus larger capacity intra-aortic balloon counterpulsation pumps. J Inv Card, in press; with permission.)

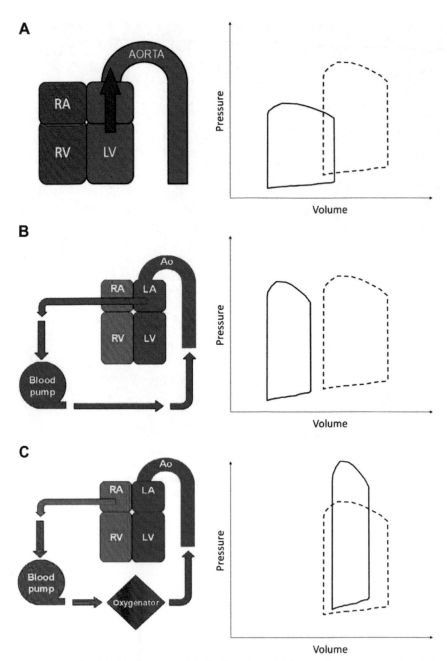

Fig. 5. Percutaneous nondurable MCS systems. (*A*) The Impella axial flow catheters are deployed in retrograde fashion across the aortic valve and directly displace blood from the LV into the proximal aorta. Immediate effects of the Impella activation include reduced left ventricular pressure and volume as shown by pressure-volume (PV) loops. (*B*) The TandemHeart centrifugal flow pump displaces oxygenated blood from the left atrium (LA) to a femoral artery, thereby reducing left ventricular preload. The net effect of immediate TandemHeart activation is a reduction in total LV volume and native left ventricular stroke volume (width of the PV loop). (*C*) Venoarterial extracorporeal membrane oxygenation (VA-ECMO) displaces venous blood from the right atrium (RA) through an extracorporeal centrifugal pump and oxygenator, then returns oxygenated blood into the femoral artery. The immediate effect of VA-ECMO without a left ventricular decompression mechanism is an increase in left ventricular pressures and a reduction in left ventricular stroke volume.

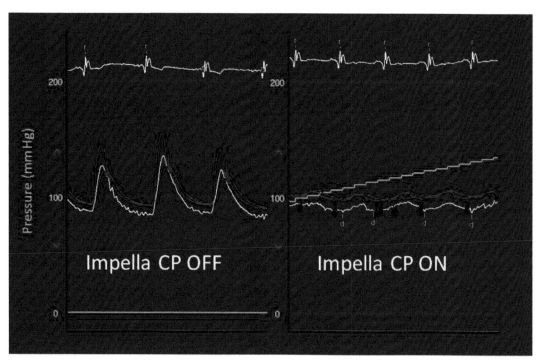

Fig. 6. Hemodynamic tracings of continuous flow nondurable MCS. A femoral artery tracing shows that activation of the Impella CP device in a patient with impaired left ventricular function leads to minimally pulsatile arterial flow.

flow in a preclinical model of acute left ventricular injury. Consistent with this observation, we recently reported that activation of the Impella CP device generated 3.1 L/min of flow and reduced LVSW by 32% in a bovine model of AMI.[35]

The safety of the Impella 2.5 LP device has been well established by 2 large registries.[36,37] The clinical utility of the Impella 2.5 LP was first studied in the ISAR-Shock (Efficacy Study of LV Assist Device to Treat Patients With Cardiogenic Shock) study, which randomized a small number of patients (n = 13/group) presenting with AMI and cardiogenic shock to the Impella 2.5 LP or IABP.[38] Acute improvement in cardiac index was greater with the Impella 2.5 LP device compared with IABP (0.49 ± 0.46 L/min/m^2 compared with a change of 0.11 ± 0.31 L/min/m^2, Impella 2.5 LP vs IABP; $P<.01$), but in-hospital mortality and 2-year follow-up data showed no significant difference between the two arms. A more recent analysis of the USPella registry reported improved survival to hospital discharge with implantation of an Impella device immediately before compared with after coronary revascularization in AMI and cardiogenic shock.[36] In this registry analysis, mean door-to-balloon time was delayed by 60 minutes in patients receiving the Impella device before versus after primary reperfusion. For patients with heart failure undergoing elective PCI, the PROTECT II study randomized patients to the Impella 2.5 LP or IABP before PCI.[27]

The trial was terminated early because of expected futility of the 30-day major adverse event primary end point. Subsequent analysis of the trial has shown potentially important benefits favoring Impella support associated with more complete revascularization and 90-day major adverse events.

Few studies have examined the utility of the Impella 5.0 device. RECOVER-I was a prospective, single-arm feasibility study of the Impella 5.0 device for postcardiotomy cardiogenic shock.[39] The Impella 5.0 significantly improved cardiac index from 1.65 to 2.7 L/min/m^2 ($P<.01$) and mean arterial pressure (71–83 mm Hg), while reducing pulmonary artery diastolic pressure (28–20 mm Hg; $P<.01$). Ninety-three percent of patients survived to hospital discharge. A larger retrospective analysis of Impella use in cardiogenic shock included 37 of 47 total patients receiving an Impella 5.0 pump. In this study, 1-year survival was 71.8% for postcardiotomy cardiogenic shock and 42.9% for patients with shock complicating AMI or dilated cardiomyopathy.[40]

THE TANDEMHEART LEFT ATRIAL TO FEMORAL ARTERY CENTRIFUGAL PUMP

The TandemHeart device is an extracorporeal centrifugal flow pump that reduces left ventricular preload by transferring oxygenated blood from the left atrium (LA) to the descending aorta via 2 cannulas: a 21-Fr transseptal inflow cannula in the LA and an arterial outflow cannula in the femoral artery (see **Fig. 5**). The TandemHeart pump can provide 3.0 to 5.0 L/min of flow via percutaneous application depending on the size of the outflow (arterial) cannula, which can range from 15-Fr to 19-Fr in clinical application.[41] Prior reports have shown that positioning of the outflow cannula affects the magnitude of left ventricular unloading. Specifically, LA to ascending aortic bypass increases LVSW, whereas LA to descending aortic bypass greatly reduces LVSW. In theory, by transferring blood volume from the LA to the arterial system, the Tandem-Heart device pressurizes the aorta.[42] In the ascending aortic position, this increase in afterload limits the magnitude of left ventricular unloading.[43] In the descending aorta, the increase in afterload is mitigated by retrograde perfusion of runoff vessels, including the mesenteric, renal, and great vessels of the aortic arch, thereby allowing a reported 66% reduction in LVSW.[44] Consistent with this study, we recently reported that activation of the TandemHeart pump at 5500 rotations per minute (RPM) with an 17-Fr arterial cannula generates 3.1 L/min of flow and reduces LVSW by 38%, whereas maximal activation at 7500 RPM generates 4.4 L/min of flow and reduces LVSW by 67% in a bovine model of AMI.[34] In contrast with the Impella CP, the primary effect of the TandemHeart was a reduction in native left ventricular stroke volume leading to reduced LVSW.

The safety and efficacy of the TandemHeart assist device compared with IABP use was clinically assessed in small multicenter randomized trials in which the TandemHeart device significantly improved hemodynamic parameters with no mortality benefit compared with IABP.[45,46] The largest data series with TandemHeart was reported by Kar and colleagues,[36] who studied the Tandem-Heart in 117 patients with severe cardiogenic shock refractory to IABP and pressor support. The TandemHeart device improved mean arterial pressure, pulmonary capillary wedge pressure, mixed venous oxygen saturation, and end-organ perfusion. In this study of critically ill patients with advanced heart failure and end-stage shock, only 40.2% of patients died within 30 days after device implantation.[38] An important meta-analysis of smaller studies evaluating these continuous flow devices for cardiogenic shock showed improved hemodynamic profiles associated with the Impella and TandemHeart devices compared with IABP; however, it showed no difference in short-term mortality.[47]

VENOARTERIAL EXTRACORPOREAL MEMBRANE OXYGENATION

Venoarterial extracorporeal membrane oxygenation (VA-ECMO) is commonly used to improve systemic oxygenation during cardiorespiratory

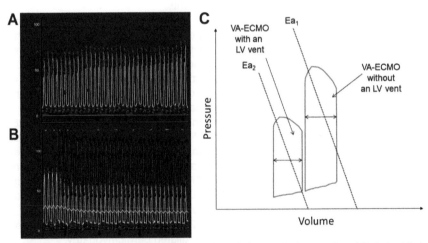

Fig. 7. Hemodynamic profile of VA-ECMO with and without left ventricular venting. (A) A double-lumen pigtail catheter during activation of VA-ECMO shows increased left ventricular systolic pressure and reduced aortic pulse pressure. (B) Initiation of an IABP with VA-ECMO shows reduced left ventricular systolic pressure (venting) and increased aortic diastolic pressure. (C) Venting of the LV with an IABP, Impella device, or transseptal left atrial cannula during VA-ECMO support reduces left ventricular end-systolic pressure and end-diastolic volume. Ea1, arterial elastance condition 1; Ea2, arterial elastance condition two. Conditions are labelled in the figure. (From Aghili N, Kang S, Kapur NK. The fundamentals of extracorporeal membrane oxygenation. Minerva Cardioangiol, in press; with permission.)

collapse or biventricular failure. When deployed percutaneously, an extracorporeal centrifugal pump (ie, TandemHeart, Centrimag, Rotaflow, or Biomedicus pumps) displaces venous blood from the right atrium (RA) through an oxygenator into an artery (most commonly the femoral artery) (see **Fig. 5**). As a result, VA-ECMO reduces both right and left ventricular volumes with a concomitant increase in mean arterial pressure and both left ventricular systolic and diastolic pressures. The potential risk of increased left ventricular afterload is progressive acute lung injury leading to worse outcomes.[48] This increase in left ventricular afterload or wall stress occurs in contrast with the Impella or TandemHeart devices because there is no direct venting of the LV with VA-ECMO (**Fig. 7**). Several approaches to vent the LV can be considered (**Table 1**).

Most clinical studies of VA-ECMO in cardiogenic shock involve extracorporeal life support (ECLS) for cardiac arrest. These data suggest a potential benefit of VA-ECMO if door-to-ECLS times are less than 30 minutes, which has led to growing interest in the application of VA-ECMO in the field by specialized teams of first responders.[49] A systematic review of the published literature for VA-ECMO identified 67 articles between 1966 and 2008 and reported a median survival of 41% (range, 13%–78%) for cardiogenic shock.[50] The best median survival was associated with VA-ECMO use in myocarditis (73%; range, 40%–83%).

EMERGING NONDURABLE MECHANICAL CIRCULATORY SUPPORT OPTIONS FOR RIGHT VENTRICULAR FAILURE

Right ventricular failure is a major cause of morbidity and mortality for patients with congestive heart failure. Causes of right ventricular failure can be categorized into 3 main groups: (1) direct right ventricular myocyte injury as a result of MI or myocarditis; (2) volume overload secondary to right-sided valvular insufficiency or after placement of an LVAD; and (3) pressure overload caused by pulmonary hypertension, pulmonic valve stenosis, or a pulmonary embolus. Irrespective of the underlying cause, right ventricular dysfunction is associated with higher morbidity and short-term mortality in patients with advanced heart failure.[51–58]

Contemporary management of right ventricular failure includes reversal of the primary cause, volume resuscitation, inotropic support, and pulmonary vasodilation, which serve to maintain right ventricular preload, enhance right ventricular contractility, and reduce right ventricular afterload respectively.[59] In refractory right ventricular failure, treatment options are limited to surgical right ventricular assist devices (RVADs), VA-ECMO, atrial septostomy, and cardiac transplantation. Emerging nondurable MCS options for right ventricular failure include the TandemHeart pump and the axial flow Impella RP catheter (under investigation).

The TandemHeart pump can be used as a right ventricular support system by placing a 21-Fr to 28-Fr single-stage or multistage cannula across the RA and a 21-Fr outflow cannula into the main pulmonary artery (MPA) (**Fig. 8**, Video 1). The outflow cannula can be deployed via the femoral vein or via the internal jugular vein in patients with large torso height. Since 2006, the TandemHeart RVAD (TH-RVAD) has been implanted for right ventricular failure in the setting of AMI,[60] post-LVAD implantation,[61] severe pulmonary hypertension,[62] and cardiac rejection after orthotopic heart transplantation.[63]

We previously reported our single-center experience with fully percutaneous deployment of the TH-RVSD in 9 patients with medically refractory right ventricular failure and identified that, compared with preprocedural values, mean arterial pressure (57 ± 7 vs 75 ± 19 mm Hg; $P<.05$), right atrial pressure (22 ± 3 vs 15 ± 6 mm Hg; $P<.05$), cardiac index (1.5 ± 0.4 vs 2.3 ± 0.5 L/min/m2; $P<.05$), mixed venous oxygen saturation (40 ± 14 vs 58 ± 4%; $P<.05$), and right ventricular stroke work (3.4 ± 3.9 vs 9.7 ± 6.8 g*m/beat; $P<.05$) improved significantly within 24 hours of TH-RVSD implantation.[64] In-hospital mortality among 9 patients was 44% (n = 4). Time from admission to TH-RVSD placement was lower in subjects who survived to hospital discharge (0.9 ± 0.8 days vs 4.8 ± 3.5 days, $P = .04$, survivors vs nonsurvivors). In this report, no mechanical

Table 1
Left heart decompression strategies with VA-ECMO

Left Heart Decompression Strategies During VA-ECMO	
Percutaneous	IABP
	Impella axial flow catheter
	Transseptal left ventricular cannulation
	Transseptal LA cannulation
	Atrial septostomy
Surgical	Direct left ventricular apical cannulation
	Direct LA cannulation
Noninvasive	Inotropic support
	Reducing VA-ECMO flow

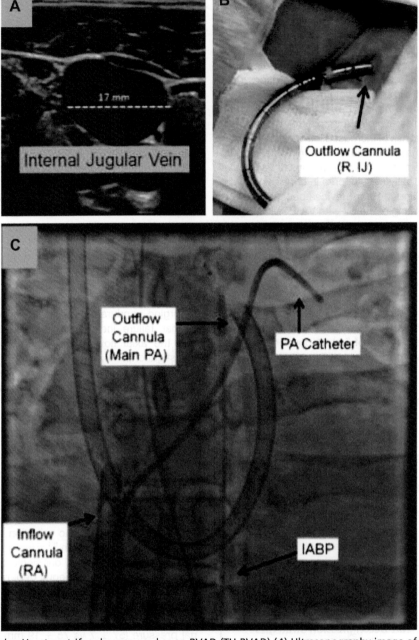

Fig. 8. A TandemHeart centrifugal pump used as an RVAD (TH-RVAD) (*A*) Ultrasonography image of the right internal jugular (IJ) vein before deployment of a TH-RVAD. (*B*) Appearance of the incision site and cannula placement in the right IJ vein. (*C*) Final fluoroscopic image of the TH-RVAD inflow and outflow cannulas in the MPA and RA. A pulmonary artery (PA) catheter and IABP are also shown.

complications were observed during or after device implantation, suggesting that TH-RVSD is clinically feasible and may not be associated with excess risk.

The TandemHeart in Right Ventricular support (THRIVE) study was a retrospective, observational registry of 46 patients receiving a TH-RVAD for right ventricular failure in 8 tertiary care centers in the United States.[65] The central finding of this study was that implantation of the TH-RVAD is clinically feasible via both surgical and percutaneous routes and is associated with acute hemodynamic improvement in right ventricular failure across a broad variety of clinical presentations.

In-hospital mortality varied widely among different indications for mechanical right ventricular support and was lowest among patients with right ventricular failure in the setting of AMI or after LVAD implantation. Increased age, biventricular failure, and Thrombolysis in Myocardial Infarction (TIMI) major bleeding were more commonly observed in patients not surviving to hospital discharge.

Because the TH-RVAD provides centrifugal flow from the RA to MPA, penetration of cannulas into the heart is required to bypass a poorly functioning right ventricle. Close monitoring for evidence of cannula migration is essential and can be prevented by marking cannula depths at the skin incision site, minimizing patient mobility, and stabilizing cannulas during patient transport. Echocardiographic and daily chest radiographs to confirm cannula position also reduce the likelihood of cannula migration. Antegrade migration into a secondary branch of the pulmonary arteries could present as hypoxic respiratory failure, hemothorax, hemoptysis, decreased cardiac output, and an acute decrease in TH-RVAD flows. Retrograde migration into the right ventricle may result in decreased cardiac output caused by tricuspid regurgitation, reduced TH-RVAD flows, or ventricular arrhythmia. Although antegrade or retrograde cannula migration are possible, no institutions in the THRIVE study reported migration as a device-associated complication. TIMI major bleeding was the most common complication associated with the TH-RVSD and is likely secondary to the need for continuous anticoagulation and sheathless deployment of the device cannulas. Bleeding is best controlled by close monitoring of anticoagulation and minimizing patient movement while on support. Mechanical complications associated with the TH-RVSD were rare and included isolated cases of injury to the MPA during surgical deployment only and an isolated case of retroperitoneal bleed associated with peripheral venous cannulation. The development of deep venous thrombosis was reported in 3 cases despite required anticoagulation during device support and may be caused by severe multiorgan dysfunction or partial obstruction of venous flow by cannulas in the inferior vena cava.

The more recent Impella RP (Abiomed Inc) axial flow catheter is a 22-Fr motor mounted onto an 11-Fr catheter for single-access venous delivery of the pump into the MPA (Video 2).[66] Blood is displaced from the lower RA and inferior vena cava to the MPA at estimated flow rates of 4 L/min. The Impella RP is currently undergoing investigation as a support option for right ventricular failure in the Recover Right prospective trial. Cohort A patients developed right ventricular failure after LVAD implantation and cohort B includes patients with right ventricular MI or postcardiotomy right ventricular failure.[67] The primary end point of the study was survival at 30 days or hospital discharge or discharge to the next therapy, including cardiac transplantation or durable RVAD implantation.

Table 2
Decision making: nondurable MCS device-specific characteristics

	Deployment <I h	Percutaneous	Surgical Access	Ambulatory Support (wk)	Bedside Deployment	Oxygenation
IABP	Yes	Yes	No	No/yes	Yes	No
Impella CP	Yes	Yes	No	No	No	No
Impella 5.0 (axillary)	No	No	Yes	Yes	No	No
Impella RP (investigational)	Yes	Yes	No	No	No	No
TandemHeart LVAD	Yes	Yes	No	No	No	Yes
TandemHeart RVAD	Yes	Yes	No	No	No	Yes
Centrimag LVAD (surgical)	No	No	Yes	Yes	Yes	Yes
VA-ECMO	Yes	Yes	No	No	Yes	Yes

Table 3
Decision making: clinical applications of percutaneously deployed nondurable MCS devices in advanced heart failure

| | Advanced Heart Failure/Cardiogenic Shock (Refractory to IABP or ≥1 inotrope) | | | | | | | | | | | |
| | LV Failure | | | Right Ventricular Failure | | Biventricular Failure | | | Cardiopulmonary Failure | | AMI Killip IV MI | |
	Recovery	Decision	DT-LVAD	Recovery	Decision	Recovery	Decision	DT-LVAD	Recovery	Decision	LV	RV
Impella CP	X	X	X	—	—	X	X	X	—	—	X	—
Impella 5.0 (Axillary)	X	X	X	—	—	X	X	X	—	—	—	—
Impella RP (investigational)	—	—	—	X	X	X	X	X	—	—	—	X
TandemHeart LVAD	X	X	X	—	—	X	X	X	X	X	X	—
TandemHeart RVAD	—	—	—	X	X	X	X	X	X	X	—	X
VA-ECMO	—	—	—	X	X	X + vent*	X + vent*	X + vent*	X + vent*	X + vent*	—	—

Abbreviations: DT-LVAD, destination therapy- LVAD; MI, myocardial infarction; RV, right ventricle.
* with the addition of a venting mechanism to reduce left ventricular pressure.

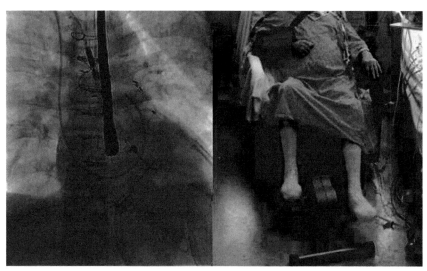

Fig. 9. Percutaneous implantation of the Impella 5.0 allows improved patient mobility. A fluoroscopic image of the Impella 5.0 device implanted via the right axillary artery is shown. A patient on impella 5.0 support is shown sitting in a chair using an exercise cycle.

ALGORITHMS FOR NONDURABLE MECHANICAL CIRCULATORY SUPPORT USE

The growing field of nondurable MCS is being driven by an increasing population of patients with advanced heart failure, improving durable MCS options, and more demand for higher risk interventional and electrophysiology procedures. However, uniform guidelines for the application of nondurable MCS are lacking despite an increasing variety of devices and device applications. Optimal MCS use depends heavily on device and patient characteristics (**Tables 2** and **3**). A fundamental knowledge of each device's hemodynamic effects, versatility, and capabilities is critical to optimal patient outcomes.

EMERGING TECHNOLOGIES AND FUTURE DIRECTIONS

Several novel approaches to short-term (hours to days) and intermediate-term (days to weeks) MCS are actively being explored. The most recent device to be tested in humans is the percutaneous heart pump (PHP; Thoratec Corp), which is an investigational axial flow catheter that can be deployed into the LV via a 12-Fr arterial sheath. The PHP contains a collapsible 24-Fr impeller within a self-expanding cannula that generates a reported 4 to 5 L of flow per minute. The 24-Fr impeller can then be retracted and removed via the femoral artery.

In addition to advances in engineering, the growing application of nondurable MCS is leading to new questions for patients with advanced heart failure. First, can nondurable MCS devices be used to optimize patients before durable MCS surgery?[68] Second, can patients ambulate with a nondurable MCS and does this lead to improved total body conditioning and open the potential for recovering native heart function (**Fig. 9**), thereby obviating a durable MCS device?[69] Third, can nondurable MCS devices reduce the burden of heart failure by reducing myocardial damage during an AMI?[70–72]

SUMMARY

Advances in durable MCS technology have redefined the term medical futility in heart failure and prepared the way for more supportive therapies for patients with New York Heart Association class III and IV symptoms. As a result, the number of LVAD recipients has also grown over the past decade. This increasing population of patients with heart failure spurred demand for nondurable MCS options to manage medically refractory heart failure. Percutaneously delivered MCS devices have evolved over the past 30 years to now include pulsatile, axial flow, and centrifugal flow options that can be rapidly deployed in patients with advanced heart failure and cardiogenic shock. Because these devices are commonly deployed by interventional cardiologists, the approach to patients with advanced heart failure now requires a multidisciplinary understanding of an individual's hemodynamic condition and candidacy for advanced heart failure therapies, including high-risk intervention, surgical ventricular assist devices, or cardiac transplantation.

SUPPLEMENTARY DATA

Supplementary data related to this article can be found online at http://dx.doi.org/10.1016/j.hfc.2014.12.012.

REFERENCES

1. Roger VL, Go AS, Lloyd-Jones DM, et al. Heart disease and stroke statistics–2012 update: a report from the American Heart Association. Circulation 2012;125(1):e2–220.

2. Heidenreich PA, Albert NM, Allen LA, et al. Forecasting the impact of heart failure in the United States: a policy statement from the American Heart Association. Circ Heart Fail 2013;6(3):606–19.

3. Kirklin JK, Naftel DC, Pagani FD, et al. Sixth INTERMACS annual report: a 10,000-patient database. J Heart Lung Transplant 2014;33:555–64.

4. Stretch R, Sauer CM, Yuh DD, et al. National trends in the utilization of short-term mechanical circulatory support: incidence, outcomes, and cost analysis. J Am Coll Cardiol 2014;64(14):1407–15.

5. Cohen M, Urban P, Christenson JT, et al. Intra-aortic balloon counterpulsation in US and non-US centres: results of the benchmark registry. Eur Heart J 2003; 24(19):1763–70.

6. Stone GW, Ohman EM, Miller MF, et al. Contemporary utilization and outcomes of intra-aortic balloon counterpulsation in acute myocardial infarction: the benchmark registry. J Am Coll Cardiol 2003;41(11): 1940–5.

7. Williams DO, Korr KS, Gewirtz H, et al. The effect of intraaortic balloon counterpulsation on regional myocardial blood flow and oxygen consumption in the presence of coronary artery stenosis in patients with unstable angina. Circulation 1982;66(3):593–7.

8. Kern MJ, Aguirre F, Bach R, et al. Augmentation of coronary blood flow by intra-aortic balloon pumping in patients after coronary angioplasty. Circulation 1993;87(2):500–11.

9. Kern MJ, Aguirre FV, Tatineni S, et al. Enhanced coronary blood flow velocity during intraaortic balloon counterpulsation in critically ill patients. J Am Coll Cardiol 1993;21(2):359–68.

10. Braunwald E, Sarnoff SJ, Case RB, et al. Hemodynamic determinants of coronary flow: effect of changes in aortic pressure and cardiac output on the relationship between myocardial oxygen consumption and coronary flow. Am J Physiol 1958; 192(1):157–63.

11. Sarnoff SJ, Braunwald E, Welch GH, et al. Hemodynamic determinants of oxygen consumption of the heart with special reference to the tension-time index. Am J Physiol 1958;192(1):148–56.

12. Sarnoff SJ, Case RB, Welch GH Jr, et al. Performance characteristics and oxygen debt in a nonfailing, metabolically supported, isolated heart preparation. Am J Physiol 1958;192(1):141–7.

13. Welch GH Jr, Braunwald E, Case RB, et al. The effect of mephentermine sulfate on myocardial oxygen consumption, myocardial efficiency and peripheral vascular resistance. Am J Med 1958;24(6):871–81.

14. Schreuder JJ, Castiglioni A, Donelli A, et al. Automatic intraaortic balloon pump timing using an intra-beat dicrotic notch prediction algorithm. Ann Thorac Surg 2005;79(3):1017–22.

15. Schreuder JJ, Maisano F, Donelli A, et al. Beat-to-beat effects of intraaortic balloon pump timing on left ventricular performance in patients with low ejection fraction. Ann Thorac Surg 2005;79(3):872–80.

16. Majithia A, Jumean M, Shih H, et al. The hemodynamic effects of the MEGA intra-aortic balloon counterpulsation pump. J Heart Lung Transplant 2013; 32(4S):S226.

17. Kapur NK, Paruchuri V, Majithia A, et al. Hemodynamic effects of standard versus larger capacity intra-aortic balloon counterpulsation pumps. J Inv Card, in press.

18. Charitos CE, Nanas JN, Kontoyiannis DA, et al. The efficacy of the high volume counterpulsation technique at very low levels of aortic pressure. J Cardiovasc Surg (Torino) 1998;39(5):625–32.

19. Weber KT, Janicki JS, Walker AA. Intra-aortic balloon pumping: an analysis of several variables affecting balloon performance. Trans Am Soc Artif Intern Organs 1972;18(0):486–92.

20. Papaioannou TG, Mathioulakis DS, Nanas JN, et al. Arterial compliance is a main variable determining the effectiveness of intra-aortic balloon counterpulsation: quantitative data from an in vitro study. Med Eng Phys 2002;24(4):279–84.

21. Stamatelopoulos SF, Nanas JN, Saridakis NS, et al. Treating severe cardiogenic shock by large counterpulsation volumes. Ann Thorac Surg 1996;62(4): 1110–7.

22. Ferguson JJ 3rd, Cohen M, Freedman RJ Jr, et al. The current practice of intra-aortic balloon counterpulsation: results from the benchmark registry. J Am Coll Cardiol 2001;38(5):1456–62.

23. Eltchaninoff H, Dimas AP, Whitlow PL. Complications associated with percutaneous placement and use of intraaortic balloon counterpulsation. Am J Cardiol 1993;71(4):328–32.

24. Erdogan HB, Goksedef D, Erentug V, et al. In which patients should sheathless IABP be used? An analysis of vascular complications in 1211 cases. J Card Surg 2006;21(4):342–6.

25. Abdel-Wahab M, Saad M, Kynast J, et al. Comparison of hospital mortality with intra-aortic balloon counterpulsation insertion before versus after primary percutaneous coronary intervention for cardiogenic shock complicating acute myocardial infarction. Am J Cardiol 2010;105(7):967–71.

26. Curtis JP, Rathore SS, Wang Y, et al. Use and effectiveness of intra-aortic balloon pumps among patients undergoing high risk percutaneous coronary intervention: insights from the national cardiovascular data registry. Circ Cardiovasc Qual Outcomes 2012;5(1):21–30.

27. Patel MR, Smalling RW, Thiele H, et al. Intra-aortic balloon counterpulsation and infarct size in patients with acute anterior myocardial infarction without shock: the CRISP AMI randomized trial. JAMA 2011;306(12):1329–37.

28. Thiele H, Schuler G, Neumann FJ, et al. Intraaortic balloon counterpulsation in acute myocardial infarction complicated by cardiogenic shock: design and rationale of the Intraaortic Balloon Pump in Cardiogenic Shock II (IABP-SHOCK II) trial. Am Heart J 2012;163(6):938–45.

29. O'Neill WW, Kleiman NS, Moses J, et al. A prospective, randomized clinical trial of hemodynamic support with Impella 2.5 versus intra-aortic balloon pump in patients undergoing high-risk percutaneous coronary intervention: the PROTECT II study. Circulation 2012;126(14):1717–27.

30. Perera D, Stables R, Clayton T, et al. Long-term mortality data from the balloon pump-assisted coronary intervention study (BCIS-1): a randomized, controlled trial of elective balloon counterpulsation during high-risk percutaneous coronary intervention. Circulation 2013;127(2):207–12.

31. Perera D, Stables R, Thomas M, et al. Elective intra-aortic balloon counterpulsation during high-risk percutaneous coronary intervention: a randomized controlled trial. JAMA 2010;304(8): 867–74.

32. Valgimigli M, Steendijk P, Serruys PW, et al. Use of Impella Recover(R) LP 2.5 left ventricular assist device during high-risk percutaneous coronary interventions; clinical, haemodynamic and biochemical findings. EuroIntervention 2006;2:91–100.

33. Remmelink M, Sjauw KD, Henriques JP, et al. Effects of mechanical left ventricular unloading by Impella on left ventricular dynamics in high-risk and primary percutaneous coronary intervention patients. Catheter Cardiovasc Interv 2010;75: 187–94.

34. Sauren LD, Accord RE, Hamzeh K, et al. Combined Impella and intra-aortic balloon pump support to improve both ventricular unloading and coronary blood flow for myocardial recovery: an experimental study. Artif Organs 2007;31:839–42.

35. Kapur NK, Paruchuri V, Pham DT, et al. Hemodynamic effects of left atrial or left ventricular cannulation for acute circulatory support in a bovine model of left heart injury. ASAIO J 2014. [Epub ahead of print].

36. Sjauw KD, Konorza T, Erbel R, et al. Supported high-risk percutaneous coronary intervention with the Impella 2.5 device the Europella registry. J Am Coll Cardiol 2009;54(25):2430–4.

37. Maini B, Naidu SS, Mulukutla S, et al. Real-world use of the Impella 2.5 circulatory support system in complex high-risk percutaneous coronary intervention: The USpella Registry. Catheter Cardiovasc Interv 2012;80(5):717–25.

38. Seyfarth M, Sibbing D, Bauer I, et al. A randomized clinical trial to evaluate the safety and efficacy of a percutaneous left ventricular assist device versus intraaortic balloon pumping for treatment of cardiogenic shock caused by myocardial infarction. J Am Coll Cardiol 2008;52:1584–8.

39. Griffith BP, Anderson MB, Samuels LE, et al. The RECOVER I: a multicenter prospective study of Impella 5.0/LD for postcardiotomy circulatory support. J Thorac Cardiovasc Surg 2013;145:548–54.

40. Lemaire A, Anderson MB, Lee LY, et al. The Impella device for acute mechanical circulatory support in patients in cardiogenic shock. Ann Thorac Surg 2014;97(1):133–8.

41. Kar B, Gregoric ID, Basra SS, et al. The percutaneous ventricular assist device in severe refractory cardiogenic shock. J Am Coll Cardiol 2011;57: 688–96.

42. Burkhoff D, Naidu SS. The science behind percutaneous hemodynamic support: a review and comparison of support strategies. Catheter Cardiovasc Interv 2012;80:816–29.

43. Kono S, Nishimura K, Nishina T, et al. Autosynchronized systolic unloading during left ventricular assist with a centrifugal pump. J Thorac Cardiovasc Surg 2003;125:353–60.

44. Goldstein AH, Pacella JJ, Clark RE. Predictable reduction in left ventricular stroke work and oxygen utilization with an implantable centrifugal pump. Ann Thorac Surg 1994;58:1018–24.

45. Burkhoff D, Cohen H, Brunckhorst C, et al. A randomized multicenter clinical study to evaluate the safety and efficacy of the TandemHeart percutaneous ventricular assist device versus conventional therapy with intraaortic balloon pumping for treatment of cardiogenic shock. Am Heart J 2006;152: e1–8.

46. Thiele H, Sick P, Boudriot E, et al. Randomized comparison of intra-aortic balloon support versus a percutaneous left ventricular assist device in patients with revascularized acute myocardial infarction complicated by cardiogenic shock. Eur Heart J 2005;26:1276–83.

47. Cheng JM, den Uil CA, Hoeks SE, et al. Percutaneous left ventricular assist devices vs. intra-aortic balloon pump counterpulsation for treatment of cardiogenic shock: a meta-analysis of controlled trials. Eur Heart J 2009;30(17):2102–8.

48. Boulate D, Luyt CE, Pozzi M, et al. Acute lung injury after mechanical circulatory support implantation in

patients on extracorporeal life support: an unrecognized problem. Eur J Cardiothorac Surg 2013;44(3): 544–50.

49. Leick J, Liebetrau C, Szardien S, et al. Door-to-implantation time of extracorporeal life support systems predicts mortality in patients with out-of-hospital cardiac arrest. Clin Res Cardiol 2013;102:661–9.

50. Allen S, Holena D, McCunn M, et al. A review of the fundamental principles and evidence base in the use of extracorporeal membrane oxygenation (ECMO) in critically ill adult patients. J Intensive Care Med 2011;26(1):13–26.

51. Ghio S, Gavazzi A, Campana C, et al. Independent and additive prognostic value of right ventricular systolic function and pulmonary artery pressure in patients with chronic heart failure. J Am Coll Cardiol 2001;37:183–8.

52. Zehender M, Kasper W, Kauder E, et al. Right ventricular infarction as an independent predictor of prognosis after acute inferior myocardial infarction. N Engl J Med 1993;328:981–8.

53. Jacobs AK, Leopold JA, Bates E, et al. Cardiogenic shock caused by right ventricular infarction: a report from the SHOCK registry. J Am Coll Cardiol 2003;41: 1273–9.

54. Budweiser S, Jörres RA, Riedl T, et al. Predictors of survival in COPD patients with chronic hypercapnic respiratory failure receiving noninvasive home ventilation. Chest 2007;131(6):1650–8.

55. Benza RL, Miller DP, Gomberg-Maitland M, et al. Predicting survival in pulmonary arterial hypertension: insights from the Registry to Evaluate Early and Long-Term Pulmonary Arterial Hypertension Disease Management (REVEAL). Circulation 2010; 122:164–72.

56. Haddad F, Peterson T, Fuh E, et al. Characteristics and outcome after hospitalization for acute right heart failure in patients with pulmonary arterial hypertension. Circ Heart Fail 2011;4:692–9.

57. Apostolakis S, Konstantinides S. The right ventricle in health and disease: insights into physiology, pathophysiology and diagnostic management. Cardiology 2012;121(4):263–73.

58. Sanchez O, Planquette B, Roux A, et al. Triaging in pulmonary embolism. Semin Respir Crit Care Med 2012;33:156–62.

59. Greyson CR. Pathophysiology of right ventricular failure. Crit Care Med 2008;36:S57–65.

60. Atiemo AD, Conte JV, Heldman AW. Resuscitation and recovery from acute right ventricular failure using a percutaneous right ventricular assist device. Catheter Cardiovasc Interv 2006;68(1):78–82.

61. Takagaki M, Wurzer C, Wade R, et al. Successful conversion of TandemHeart left ventricular assist device to right ventricular assist device after implantation of a HeartMate XVE. Ann Thorac Surg 2008; 86:1677–9.

62. Rajdev S, Benza R, Misra V. Use of tandem heart as a temporary hemodynamic support option for severe pulmonary artery hypertension complicated by cardiogenic shock. J Invasive Cardiol 2007; 19(8):E226–9.

63. Bajona P, Salizzoni S, Brann SH, et al. Prolonged use of right ventricular assist device for refractory graft failure following orthotopic heart transplantation. J Thorac Cardiovasc Surg 2010;139(3):e53–4.

64. Kapur NK, Paruchuri V, Korabathina R, et al. Effects of a percutaneous mechanical circulatory support device for medically refractory right ventricular failure. J Heart Lung Transplant 2011;30(12):1360–7.

65. Kapur NK, Paruchuri V, Jagannathan A, et al. Mechanical circulatory support for right ventricular failure: the TandemHeart in RIght VEntricular support (THRIVE) Registry. JACC Heart Fail 2013; 1(2):127–34.

66. Cheung AW, White CW, Davis MK, et al. Short-term mechanical circulatory support for recovery from acute right ventricular failure: clinical outcomes. J Heart Lung Transplant 2014;33(8):794–9.

67. The use of Impella RP support system in patients with right heart failure. Available at: http://clinicaltrials.gov/show/NCT01777607. Accessed October 27, 2014.

68. Rajagopalan N, Yanagida R, Hoopes CW. Insertion of Impella 5.0 to improve candidacy for HeartMate II left ventricular assist device placement. J Invasive Cardiol 2014;26(4):E40–1.

69. Estep JD, Cordero-Reyes AM, Bhimaraj A, et al. Percutaneous placement of an intra-aortic balloon pump in the left axillary/subclavian position provides safe, ambulatory long-term support as bridge to heart transplantation. JACC Heart Fail 2013;1(5): 382–8.

70. Smalling RW, Cassidy DB, Barrett R, et al. Improved regional myocardial blood flow, left ventricular unloading, and infarct salvage using an axial-flow, transvalvular left ventricular assist device. A comparison with intra-aortic balloon counterpulsation and reperfusion alone in a canine infarction model. Circulation 1992;85:1152–9.

71. Meyns B, Stolinski J, Leunens V, et al. Left ventricular support by catheter-mounted axial flow pump reduces infarct size. J Am Coll Cardiol 2003;41: 1087–95.

72. Kapur NK, Paruchuri V, Urbano-Morales JA, et al. Mechanically unloading the left ventricle before coronary reperfusion reduces left ventricular wall stress and myocardial infarct size. Circulation 2013;128(4): 328–36.

Transcatheter Aortic Valve Replacement for Patients with Heart Failure

Dominique Himbert, MD*, Alec Vahanian, MD

KEYWORDS

- Heart failure • TAVR • Valve replacement • Aortic stenosis

KEY POINTS

- Heart failure is frequent in patients referred for transcatheter aortic valve replacement (TAVR) and constitutes an adverse prognostic factor.
- Heart failure diagnosis may be difficult owing to confounding conditions in elderly patients with co-morbidities and require multimodality imaging to ascertain the severity of aortic stenosis (AS) and its relationship with symptoms.
- In the future, efforts should be made to better identify AS patients at high risk of developing heart failure or at its early stages.
- Early intervention and patient safety are important factors to consider in seeking to offer patients the most suitable conditions for a full postoperative recovery.

INTRODUCTION

The first transcatheter aortic valve replacement (TAVR) was performed in 2002 by Alain Cribier (Rouen, France) on a compassionate basis in a patient with cardiogenic shock owing to end-stage aortic stenosis (AS).[1,2] Since then, more than 150,000 patients have undergone TAVR around the world. TAVR is now considered the treatment of choice for inoperable patients with severe AS and an attractive alternative option in those at high surgical risk. The large majority of candidates to TAVR suffer various degrees of heart failure. The aim of this review was to present the specific features of patients with severe heart failure undergoing TAVR, focusing on diagnostic, management, and prognostic issues in this high-risk population.

PATHOPHYSIOLOGY

Understanding the pathophysiology of heart failure in patients with severe AS is crucial to reach adequate therapeutic decisions, to determine timely and avoid futile interventions. The most important point is to differentiate between primary heart failure, in relation with AS, and heart failure secondary to other causes, such as severe ischemic cardiomyopathy with large sequelae of myocardial infarction. If cardiac failure and depressed left ventricular function are predominantly caused by excessive afterload (afterload mismatch), the probability of left ventricular recovery after TAVR is high, provided that intervention is performed in a timely manner.[3–5] Conversely, improvement in left ventricular function after intervention is uncertain if the primary cause is scarring owing to extensive myocardial infarction or cardiomyopathy, which may render TAVR futile. In addition, the presence of worsening factors, such as anemia, atrial fibrillation, and pulmonary infection, should be investigated systematically and corrected before starting the decision process.

PREVALENCE

Because patients with severe AS complicated by congestive heart failure represent a population at

Department of Cardiology, Bichat-Claude Bernard Hospital, Assistance Publique Hôpitaux de Paris, 46 Rue Henri Huchard, Paris 75018, France
* Corresponding author.
E-mail address: dominique.himbert@bch.aphp.fr

Heart Failure Clin 11 (2015) 231–242
http://dx.doi.org/10.1016/j.hfc.2014.12.003
1551-7136/15/$ – see front matter © 2015 Elsevier Inc. All rights reserved.

high risk for surgery, they are often considered for TAVR. The various parameters of heart failure (New York Heart Association [NYHA] functional class III/IV, left ventricular dysfunction, pulmonary hypertension, critical hemodynamic state) are taken into account by the Society of Thoracic Surgeons predictive risk score and by the Euro-SCORE I and II.[6–8]

Table 1 presents the main parameters of heart failure in recent TAVR trials and registries.[9–16] The vast majority of the patients have severe symptoms of heart failure reflected by NYHA functional classes III to IV. Their proportion is between 75% and 85% in real-life registries, but exceeds 90% in trials including patients who are deemed inoperable or at extreme risk. This severe functional status contrasts with the preserved mean left ventricular ejection fraction (LVEF), which is consistently reported as between 50% and 55% in all TAVR cohorts. The prevalence of left ventricular systolic dysfunction among patients with severe AS treated with TAVR ranges between 6% and 11%, considering a cutoff value of LVEF of $\leq$30%, and between 27% and 46%, if LVEF is between 30% and 50%.[14,17,18] The small proportion of patients with severely depressed LVEF represents a particularly high-risk subgroup, with specific therapeutic and prognostic issues.[19–22] The presence of pulmonary hypertension (usually defined by a systolic pulmonary artery pressure $\geq$60 mm Hg) is not systematically reported and seems much more variable, being encountered in 15% to 40% of patients.

However, the evaluation of the prevalence of heart failure in TAVR patients may be rendered uncertain by the difficulties of its diagnosis in such an aged population frequently suffering from confounding comorbidities.

DIAGNOSIS

The diagnosis of heart failure may be done in 2 different settings. Usually, symptoms or physical signs of congestive heart failure are detected during the follow-up of patients with known AS. However, in many instances, the occurrence of an acute pulmonary edema or cardiogenic shock in a given patient is related to the presence of undiagnosed AS by echocardiographic examination.

Dyspnea is the main symptom of heart failure in patients with severe AS. However, in elderly patients, it may be owing to many other causes, such as respiratory failure, overweight, or muscle loss, or underreported owing to cognitive deterioration or limitation of activity.

The second point of the diagnosis is to establish the relationship between symptoms and AS. The answer requires a thorough clinical examination with a particular emphasis on medical history and timing of the appearance and worsening of symptoms, also involving the family and close relations of the patient. Physical signs of heart failure, such as pulmonary rales and leg edema, may be difficult to interpret in many cases.

Echocardiography is, of course, the key examination to assess the severity of AS and to identify the presence of parameters associated with heart failure, such as low LVEF, low cardiac output, and pulmonary hypertension.[19,20,22–30] However, accurate assessment is sometimes challenging. Severe AS with small aortic valve area (<1.0 cm^2) and low transvalvular gradients is not uncommon

Table 1
Parameters of heart failure in transcatheter aortic valve replacement trials and registries

Trial or Registry	NYHA III/IV (%)		LVEF (Mean ± SD, %)		Pulmonary Hypertension (Mean ± SD, %)
PARTNER B[9]	92		54 ± 13		42
FRANCE 2[10]	76		53 ± 14		20
CoreValve ADVANCE[11]	80		53 ± 14		13
CoreValve US Pivotal Extreme Risk[12]	92		NA		NA
CoreValve US Pivotal High Risk[13]	86		NA		NA
GARY[14]	85		NA		40
PARTNER II Inoperable[15]	97		53 ± 13		25
CHOICE Trial[16]	BEV 80	SEV 82	BEV 53 ± 14	SEV 55 ± 12	NA

Abbreviations: BEV, balloon expandable valve; GARY, German Aortic Valve Registry; LVEF, left ventricular ejection fraction; NA, not applicable; NYHA, New York Heart Association; SD, standard deviation; SEV, self-expandable valve; US, United States.
Data from Refs.[9–16]

in daily clinical practice. According to recent guidelines, severe AS is defined as an aortic valve area of less than 1 cm^2, a mean gradient of greater than 40 mm Hg, and a maximum jet velocity of greater than 4 m/s.[5,31] However, many patients have discordant findings, mostly with small aortic valve area, but with low gradients. This situation raises uncertainty with regard to the severity of AS, as well as the indication for intervention. The entity of severe AS with a low transvalvular gradient was first recognized in patients with reduced LVEF.[3] In such patients, a small valve area does not definitely confirm severe AS, because mildly to moderately diseased valves may not open fully (secondary to the reduced left ventricular function), resulting in a small valve area (pseudosevere AS), which is not an indication for intervention. Low-dose dobutamine stress echocardiography may be helpful to distinguish severe AS from pseudosevere AS. In severe AS, the valve area changes minimally during low-dose dobutamine echocardiography, but the gradient increases significantly (mean gradient >40 mm Hg). More recently, the possibility of severe AS in patients with an aortic valve area of less than 1.0 cm^2 and a mean gradient of less than 40 mm Hg, despite preserved LVEF, has been suggested, introducing the new entity of paradoxic low-flow (stroke volume index ≤35 mL/m^2), low-gradient AS.[32] The management of this subset of AS patients remains challenging. When confronted with this entity, the following steps should be taken. First, potential errors in the measurement of gradient, stroke volume index, and aortic valve area should be excluded. Second, to eliminate the confounding effect of small body size, calculation of the indexed aortic valve area may be helpful. A value of less than 0.6 cm^2/m^2 indicates severe AS. Finally, establishing whether the global hemodynamic load is severely increased (ie, valvuloarterial impedance) may be helpful.[33] Corroborating methods are useful in cases where echocardiography is technically challenging or inconclusive because of discordant evaluation of severity. Particular attention has been given recently to the evaluation of the degree of valve calcification. Recent studies have emphasized the use of multidetector CT for the quantification of valvular calcification.[34,35] Aortic valve calcification load identifies severe AS accurately (sensitivity, 86%; specificity, 79%) in men (calcium score threshold ≥2065 arbitrary units [AU]) and in women (threshold ≥1275 AU). When applied to low-flow, low-gradient AS, these criteria showed that at least one-half of the patients had severe AS, irrespective of flow. Multidetector CT has the advantage of being a reproducible technique,

which is flow independent. Currently, multidetector CT and low-dose dobutamine echocardiography should not be considered as competitive, but rather as complementary techniques (**Fig. 1**). Further studies comparing diagnostic strategies and outcome in patients with low-flow, low-gradient AS are needed to optimally identify and manage these patients.

Finally, the degree of elevation of biomarkers of cardiac failure, mainly the brain natriuretic peptide (BNP) or the N-terminal pro-BNP correlates with the severity of AS, facilitates the diagnosis of cardiac failure and provides useful prognostic information.[36–40]

PROGNOSIS

The first step of patients' prognostic evaluation is to distinguish those in whom heart failure is related to coronary artery disease or other causes and those in whom it is related to afterload mismatch owing to severe AS. In the former, the prognosis may not be substantially improved by TAVR. In the latter, the probability of left ventricular recovery and clinical improvement is high.

The prognostic impact of heart failure in patients undergoing TAVR has been studied extensively in registries. However, the conclusions drawn from these studies need to be tempered by the fact that the most severe patients have been excluded systematically from large, randomized trials. The literature can be classified according to the criteria taken into account, mainly clinical, echocardiographic, or biological.

Clinical Heart Failure

The presence of clinical signs of heart failure has a negative impact on patients' outcomes after TAVR performed in routine clinical practice. In the FRANCE 2 registry,[41] NYHA class IV, critical hemodynamic state, and history of more than 1 recent pulmonary edema were 3 major predictors of 1-year mortality, beside others such as age ≥80 years, low body mass index, dialysis, and transapical approach (**Table 2**). Based on these findings, a score has been elaborated to assess the individual risk of patients undergoing TAVR, in whom the weight of heart failure parameters accounts for one-third of the whole scoring (8/24; **Fig. 2**). The C-index was 0.67 for the score in the development cohort and 0.59 in the validation cohort. There was a good concordance between predicted and observed 30-day mortality rates in the development and validation cohorts. The moderate discrimination was, however, a limitation for the accurate identification of high-risk patients.

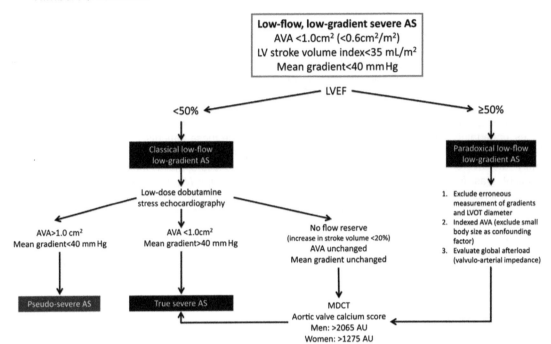

Fig. 1. Evaluation of patients with low-flow, low-gradient severe AS. AS, aortic stenosis; AU, arbitrary units; AVA, aortic valve area; LV, left ventricular; LVEF, left ventricular ejection fraction; LVOT, left ventricular outflow tract; MDCT, multidetector row CT. (*Data from* Bax JJ, Delgado V, Bapat V, et al. Open issues in transcatheter aortic valve implantation. Part 1: patient selection and treatment strategy for transcatheter aortic valve implantation. Eur Heart J 2014;35:2627–38.)

Table 2
FRANCE 2: predictors of 30-day mortality

	Adjusted OR (95% CI)	P	Points for Score (/19)
Age (y)			
<80	1		0
≥80	1.42 (1.01–1.99)	.04	1
Body mass index (kg/m²)			
≥30	1		0
18.5–29.9	1.63 (1.05–2.53)	.03	2
<18.5	2.44 (1.13–5.29)	.02	3
NYHA class IV	1.66 (1.16–2.39)	.006	2
Pulmonary hypertension (sPAP ≥60 mm Hg)	1.43 (1.05–1.93)	.02	1
Critical state[a]	2.64 (1.56–4.46)	.0003	3
Respiratory insufficiency and APE			
No respiratory insufficiency and <2 APE last year	1		0
Respiratory insufficiency or ≥2 APE last year	2.06 (1.54–2.74)	<.0001	2
Dialysis	3.33 (1.68–6.57)	.0005	4
Approach			
Transfemoral or subclavian			0
Transapical	2.02 (1.46–2.81)	<.0001	2
Other	2.44 (1.24–4.79)	.01	3

Abbreviations: APE, acute pulmonary edema; NYHA, New York Heart Association; sPAP, systolic pulmonary artery pressure.
[a] Definition according to the EuroSCORE.

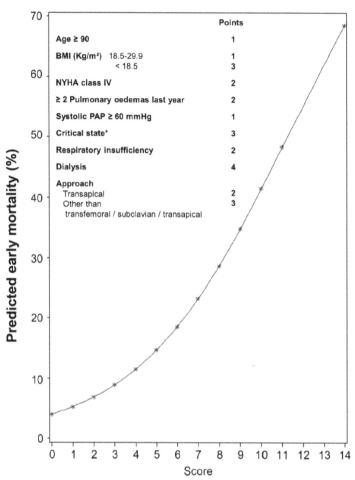

Fig. 2. Relationship between the score value and predicted early mortality after transcatheter aortic valve replacement. BMI, body mass index; PAP, pulmonary artery pressure. * Definition according to the EuroSCORE.

The results from the German Transcatheter Aortic Valve Interventions Registry are similar.[14] Overall 1-year mortality was 10% among the 1391 patients included in the registry. Previous cardiac decompensation ($P = .0061$), NYHA class IV ($P = .0254$), and low-gradient AS ($P = .0008$) were 3 independent pre-intervention predictors of 1-year mortality. In the Canadian experience on TAVR in patients at very high or prohibitive surgical risk, pulmonary hypertension and need for hemodynamic support were predictors of cumulative late mortality.[42] In an Italian multicenter study on results after TAVR in patients with severe left ventricular dysfunction, the main predictor of cumulative mortality was congestive heart failure, associated with the logistic EuroSCORE and post-implantation moderate to severe periprosthetic leakage.[23] The same findings are reported in most papers on transcatheter aortic valve implantation cohorts.

Echocardiographic Signs of Heart Failure

LVEF is an important prognostic factor and is included in current operative risk scores.[6–8] Despite important limitations, these scores are commonly used for patients' risk stratification and orientation toward either conventional surgery or TAVR, on top of the multidisciplinary heart team judgment.

Table 3 summarizes the impact of the main echocardiographic parameters of heart failure on survival after TAVR.[19–25,28,29] Overall, most findings suggest that low LVEF, low flow, and low gradient are adverse prognostic factors. However, the association between left ventricular systolic dysfunction and TAVR procedural risks remains controversial.[18,29,43–46] Although some studies have shown an increased procedural risk among patients with low LVEF, other series have not confirmed this association. For example, in the

Table 3
Impact of echocardiographic parameters of heart failure on survival after transcatheter aortic valve replacement

Study	LVEF (%)	Low Flow	Low Gradient (mm Hg)	Survival (%)
Fraccaro et al,[23] 2012	≤35 vs >35			1-y: 69 vs 87 (P<.001)
Van der Boon et al,[19] 2012	≤35 vs >35	+	+	30-d: 91.4 vs 97.0 (P = .21)
O'Sullivan et al,[21] 2013	≥50 vs <40	+	+	1-y: 79.5 vs 75.5 (P = .67)
Elhmidi et al,[28] 2014	<35	+	+ vs −	1-y: 62.2 vs 86.7 (P = .01)
Biner et al,[24] 2014	Preserved		+ vs −	2-y: 68 ± 8 vs 77 ± 5 (P = .3)
Gotzmann et al,[20] 2012	>50 vs ≤50		>40 vs ≤40	1-y (P = .007) >50/>40 >50/<40 <50/>40 <50/<40 86 78 73 61
Ben Dor et al,[25] 2012	<40		>40 vs ≤40	Follow-up: 59 vs 46.2 (P = .01)
Le Ven et al,[29] 2013		+ vs −		2-y: 64.7 vs 69.1 (P = .005)

Abbreviation: LVEF, left ventricular ejection fraction.
  Data from Refs.[19–21,23–25,28,29]

Italian registry including 663 patients undergoing TAVR with the CoreValve system, a LVEF of less than 40% was independently associated with early mortality.[46] In contrast, data from the Pilot European Sentinel registry, including 4571 patients with 5.7% having an LVEF of less than 30%, did not demonstrate this association.[17] Furthermore, it has been suggested that LVEF may not reflect the extent of myocardial dysfunction in patients with severe AS and concentric left ventricular hypertrophy, whereas stroke volume may be a more comprehensive parameter of the effects of increased afterload on the left ventricular. The recent subanalysis of the PARTNER trial including all cohorts showed that only low- flow (stroke volume index ≤35 mL/m^2) was independently associated with 2-year mortality, whereas low gradient and low LVEF were not associated with 2-year mortality.[47] However, these parameters may interact and render interpretation of data complex. The presence of low gradients seems to be more deleterious in patients with reduced LVEF than in those with preserved LVEF. In patients with low-flow, low-gradient AS, the presence of low LVEF does not have a significant impact on survival, in contrast with those with preserved LVEF. TAVR has been associated with significant improvement in LVEF at follow-up.[23,48–50] The majority of series have shown a significant improvement in LVEF early after TAVR (before hospital discharge), which is generally followed by a gradual and sustained improvement at the 1-year follow-up. This improvement in LVEF is associated with a significant and durable improvement in symptoms, functional class, and quality of life.[20,23] The degree of LVEF improvement is highly variable and depends on several factors. Compared with surgical aortic valve replacement (SAVR), LVEF improves more after TAVR.[50] In the randomized PARTNER cohort A trial, LVEF improved earlier with TAVR, although there was no difference between groups at 2 years.[43] It has been suggested that a greater improvement in left ventricular function might be expected with TAVR, because this is a less invasive procedure that may minimize myocardial injury and transcatheter aortic valves have superior hemodynamic performance.[51] Other factors associated with changes in LVEF after TAVR include a lower mean aortic valve gradient and a higher baseline LVEF, previous permanent pacemaker, new onset of a left bundle branch block, and pacemaker implantation after TAVR.[24,52] Transcatheter aortic valve implantation access (transfemoral vs transapical) has also been associated with LVEF improvement in univariate analysis. Elmariah and colleagues[53] showed that transfemoral access was an unadjusted predictor of LVEF improvement, whereas transapical access was not.

Beside baseline left ventricular function, the analysis of contractile reserve using dobutamine stress hemodynamics adds substantial prognostic information in patients with low-gradient AS. A contractile reserve (defined by an increase in stroke volume ≥20% with dobutamine) is present in the majority of patients who survive after surgical aortic valve replacement, but does not predict the absence of LVEF recovery, which supports the concept that interventions, including TAVR, should not be contraindicated on the basis of absence of contractile reserve alone.[4,54] Also, analysis of left ventricular function using the global left ventricular longitudinal systolic strain may add prognostic information, the greatest improvements in global left ventricular longitudinal systolic strain after TAVR being correlated with the lowest mortality rates.[55] Finally, although left ventricular dysfunction alone may not be sufficient to refer patients for TAVR instead of surgery,[56] it seems that TAVR can be performed in patients with left ventricular dysfunction with a modest risk and is associated with marked symptomatic and survival benefits.

Beside left ventricular dysfunction, pulmonary hypertension is an important parameter of heart failure to be considered. Pulmonary hypertension is a well-known parameter of high surgical risk and is also a predictor of early and mid-term mortality after TAVR.[41,57,58] Because it usually indicates advanced aortic valve disease, it may be interpreted as an incentive to consider earlier correction of severe AS. In the context of severe pulmonary hypertension, right ventricular dysfunction has the same negative prognostic impact.[59] However, taken in isolation, right ventricular dysfunction has been reported not to impair adversely immediate or follow-up survival during medium-term follow-up after TAVR.[60]

Biological Markers of Heart Failure

Pro-BNP and N-terminal–proBNP have been found to correlate with the severity of AS and to provide information in AS patients undergoing surgical aortic valve replacement.[61] There is growing evidence that these markers also offer independent prognostic information on candidates to TAVR and should be included in their risk stratification before the procedure (**Table 4**).[36–40] In the large series of Clavel and colleagues,[36] the correlation between higher mortality and higher BNP clinical activation has been found even in asymptomatic patients. This probably does not imply that TAVR should be considered in asymptomatic AS patients but emphasizes the importance of appropriate clinical interpretation of BNP levels in managing these patients.

TREATMENT

In the majority of cases, the management of patients with compensated stable heart failure during TAVR does not raise very specific issues, even when associated with severe left ventricular dysfunction. As for all TAVR procedures, but even more in such high-risk patients, the constant presence in the catheterization laboratory of a skilled anesthesiology team is essential to closely monitor the hemodynamic state of the patient and react immediately to any event or complication. When possible, locoregional anesthesia with conscious sedation should be considered as the first option to avoid the hemodynamic instability induced by general anesthesia. Rapid ventricular pacing runs should be avoided or kept as short as possible, and not repeated until full and stable aortic pressure recovery is observed.

In contrast, the management of patients with decompensated, unstable, or critical hemodynamic state, including the extreme condition represented by cardiogenic shock, should follow different strategies. In such settings, patients require urgent or emergent interventions and cannot afford to undergo the screening process. Several studies emphasized the clinical benefit of bridge percutaneous balloon aortic valvuloplasty in those patients with temporary contraindications to TAVR.[62–65] Such a strategy may contribute to stabilizing the hemodynamic status of patients, improve their left ventricular function, and allow

---

Table 4
Impact of biological markers of heart failure on survival after transcatheter aortic valve replacement

	Marker	Outcome
Elhmidi et al,[37] 2013	High baseline NT-proBNP	1-y mortality HR, 1.02; 95% CI, 1.01–1.05; $P = .006$
Lopez-Otero et al,[38] 2013	High Log transform Pro-BNP	Long-term mortality HR, 11; CI, 1.51–81.3; $P = .018$
Clavel et al,[36] 2013	BNP Normal vs ×2 vs ×3 vs ≥3	8-y survival 62 ± 3 vs 44 ± 3 vs 25 ± 4 vs 15 ± 2
Ribeiro et al,[39] 2014	High baseline NT-proBNP	Long-term mortality (overall and CV) $P<.01$
Giordana et al,[40] 2014	High Pro-BNP	1-y mortality OR, 5.4%; 95% CI, 1.7–16.5

Abbreviations: BNP, pro-hormone B-type natriuretic peptide; CV, cardiovascular; HR, hazard ratio; NT, N-terminal.
Data from Refs.[36–40]

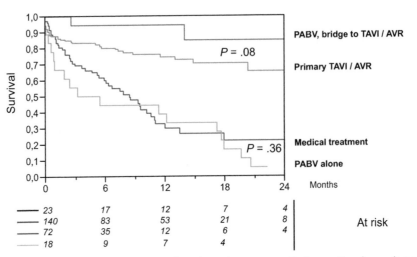

Fig. 3. Compared clinical outcomes in patients undergoing primary transcatheter aortic valve replacement (TAVR) or SAVR, TAVR or SAVR after bridge percutaneous balloon aortic valvuloplasty (PABV) because of a temporary contraindication, PABV alone and medical treatment. AVR, aortic valve replacement; TAVI, transcatheter aortic valve implantation.

for considering an elective, standard TAVR procedure, which may lead to results similar to those observed after primary TAVR in lower risk patients **(Fig. 3)**. To avoid the risk of severe heart failure recurrence and to perform TAVR in the safest conditions, the latter should be considered early after clinical recovery, without waiting for tight aortic valve restenosis or worsening of symptoms.

However, a small number of isolated cases or short series of patients with cardiogenic shock or hemodynamic instability undergoing TAVR have been reported over the last few years **(Table 5)**.[59,66–71] The prophylactic use of cardiopulmonary support seems desirable and is associated with an acceptable immediate outcome. However, owing to the small number of cases published, their heterogeneity and the probable underreporting of negative experiences, these results should be interpreted with caution and today no definite conclusion can be drawn on the real safety and effectiveness of TAVR in cardiogenic shock patients.

Despite the recovery in systolic left ventricular function usually observed after TAVR in patients with baseline low LVEF, this favorable evolution may be hampered by the occurrence of left bundle branch block induced by TAVR. In the PARTNER trial, new left bundle branch block was not associated with significant differences in 1-year mortality, cardiovascular mortality, repeat hospitalization,

Table 5
Recent cases of transcatheter aortic valve replacement performed in patients with cardiogenic shock or unstable hemodynamic state

	n	Cardiocirculatory Support	Immediate Outcome
Fudim et al,[66] 2013	2	0	Alive
Pilgrim et al,[67] 2013	1	0	Alive
Pasic et al,[68] 2012	1	0	Alive
Husser et al,[69] 2013	18	Prophylactic (n = 9) or emergency (n = 9) ECMO	30-d mortality Prophylactic ECMO: 0% Emergency ECMO: 44%
Seco et al,[59] 2014	8	Prophylactic ECMO	Alive
Pizzighini et al,[70] 2014	1	0	Alive
Drews et al,[71] 2014	23	Prophylactic F-F CPB	30-d mortality: 28.6%

Abbreviations: CPB, cardiopulmonary bypass; ECMO, extracorporeal membrane oxygenator; F-F, femorofemoral.
Data from Refs.[59,66–70]

stroke, or myocardial infarction. However, it was associated with the failure of LVEF improvement after TAVR, which remained lower at 6 months to 1 year (52.8 vs 58.1%; P <.001).[52] In such cases, cardiac resynchronization therapy can be effective to improve systolic left ventricular function and avoid recurrence of heart failure.[72,73]

Finally, TAVR can be used for very specific indications regarding patients with end-stage heart failure treated by left ventricular assist devices. New-onset aortic regurgitation can be encountered in these patients, in particular when they are treated by continuous flow devices. To avoid high-risk reoperations, TAVR can be considered and the reported experiences demonstrate that it is feasible and can be a reasonable option to treat aortic regurgitation induced by left ventricular assist device implantation.[74,75]

SUMMARY

Heart failure is frequent in patients referred for TAVR and constitutes an adverse prognostic factor. Its diagnosis may be difficult owing to confounding conditions in elderly patients with comorbidities and require multimodality imaging to ascertain the severity of AS and its relationship with symptoms. In the future, efforts should be made to better identify AS patients at high risk of developing heart failure or at its early stages, to be able to intervene as early and safely as possible and offer them the most suitable conditions for a full postoperative recovery.

REFERENCES

1. Cribier A, Eltchaninoff H, Bash A, et al. Percutaneous transcatheter implantation of an aortic valve prosthesis for calcific aortic stenosis: first human case description. Circulation 2002;106:3006–8.
2. Cribier A, Eltchaninoff H, Tron C, et al. Early experience with percutaneous transcatheter implantation of heart valve prosthesis for the treatment of end-stage inoperable patients with calcific aortic stenosis. J Am Coll Cardiol 2004;43:698–703.
3. Monin JL, Quere JP, Monchi M, et al. Low-gradient aortic stenosis: operative risk stratification and predictors for long-term outcome: a multicenter study using dobutamine stress hemodynamics. Circulation 2003;108:319–24.
4. Tribouilloy C, Lévy F, Rusinaru D, et al. Outcome after aortic valve replacement for low-flow/low-gradient aortic stenosis without contractile reserve on dobutamine stress echocardiography. J Am Coll Cardiol 2009;53:1865–73.
5. Vahanian A, Alfieri O, Andreotti F, et al. Guidelines on the management of valvular heart disease (version 2012): The Joint Task Force on the Management of Valvular Heart Disease of the European Society of Cardiology (ESC) and the European Association for Cardio-Thoracic Surgery (EACTS). Eur Heart J 2012;33:2451–96.
6. STS National Database Risk Calculator. Available at: http://www.sts.org/sections/stsnationaldatabase/riskcalculator. Accessed December, 2013.
7. Roques F, Nashef SA, Michel P, et al. Risk factors and outcome in European cardiac surgery: analysis of the EuroSCORE multinational database of 19030 patients. Eur J Cardiothorac Surg 1999;15:816–22.
8. Nashef SA, Roques F, Sharples LD, et al. EuroSCORE II. Eur J Cardiothorac Surg 2012;41:734–44.
9. Leon MB, Smith CR, Mack M, et al, PARTNER Trial Investigators. Transcatheter aortic-valve implantation for aortic stenosis in patients who cannot undergo surgery. N Engl J Med 2010;363:1597–607.
10. Gilard M, Eltchaninoff H, Iung B, et al, FRANCE 2 Investigators. Registry of transcatheter aortic-valve implantation in high-risk patients. N Engl J Med 2012;366:1705–15.
11. Linke A, Wenaweser P, Gerckens U, et al, ADVANCE Study Investigators. Treatment of aortic stenosis with a self-expanding transcatheter valve: the International Multi-centre ADVANCE Study. Eur Heart J 2014;35:2672–84.
12. Yakubov, on behalf of the CoreValve US Investigators. CoreValve US Pivotal Trial, Extreme risk iliofemoral. Study results [abstract]. Washington, TCT 2014.
13. Adams DH, Popma JJ, Reardon MJ, et al, U.S. CoreValve Clinical Investigators. Transcatheter aortic-valve replacement with a self-expanding prosthesis. N Engl J Med 2014;370:1790–8.
14. Hamm CW, Möllmann H, Holzhey D, et al, GARY-Executive Board. The German Aortic Valve Registry (GARY): in-hospital outcome. Eur Heart J 2014;35:1588–98.
15. Leon MB, on behalf of the PARTNER Trial Investigators. A randomized evaluation of the SAPIEN XT transcatheter valve system in patients with aortic stenosis who are not candidates for surgery: PARTNER II, inoperable cohort. ACC. San Francisco, March 9-11, 2013.
16. Abdel-Wahab M, Mehilli J, Frerker C, et al, CHOICE Investigators. Comparison of balloon-expandable vs self-expandable valves in patients undergoing transcatheter aortic valve replacement: the CHOICE randomized clinical trial. JAMA 2014;311:1503–14.
17. Di Mario C, Eltchaninoff H, Moat N, et al. The 2011–12 pilot European Sentinel Registry of Transcatheter Aortic Valve Implantation: in-hospital results in 4,571 patients. EuroIntervention 2013;8:1362–71.
18. Moat NE, Ludman P, de Belder MA, et al. Long-term outcomes after transcatheter aortic valve implantation in high-risk patients with severe aortic stenosis: the U.K. TAVI (United Kingdom Transcatheter Aortic

Valve Implantation) Registry. J Am Coll Cardiol 2011; 58:2130–8.

19. van der Boon RM, Nuis RJ, Van Mieghem NM, et al. Clinical outcome following Transcatheter Aortic Valve Implantation in patients with impaired left ventricular systolic function. Catheter Cardiovasc Interv 2012;79:702–10.

20. Gotzmann M, Rahlmann P, Hehnen T, et al. Heart failure in severe aortic valve stenosis: prognostic impact of left ventricular ejection fraction and mean gradient on outcome after transcatheter aortic valve implantation. Eur J Heart Fail 2012;14:1155–62.

21. O'Sullivan CJ, Stortecky S, Heg D, et al. Clinical outcomes of patients with low-flow, low-gradient, severe aortic stenosis and either preserved or reduced ejection fraction undergoing transcatheter aortic valve implantation. Eur Heart J 2013;34:3437–50.

22. Sannino A, Gargiulo G, Schiattarella GG, et al. Increased mortality after transcatheter aortic valve implantation (TAVI) in patients with severe aortic stenosis and low ejection fraction: a meta-analysis of 6898 patients. Int J Cardiol 2014;176:32–9.

23. Fraccaro C, Al-Lamee R, Tarantini G, et al. Transcatheter aortic valve implantation in patients with severe left ventricular dysfunction: immediate and mid-term results, a multicenter study. Circ Cardiovasc Interv 2012;5:253–60.

24. Biner S, Birati EY, Topilsky Y, et al. Outcome of transcatheter aortic valve implantation in patients with low-gradient severe aortic stenosis and preserved left ventricular ejection fraction. Am J Cardiol 2014; 113:348–54.

25. Ben-Dor I, Maluenda G, Iyasu GD, et al. Comparison of outcome of higher versus lower transvalvular gradients in patients with severe aortic stenosis and low (<40%) left ventricular ejection fraction. Am J Cardiol 2012;109:1031–7.

26. Clavel MA, Pibarot P. Assessment of low-flow, low gradient aortic stenosis: multimodality imaging is the key to success. EuroIntervention 2014;10:U52–60.

27. Clavel MA, Pibarot P, Dumesnil JG. Paradoxical low flow aortic valve stenosis: incidence, evaluation, and clinical significance. Curr Cardiol Rep 2014;16:431.

28. Elhmidi Y, Piazza N, Krane M, et al. Clinical presentation and outcomes after transcatheter aortic valve implantation in patients with low flow/low gradient severe aortic stenosis. Catheter Cardiovasc Interv 2014;84:283–90.

29. Le Ven F, Freeman M, Webb J, et al. Impact of low flow on the outcome of high-risk patients undergoing transcatheter aortic valve replacement. J Am Coll Cardiol 2013;62:782–8.

30. Bax JJ, Delgado V, Bapat V, et al. Open issues in transcatheter aortic valve implantation. Part 1: patient selection and treatment strategy for transcatheter aortic valve implantation. Eur Heart J 2014;35: 2627–38.

31. Nishimura RA, Otto CM, Bonow RO, et al. 2014 AHA/ACC guideline for the management of patients with valvular heart disease: a report of the American College of Cardiology/American Heart Association Task Force on Practice Guidelines. Circulation 2014;129: e521–643.

32. Clavel MA, Dumesnil JG, Capoulade R, et al. Outcome of patients with aortic stenosis, small valve area, and low-flow, low-gradient despite preserved left ventricular ejection fraction. J Am Coll Cardiol 2012;60:1259–67.

33. Dumesnil JG, Pibarot P, Carabello B. Paradoxical low flow and/or low gradient severe aortic stenosis despite preserved left ventricular ejection fraction: implications for diagnosis and treatment. Eur Heart J 2010;31:281–9.

34. Cueff C, Serfaty JM, Cimadevilla C, et al. Measurement of aortic valve calcification using multislice computed tomography: correlation with haemodynamic severity of aortic stenosis and clinical implication for patients with low ejection fraction. Heart 2011;97:721–6.

35. Clavel MA, Messika-Zeitoun D, Pibarot P, et al. The complex nature of discordant severe calcified aortic valve disease grading: new insights from combined Doppler-Echocardiographic and Computed Tomographic Study. J Am Coll Cardiol 2013;62:2329–38.

36. Clavel MA, Malouf J, Michelena HI, et al. B-type natriuretic peptide clinical activation in aortic stenosis: impact on long-term survival. J Am Coll Cardiol 2014;63:2016–25.

37. Elhmidi Y, Bleiziffer S, Piazza N, et al. The evolution and prognostic value of N-terminal brain natriuretic peptide in predicting 1-year mortality in patients following transcatheter aortic valve implantation. J Invasive Cardiol 2013;25:38–44.

38. López-Otero D, Trillo-Nouche R, Gude F, et al. Pro B-type natriuretic peptide plasma value: a new criterion for the prediction of short- and long-term outcomes after transcatheter aortic valve implantation. Int J Cardiol 2013;168:1264–8.

39. Ribeiro HB, Urena M, Le Ven F, et al. Long-term prognostic value and serial changes of plasma N-terminal prohormone B-type natriuretic peptide in patients undergoing transcatheter aortic valve implantation. Am J Cardiol 2014;113:851–9.

40. Giordana F, D'Ascenzo F, Nijhoff F, et al. Meta-analysis of predictors of all-cause mortality after transcatheter aortic valve implantation. Am J Cardiol 2014;114 [pii:S0002-9149(14) 01603–8].

41. Iung B, Laouénan C, Himbert D, et al, FRANCE 2 Investigators. Predictive factors of early mortality after transcatheter aortic valve implantation: individual risk assessment using a simple score. Heart 2014; 100:1016–23.

42. Rodés-Cabau J, Webb JG, Cheung A, et al. Transcatheter aortic valve implantation for the treatment

of severe symptomatic aortic stenosis in patients at very high or prohibitive surgical risk: acute and late outcomes of the multicenter Canadian experience. J Am Coll Cardiol 2010;55:1080–90.

43. Hahn RT, Pibarot P, Stewart WJ, et al. Comparison of transcatheter and surgical aortic valve replacement in severe aortic stenosis: a longitudinal study of echocardiography parameters in cohort A of the PARTNER trial (placement of aortic transcatheter valves). J Am Coll Cardiol 2013;61:2514–21.

44. Kodali SK, Williams MR, Smith CR, et al. Two-year outcomes after transcatheter or surgical aortic-valve replacement. N Engl J Med 2012;366:1686–95.

45. Lauten A, Zahn R, Horack M, et al. Transcatheter aortic valve implantation in patients with low-flow, low-gradient aortic stenosis. JACC Cardiovasc Interv 2012;5:552–9.

46. Tamburino C, Capodanno D, Ramondo A, et al. Incidence and predictors of early and late mortality after transcatheter aortic valve implantation in 663 patients with severe aortic stenosis. Circulation 2011;123:299–308.

47. Herrmann HC, Pibarot P, Hueter I, et al. Predictors of mortality and outcomes of therapy in low-flow severe aortic stenosis: a Placement of Aortic Transcatheter Valves (PARTNER) trial analysis. Circulation 2013;127:2316–26.

48. Bauer F, Coutant V, Bernard M, et al. Patients with severe aortic stenosis and reduced ejection fraction: earlier recovery of left ventricular systolic function after transcatheter aortic valve implantation compared with surgical valve replacement. Echocardiography 2013;30:865–70.

49. Pilgrim T, Wenaweser P, Meuli F, et al. Clinical outcome of high-risk patients with severe aortic stenosis and reduced left ventricular ejection fraction undergoing medical treatment or TAVI. PLoS One 2011;6:e27556.

50. Clavel MA, Webb JG, Rodés-Cabau J, et al. Comparison between transcatheter and surgical prosthetic valve implantation in patients with severe aortic stenosis and reduced left ventricular ejection fraction. Circulation 2010;122(19):1928–36.

51. Clavel MA, Webb JG, Pibarot P, et al. Comparison of the hemodynamic performance of percutaneous and surgical bioprostheses for the treatment of severe aortic stenosis. J Am Coll Cardiol 2009;53:1883–91.

52. Nazif TM, Williams MR, Hahn RT, et al. Clinical implications of new-onset left bundle branch block after transcatheter aortic valve replacement: analysis of the PARTNER experience. Eur Heart J 2014;35:1599–607.

53. Elmariah S, Palacios IF, McAndrew T, et al. Outcomes of transcatheter and surgical aortic valve replacement in high-risk patients with aortic stenosis and left ventricular dysfunction: results from the Placement of Aortic Transcatheter Valves (PARTNER) trial (cohort A). Circ Cardiovasc Interv 2013;6:604–6.

54. Quere JP, Monin JL, Levy F, et al. Influence of preoperative left ventricular contractile reserve on postoperative ejection fraction in low-gradient aortic stenosis. Circulation 2006;113:1738–44.

55. Løgstrup BB, Andersen HR, Thuesen L, et al. Left ventricular global systolic longitudinal deformation and prognosis 1 year after femoral and apical transcatheter aortic valve implantation. J Am Soc Echocardiogr 2013;26:246–54.

56. Onorati F, D'Errigo P, Grossi C, et al, OBSERVANT Research Group. Effect of severe left ventricular systolic dysfunction on hospital outcome after transcatheter aortic valve implantation or surgical aortic valve replacement: results from a propensity-matched population of the Italian OBSERVANT multicenter study. J Thorac Cardiovasc Surg 2014;147:568–75.

57. Auffret V, Boulmier D, Oger E, et al. Predictors of 6-month poor clinical outcomes after transcatheter aortic valve implantation. Arch Cardiovasc Dis 2014;107:10–20.

58. Roselli EE, Abdel Azim A, Houghtaling PL, et al. Pulmonary hypertension is associated with worse early and late outcomes after aortic valve replacement: implications for transcatheter aortic valve replacement. J Thorac Cardiovasc Surg 2012;144:1067–74.e2.

59. Seco M, Forrest P, Jackson SA, et al. Extracorporeal membrane oxygenation for very high-risk transcatheter aortic valve implantation. Heart Lung Circ 2014;23:957–62.

60. Poliacikova P, Cockburn J, Pareek N, et al. Prognostic impact of pre-existing right ventricular dysfunction on the outcome of transcatheter aortic valve implantation. J Invasive Cardiol 2013;25:142–5.

61. Iwahashi N, Nakatani S, Umemura S, et al. Usefulness of plasma B-type natriuretic peptide in the assessment of disease severity and prediction of outcome after aortic valve replacement in patients with severe aortic stenosis. J Am Soc Echocardiogr 2011;24:984–91.

62. Sack S, Menne J, Krüger T, et al. Decompensated valve failure: the revival of balloon valvuloplasty - percutaneous valve intervention. Herz 2009;34:206–10.

63. Tissot CM, Attias D, Himbert D, et al. Reappraisal of percutaneous aortic balloon valvuloplasty as a preliminary treatment strategy in the transcatheter aortic valve implantation era. EuroIntervention 2011;7:49–56.

64. Eltchaninoff H, Durand E, Borz B, et al. Balloon aortic valvuloplasty in the era of transcatheter aortic valve replacement: acute and long-term outcomes. Am Heart J 2014;167:235–40.

65. Ussia GP, Capodanno D, Barbanti M, et al. Balloon aortic valvuloplasty for severe aortic stenosis as a bridge to high-risk transcatheter aortic valve implantation. J Invasive Cardiol 2010;22:161–6.

66. Fudim M, Markley RR, Robbins MA. Transcatheter aortic valve replacement for aortic bioprosthetic valve failure with cardiogenic shock. J Invasive Cardiol 2013;25:625–6.

67. Pilgrim T, Meier B, Wenaweser P. Emergency transcatheter aortic valve implantation for decompensated aortic stenosis. J Invasive Cardiol 2013;25:247–9.

68. Pasic M, Dreysse S, Potapov E, et al. Rescue transcatheter aortic valve implantation and simultaneous percutaneous coronary intervention on cardiopulmonary bypass in a patient with an extreme risk profile. Heart Surg Forum 2012;15:E164–6.

69. Husser O, Holzamer A, Philipp A, et al. Emergency and prophylactic use of miniaturized veno-arterial extracorporeal membrane oxygenation in transcatheter aortic valve implantation. Catheter Cardiovasc Interv 2013;82:E542–51.

70. Pizzighini S, Finet G, Obadia JF, et al. Emergent transcatheter aortic valve implantation in a patient with bicuspid aortic valve stenosis in cardiogenic shock. Ann Cardiol Angeiol (Paris) 2014 [pii:S0003-3928(14) 00057–2].

71. Drews T, Pasic M, Buz S, et al. Elective use of femoro-femoral cardiopulmonary bypass during transcatheter aortic valve implantation. Eur J Cardiothorac Surg 2014. [Epub ahead of print].

72. Meguro K, Lellouche N, Teiger E. Cardiac resynchronization therapy improved heart failure after left bundle branch block during transcatheter aortic valve implantation. J Invasive Cardiol 2012;24:132–3.

73. Osmancik P, Stros P, Herman D, et al. Cardiac resynchronization therapy implantation following transcatheter aortic valve implantation. Europace 2011;13:290–1.

74. Atkins BZ, Hashmi ZA, Ganapathi AM, et al. Surgical correction of aortic valve insufficiency after left ventricular assist device implantation. J Thorac Cardiovasc Surg 2013;146:1247–52.

75. D'Ancona G, Pasic M, Buz S, et al. TAVI for pure aortic valve insufficiency in a patient with a left ventricular assist device. Ann Thorac Surg 2012;93:e89–91.

Percutaneous Intervention for Mitral Regurgitation

Mohammad Sarraf, MD, Ted Feldman, MD, FESC, FACC, MSCAI*

KEYWORDS

- Mitral regurgitation • Mitral valve • Valve replacement • Heart failure

KEY POINTS

- Percutaneous treatment of mitral regurgitation (MR) is a promising alternative for patients with functional MR (FMR) who are not appropriate for surgery and are not responding to optimal medical therapy and cardiac resynchronization therapy.
- Unlike degenerative MR, where repair therapy is clearly preferred, the optimal approach for FMR has not been defined.
- Challenges for novel mitral repair devices are to demonstrate safety and superior efficacy to medical management in higher risk patients.
- Transcatheter mitral valve replacement is emerging as a feasible therapy, but requires significant additional clinical trials to define its place in treating heart failure related to MR.

Our understanding of mitral regurgitation (MR) as a clinical and pathophysiologic entity has evolved greatly over the last decade. As recently as in the 2006 valvular heart disease guidelines, no explicit distinction was made between degenerative and functional MR (FMR) in terms of broad management principles.[1] Today, we understand the pathogenesis, clinical course, and therapy for degenerative and FMR differ in more detail. Degenerative MR (DMR), involving a structural abnormality of the mitral leaflets, is treated as a disease of the valve itself. Typically, left ventricular (LV) dysfunction in DMR is secondary to the valvular abnormality, with heart failure (HF) as a late manifestation of disease. The presentation for many of these patients is acute HF owing to chordal rupture with acute MR. In contradistinction, FMR represents a disease of the LV with normal mitral leaflet structure and MR as a secondary or bystander abnormality. The discussion of intervention for MR in the context of HF is thus a discussion of FMR.

BACKGROUND
Mitral Regurgitation and Left Ventricular Dysfunction: Prevalence and Outcome

The true incidence of FMR is difficult to ascertain. Different studies have used varied criteria for grading of MR severity based on echocardiography. Nkomo and colleagues[2] conducted a population-based study combining the echocardiographic database from 3 studies that examined young patients in Coronary Artery Revascularisation in Diabetes (CARDIA) trial, middle-aged patients in Atherosclerosis Risk in Communities (ARIC) trial, and older adults in the Cardiovascular Health Study (CHS). The aim of the study was to assess the prevalence, distribution patterns, and consequences of moderate or severe mitral and

NorthShore University HealthSystem, Evanston, IL, USA
* Corresponding author. Cardiology Division, Evanston Hospital, Walgreen Building 3rd Floor, 2650 Ridge Avenue, Evanston, IL 60201.
E-mail address: tfeldman@tfeldman.org

Heart Failure Clin 11 (2015) 243–259
http://dx.doi.org/10.1016/j.hfc.2014.12.004
1551-7136/15/$ – see front matter © 2015 Elsevier Inc. All rights reserved.

aortic valve disease in the general population and in Olmsted County, Minnesota. MR was the most common disease, with an incidence of less than 1% before age 54 years but increasing each decade and reaching greater than 9% after age 75 years. Similar findings were observed in the Olmsted County community with slightly higher incidence. The incidence of valve disease was similar between men and women, and between whites and blacks. Patients with MR had significantly greater LV end-diastolic volume (LVEDV) and left atrial volume. The adjusted mortality risk ratio was 1.36 (95% CI, 1.15–1.62; $P = .0005$) in the population and 1.75 (95% CI, 1.61–1.90; $P<.0001$) in the community. A major limitation of this study is the lack of differentiation between DMR and FMR.

A more recent analysis attempted to determine the prevalence of MR in the US population based on the digital data from the National Institutes of Health, and classified the type of MR according to Carpentier's classification (**Table 1**). This analysis estimated that MR affected more than 2.5 million people in the United States in 2000. The largest group could be classified as having Carpentier type IIIb, with restricted motion owing to LV dysfunction with ischemic or nonischemic etiology. The investigators reported the prevalence of MR owing to ischemic cardiomyopathy at 7500 to 9000 per million, and of MR owing to nonischemic etiology of cardiomyopathy at 16,250 per million.[3]

The prognosis of patients with FMR is poor. Even the slightest degree of FMR can impact the survival of patients with LV dysfunction with or without coronary artery disease.[4] The impact of FMR on survival is irrespective of age, LV ejection fraction (LVEF), sex, mitral filling pattern on echocardiogram, and New York Heart Association (NYHA) functional class.[5] FMR has a 50% composite rate of mortality and HF hospitalization at 3 years, compared with 30% in HF patients without FMR.[6] Not surprisingly, in patients with ischemic FMR, the 5-year total and cardiac mortality rates were increased (62 ± 2% and 50 ± 0%, respectively) compared with those without associated coronary artery disease (39 ± 9% and 30 ± 0%, respectively).[7] Increasing severity of FMR is a strong predictor of mortality or transplantation in patients with an EF of less than 35%[8] and associated with higher mortality rates and HF hospitalizations.[9]

PATHOPHYSIOLOGY

Normal mitral valve function depends on a balance between the closing forces of the LV, that is, LV contraction, and the tethering forces that prevent the valve from prolapsing into the left atrium.[10] The papillary muscles counterbalance the force of LV contraction on the mitral leaflets via chordae tendinae by exerting force parallel and perpendicular to the leaflets that prevents leaflet prolapse. The traditional teaching for the mechanism of FMR is that altered geometry and reduced global or regional contractility, in the presence of "normal" mitral valve leaflets, results in MR. As new data emerge, this picture seems to provide an incomplete description of the mechanism of FMR. For example, this description does not explain as to why vast majority of patients with isolated severe aortic insufficiency (AI) do not have and do not develop FMR.[11] Patients with severe AI have the largest LVEDV and LV end-systolic volume (LVESV), yet the incidence of FMR is relatively

Table 1
Carpentier's classification for mitral regurgitation

	Leaflet Motion	Lesion	Etiology
Type I	Normal	Annular dilation Leaflet tear	Dilated cardiomyopathy Endocarditis
Type II	Excess motion	Elongation owing to rupture of chordae or papillary muscles	Degenerative valve disease (Barlow's disease) Endocarditis Myocardial infarction Trauma
Type IIIa	Limited motion in systole and diastole	Leaflet fibrosis/thickening/calcification Chordal fibrosis/fusion/thickening Commissural fusion	Rheumatic heart disease Carcinoid syndrome Mitral valve apparatus calcification
Type IIIb	Limited motion in systole	Left ventricular dilatation Chordal tethering	Ischemic/nonischemic cardiomyopathy

low. Therefore, FMR is not entirely a disease of ventricular dysfunction and might be better understood in terms of the interaction of different components of the mitral apparatus, namely annular, valvular, and subvalvular interaction.[12] Furthermore, the etiology of FMR plays an important role in defining and understanding the mechanism of FMR. FMR can be owing to either ischemic or nonischemic cardiomyopathy. Therefore, the underlying disease can impact the outcomes of the patients as well as appropriate treatment strategy.

Left Ventricle

In the early stages of MR, patients tolerate the volume overload until the left atrium reaches its maximum compliance, beyond which symptoms start to develop. A vicious cycle develops, as the regurgitant volume in the left atrium returns to the LV during diastole, resulting in LV volume overload and progressive LV dilatation. Dilatation and LV dysfunction has long been considered a key element of FMR. Subsequently, chamber dilatation results in annular dilation, lateral and apical displacement of the papillary muscles, and malcoaptation of the mitral leaflets.[13] The presence of coronary artery disease, either acute or chronic, can contribute to LV remodeling, displacement of the papillary muscles, and further LV dysfunction. Patients with right coronary artery or left circumflex disease are more likely to develop posterior leaflet tethering, even in the presence of normal or low normal LVEF. Patients with left anterior descending artery disease, however, develop FMR mainly owing to reduced LV contractility and spherical shape of LV that ultimately leads to displacement of the papillary muscles.

Mitral Annulus

The mitral annulus is a complex, 3-dimensional structure defined by the integration of the tissue juncture of the left atrium, the left ventricle, and the mitral leaflets. En face, mitral annulus resembles a kidney bean, but in 3 dimensions it has a saddle-shaped structure,[14] with the anterior horn higher than posterior horn. During systole, the mitral annulus undergoes a significant dynamic decrease in size and facilitates the closure of mitral leaflets. The mitral annulus moves anteriorly during normal systolic contraction. In FMR, this anterior movement is reduced and contributes to malcoaptation of the mitral leaflets. There are also a number of substantial changes that occur with the annulus in FMR that are summarized in **Table 2**.[15]

Myocardial Dyssynchrony

Myocardial dyssynchrony results in dyssynchrony of papillary muscles, disturbing mitral leaflet closure timing that contributes to FMR. Lancellotti and colleagues[16] demonstrated worsening FMR owing to dynamic LV dyssynchrony during exercise in the absence of ischemia in patients with an LVEF of less than 45%. They showed an increasing effective regurgitant orifice (ERO) with increasing LV dispersion. There is evidence that cardiac resynchronization therapy (CRT) reduces FMR at rest[17] and with exercise.[18]

Papillary Muscle and Chordae Tendinae (Subvalvular Apparatus)

Classically, "papillary muscle dysfunction" is thought to contribute to FMR. Recent studies, however, have demonstrated that changes in LV geometry and wall motion can affect papillary muscle position and function, with resultant tension on the chordal apparatus and tethering leaflet motion during systole. This relationship is regardless of presence or absence of papillary muscle ischemia. Posterior and apical displacement of the papillary muscles also has a central role in mitral leaflet tethering and FMR.[19] Tethering of leaflets, especially the anterior leaflet, limits systolic motion of the mitral valves and counteracts the closing forces produced from ventricular contraction. This leads to apical displacement of coaptation zone of the mitral leaflets relative to the annular plane (see **Fig. 2**).[19,20] Moreover, animal[21] and clinical[22] studies have suggested that it is not the papillary muscle dysfunction

Table 2 Mitral annulus dimensions in normal human hearts and patients with dilated cardiomyopathy		
	Normal	**Dilated Cardiomyopathy**
Nonplanar mitral annulus shape	Saddle shape	Flattened
Area (cm^2)	~7–12	~11–20
Circumference (cm)	7–11	8–18
Area change diastole/systole (%)	~20–42	13–23

and/or ischemia causing FMR; rather, it is the underlying LV myocardium driving tethering of the leaflets.

Mitral Leaflets

There is growing evidence that there are significant pathologic changes that occur within the mitral leaflets in patients with FMR. Beaudoin and colleagues[11] investigated patients with isolated chronic AI with and without FMR; they demonstrated the mitral valve area to be 31% larger than in normal control subjects. However, patients with aortic regurgitation (AR) and FMR did not have the same magnitude of mitral valve enlargement (15%). The authors also demonstrated that the total valve area/leaflet closure ratio remained the strongest predictor of FMR in chronic AI patients. Patients with severe AI and without FMR have maintained a normal ratio, whereas patients who develop FMR have a reduced total valve area/leaflet closure area ratio. Chaput and colleagues[23] showed a similar relationship between total valve area/leaflet closure area in patients with inferoposterior acute myocardial infarction and patients with dilated cardiomyopathy. They found that a valve area/leaflet closure ratio of less than 1.7 strongly correlates with progression of FMR, irrespective of the etiology of FMR. In conclusion, the mitral leaflets undergo significant changes in FMR and they do not have a normal histology.

TREATMENT OF FUNCTIONAL MITRAL REGURGITATION

The management of FMR is controversial. There is considerable debate regarding the optimal approach, indications, timing of intervention, and efficacy of interventions. Treatment options include medical treatment, CRT, and nonpharmacologic interventions, mainly surgery and percutaneous interventions.

Medical Therapy

Optimal medical management, focused on LV dysfunction, is the cornerstone of therapy for all patients with FMR. The goal of therapy is to reduce LV size, improve papillary muscle geometry, and reduce tethering forces, thus improving MR. These treatments may optimize cardiac performance, reduce symptoms, and reduce mortality by unloading the LV while maintaining euvolemia. HF symptoms should be treated per guideline recommendations, irrespective of the etiology and severity of FMR. Angiotensin-converting enzyme inhibitors[24] or angiotensin receptor blockers, β-blockers,[25] aldosterone antagonists, and diuretic agents should be considered for all patients. In the absence of HF, LV dysfunction, or presence of HF symptoms, there is little evidence that vasodilators are useful for treatment of the MR. The most recent American Heart Association/American College of Cardiology Valve guideline suggests optimal medical therapy (guideline-directed medical therapy; **Fig. 1**).

Cardiac Resynchronization Therapy

CRT has been shown to improve FMR in a substantial number of patients with ischemic and nonischemic cardiomyopathy.[26] The response seems to be superior in nonischemic cardiomyopathy, compared with an ischemic etiology.[26] CRT improves the LV synchrony through multiple pathways. It improves FMR by resynchronization that translates to improve valvular and subvalvular apparatus function. It also promotes reverse remodeling of the LV, improves myocardial contractility that increases closing force of the mitral valve and reduces the leaflet tethering by improving LV geometry.[18,27–29] It is self-evident that CRT is indicated based on electrocardiographic findings and not on the severity of FMR. CRT is the only therapy widely available for FMR shown to have a favorable impact on mortality.[30]

Surgery

A surgical approach to FMR can be classified under the 2 broad categories of valvular procedures and LV myocardial reconstructive procedures. Valvular procedures include restrictive annuloplasty, mitral valve repair, and mitral valve replacement. There are numerous published articles on surgery in patients with FMR, yet most studies are retrospective and observational studies with no standard surgical approach. The execution of randomized, controlled trials in cardiac surgery has been hampered for different reasons, including bias of the referring cardiologists, lack of surgical equipoise, inadequate surgical expertise, and nuanced inclusion/exclusion criteria that detract from the applicability of the findings to patients encountered in routine practice.[31] The current standard surgical treatment is to perform a restrictive annuloplasty with a complete rigid ring to achieve a leaflet coaptation length of at least 8 mm on cardiopulmonary bypass, with complete revascularization if indicated. We review 4 recently published randomized, controlled trials.

The first trial studied the effect of adding mitral repair to coronary artery bypass graft (CABG) in patients with moderate FMR (proximal isovelocity area of 5–8 mm).[32] A restrictive annuloplasty in conjunction with CABG using a rigid annuloplasty

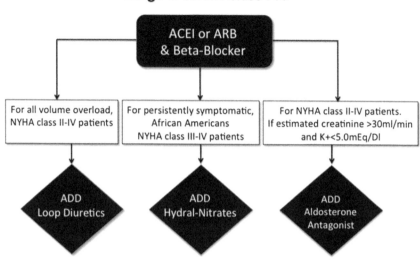

Fig. 1. Guideline-directed medical therapy (GDMT) for heart failure. ACEI, angiotensin-converting enzyme inhibitor; ARB, angiotensin receptor blocker; HFrEF, heart failure with reduced ejection fraction; LOE, level of evidence; NYHA, New York Heart Association. (*Adapted from* Nishimura RA, Otto CM, Bonow RO, et al. 2014 AHA/ACC guideline for the management of patients with valvular heart disease: executive summary: a report of the American College of Cardiology/American Heart association task force on practice guidelines. Circulation 2014;129(23):2440–92; with permission.)

ring improved NYHA functional class, promoted LV reverse remodeling, and decreased pulmonary arterial pressures compared with CABG without annuloplasty. The mean leaflet coaptation length was 8 ± 3 mm. Repair was considered successful if no or trivial MR remained on postcardiopulmonary bypass transesophageal echocardiography. No patient in the mitral valve repair arm had a recurrence of more than mild FMR at 5 years. This study was not powered to detect a difference in mortality, yet 5-year survival was 93.7 ± 3% and 88.8 ± 3% for patients in the CABG plus mitral valve repair and isolated CABG groups, respectively. The limitations of this study are the following: (1) single-center study, (2) undefined medical therapy, (3) unknown number of patients requiring CRT or previously having received CRT, and (4) nonrobust definition of FMR. Ischemic MR was defined as moderate on the basis of a proximal isovelocity area radius between 5 and 8 mm. Quantitative measures of MR severity were performed but not reported.

The Randomized Ischemic Mitral Evaluation (RIME) trial studied the impact of adding mitral valve repair to CABG in patients with more than moderate FMR and LVEF greater than 30%. Moderate FMR was defined as ERO greater than 0.2 cm², regurgitant volume of 30 to 59 mL

per beat, and vena contracta of 0.30 to 0.69 cm. Regurgitant volume was calculated by cardiac MRI. The investigators randomized 73 patients to CABG or CABG plus restrictive annuloplasty using a complete and rigid ring. Mean mitral leaflet coaptation length was 7.1 ± 1.2 mm, and technical success was defined as no or trivial MR on separation from cardiopulmonary bypass. Patients with CABG plus mitral valve repair had more perioperative morbidity, but the primary end point of peak oxygen consumption at 1 year was markedly improved in the CABG plus mitral valve repair group, compared with CABG only. Also, these patients exhibited improved LV reverse remodeling, and lower B-type natriuretic peptide levels and NYHA functional class scores. Moderate or greater FMR was observed at 1 year in 4% of patients in the CABG plus mitral valve repair group compared with 50% in the CABG-only group.[33] The limitations of this study are the following: (1) the definition of moderate FMR is not consistent with the new guidelines[34] (an ERO of greater than 0.2 cm² is considered severe in patients with FMR in the new guidelines); (2) medical therapy and CRT are not carefully identified; and (3) the perioperative morbidity was substantially greater than standard of care, which raises questions about the small sample size and how representative the centers in this study are.

A retrospective, propensity-matched analysis of patients recruited into the Surgical Treatment for Ischemic Heart Failure (STICH) trial with moderate to severe FMR and an LVEF of less than 35% has been reported recently. The addition of mitral valve annuloplasty or replacement to CABG resulted in a significantly lower risk of mortality compared with CABG alone (hazard ratio, 0.42; 95% CI, 0.21-0.88; $P = .02$). This analysis has significant limitations, mainly owing to the retrospective nature of the analysis; in addition, the mitral valve surgery was left to the discretion of the surgeon.[35]

Overall, there is a consensus that in patients with more than moderate FMR undergoing CABG, a restrictive mitral valve annuloplasty with a complete rigid ring significantly reduces the severity of FMR, improves objective and subjective assessments of HF, and promotes LV reverse remodeling. None of the current studies to date, however, show that reduction in FMR impacts the survival of patients with FMR. Currently, there are 2 ongoing clinical trials addressing this issue (www.clinicaltrials.gov, identifiers NCT00613548 and NCT00806988).

American and European guidelines recommend mitral valve repair or chordal sparing replacement for FMR, but they do not specify the operation owing to the paucity of the data. Recently, the Cardiothoracic Surgical Trials Network conducted a multicenter, randomized trial to evaluate the relative benefits and risks of repair versus replacement, with or without coronary revascularization, in patients with severe ischemic MR. The primary endpoint was the LVESV index at 12 months.[36] At 12 months, there was no difference in LVESV index between the groups. The mortality was similar between the groups. However, the recurrence of FMR was significantly higher in the repair arm compared with replacement (32.6% vs 2.3%; $P<.001$). The quality of life and functional status of patients at 1 year was similar between the groups.[36] The interpretation of this study is challenging. Although the replacement arm had markedly less MR at 12 months, it did not translate to clinical endpoints or improved quality of life and was associated with increased morbidity.

American Heart Associates/American College of Cardiology Guidelines

The recently published American Heart Associates/American College of Cardiology guidelines emphasize a comprehensive quantification of severity of MR. Furthermore, the criteria for severity of FMR has changed compared with DMR. The ERO is reduced to 0.2 cm^2 or greater for severe FMR, regurgitant volume to greater than 30 mL per beat, and regurgitant fraction to greater than 50%. These changes are important when one considers the current literature review. Virtually all recent studies with quantified severity of FMR, based on echocardiography, have used the same cutoff points for DMR that are significantly higher. These guidelines emphasize optimal medical therapy and CRT (see Cardiac Resynchronization Therapy) with class I and level of evidence A (IA). The recommendations for surgical intervention are expectedly less clear.[34] The guidelines reserve surgical approach for severely symptomatic patients or concomitant surgery other than mitral valve such, as CABG or aortic valve surgery. **Table 3** summarizes these recommendations.[34]

PERCUTANEOUS TREATMENT OF FUNCTIONAL MITRAL REGURGITATION

Over the past 2 decades, a spectrum of different technologies for percutaneous treatment of MR has been developed. They can be categorized into leaflet repair, annuloplasty, chordal implants, LV remodeling techniques, and percutaneous MV replacement. We examine some of the available and forthcoming technologies for each of these approaches (**Table 4**).[37]

Table 3
AHA/ACC guideline recommendation for surgical intervention in FMR

Recommendation	COR	LOE
MV surgery is reasonable for patients with chronic severe secondary MR (stages C and D) who are undergoing CABG or AVR	IIa	C
MV surgery may be considered for severely symptomatic patients (NYHA class III/IV) with chronic severe secondary MR (stage D)	IIb	B
MV repair may be considered for patients with chronic moderate secondary MR (stage B) who are undergoing other cardiac surgery	IIb	C

Abbreviations: ACC, American College of Cardiology; AHA, American Heart Association; AVR, aortic valve replacement; CABG, coronary artery bypass graft; COR, class of recommendation; LOE, level of evidence; MR, mitral regurgitation; MV, mitral valve.

Table 4
Percutaneous treatment technologies for mitral regurgitation

Target of Therapy	Device (Manufacturer)	Mechanism of Action
Leaflet repair	MitraClip (Abbott)	Clip-based edge-to-edge repair
	Percu Pro (Cardiosolutions)	Space-occupying in regurgitant orifice
Chordal implant	NeoChord (NeoChord)	Synthetic chordae tendineae
Indirect annuloplasty	CARILLON (Cardiac Dimensions)	Coronary sinus reshaping
	MONARC (Edwards)	Coronary sinus reshaping
	PTMA Device (Viacor)	Coronary sinus reshaping
	Mitral cerclage (NIH)	Coronary sinus–right atrial encircling
	Valcare (Valcare Medical)	Rigid "D"-shaped annuloplasty
Direct annuloplasty	Mitralign (Mitralign)	2 × 2 Plicating anchors through posterior annulus
	Accucinch (Guided Delivery Systems [GDS])	Plicating anchors on ventricular side of mitral annulus
	Cardioband (Valtech)	Plicating anchors on atrial side of mitral annulus
	QuantomCor (QuantomCor)	Radiofrequency energy shrinking annular collagen
	Milipede (Milipede)	Semirigid circumferential annular ring
Ventricular reshaping	iCoapsys	Transventricular reshaping
	BACE (Mardil)	External basal myocardial reshaping
	PARACHUTE (CardioKinetix)	Ventricular partitioning
Mitral annular anchor	M-Valve	Percutaneous anchor to allow fixation of transcatheter valve
Mitral valve replacement	Endovalve-Herrmann (Endovalve)	Valve replacement
	CardiAQ (CardiAQ)	Valve replacement
	Tiara (Neovasc)	Valve replacement
	Fortis (Edwards)	Valve replacement
	High Life Medical	Valve replacement
	Medtronic TMV (Transcutaneous Mitral Valve)	Valve replacement

Leaflet Repair: MitraClip System

Alfieri and colleagues[38] introduced an "edge-to-edge" approximation of the mitral leaflets as an alternative surgical strategy for mitral valve repair, with excellent durability and long-term results in a highly selected population.[39] The surgery was devised for DMR patients with redundant mitral valve leaflets. The MitraClip system (**Fig. 2**) mirrors the Alfieri technique by a percutaneous approach via the femoral vein. The device passes through a transseptal puncture to the left atrium. After careful maneuvering across the mitral leaflets, while avoiding grasping the chordae, the anterior and posterior leaflets is grasped at the A2–P2 segments. By closure of the device, the operator coapts the leaflets and generates a double orifice (**Fig. 3**).[40] The bridge formed between the anterior and posterior leaflets reduces the MR. It is speculated that the healing of the device by collagen deposition reduces MR even further, especially after 1 year.[41] The MitraClip system is currently the only device with CE Mark and US Food and Drug Administration approval for commercial use in patients with DMR. We review the available data on MitraClip system with a focus on FMR.

The Endovascular Valve Edge-to-Edge Repair (EVEREST II) randomized, controlled trial was conducted to evaluate the safety and effectiveness of the MitraClip compared with mitral valve surgery (repair or replacement).[40] The primary efficacy end point was freedom from death, from surgery for mitral-valve dysfunction, and from grade 3+ or 4+ MR at 12 months. The cohort of the patients included DMR (74%) and FMR (26%). The study met its primary endpoint of noninferiority of Mitra-Clip to surgery and superiority of MitraClip safety

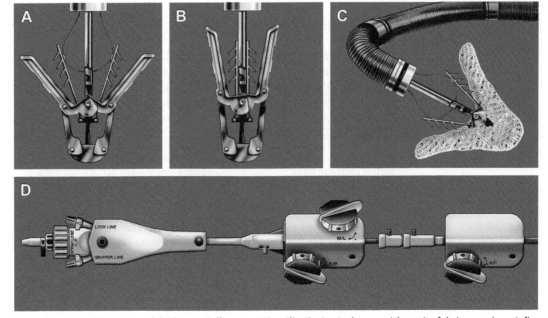

Fig. 2. The MitraClip System. (*A*) The partially open MitraClip device is shown without its fabric covering. A fine wire runs through the barbed "grippers," which is used to raise the grippers. (*B*) The device in closed configuration. (*C*) The MitraClip is attached to the clip delivery system (CDS), which protrudes from the steerable guide catheter. (*D*) Control knobs allow deflection of the guide and CDS to steer the system through the left atrium and position the MitraClip above the mitral orifice. (*From* Feldman T, Young A. Percutaneous approaches to valve repair for mitral regurgitation. J Am Coll Cardiol 2014;63:2057–68. Artwork by Craig Skaggs; with permission.)

compared with surgery.[40] The 4-year follow-up of the study presented the data on 66 patients with FMR of the 279 enrolled in the trial. The primary efficacy endpoint was not different between the MitraClip arm and surgical arm (34.1% vs 22.7%; *P* = .34), however, the patients in the MitraClip arm had a numerically higher rate of greater than 3+ MR at 4-year follow-up.[42]

The EVEREST-II High Risk Registry was a prospective, single-arm study.[43] The study enrolled 78 patients with MR (32 with DMR, 46 with FMR). The follow-up was at 12 months. The Society for

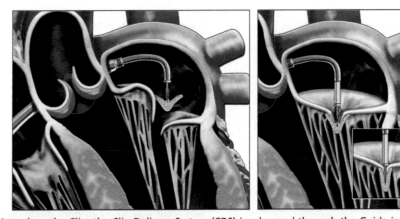

Fig. 3. To introduce the Clip, the Clip Delivery System (CDS) is advanced through the Guide into the left atrium (*left*). Under echocardiographic and fluoroscopic guidance, the Clip is aligned perpendicular to the valve plane, with the Clip Arms perpendicular to the line of coaptation. It is then advanced into the left and then slowly retracted to grasp the leaflets (*right*). The Clip is closed (*right, inset*) and, if reduction of mitral regurgitation is satisfactory, it is released. (*From* Feldman T, Young A. Percutaneous approaches to valve repair for mitral regurgitation. J Am Coll Cardiol 2014;63:2057–68. Artwork by Craig Skaggs; with permission.)

Thoracic Surgery (STS) estimated mortality and the surgical estimated mortality were 14% and 17%, respectively, whereas the actual 30-day mortality was significantly lower, at 7.7% among the total cohort. The 1-year mortality was 24%. Most patients had an NYHA functional class III of IV (89%) at baseline, but at the end of the study 78% of patients were in NYHA functional class of I or II (P<.0001). Quality of life was improved (Short Form-36 physical component score increased from 32.1 to 36.1 [P = .014] and the mental component score from 45.5 to 48.7 [P = .065]) at 1 year. The annual rate of HF related admission in surviving patients with matched data decreased from 0.59 to 0.32 (P = .034). At 12 months, 12 of 46 FMR patients (26%) and 7 of 32 DMR patients (22%) died. At 1 year, 79% of the FMR and 75% of the DMR patients had residual MR of 2+ or higher on core laboratory echocardiograms. Improvement to NYHA functional class I or II at 1 year was similar and sustained between the FMR (74%) and DMR (75%). LV reverse remodeling analysis based on the echocardiographic measurements was obtained in 54 patients. Among 20 patients with DMR with available data, there was a significant 15% reduction in LEDV at 12 months (P<.0002) when compared with baseline with no change in LVESV. Similar data were available on 34 patients with FMR, who had a 20% reduction in LVEDV (P<.0001) and 15% reduction in LVESV (P<.0002). Diastolic and systolic septal–lateral annular dimensions were significantly lesser at 1 year in FMR patients, but there was no difference in the DMR, with a trend toward smaller dimensions.[43] The clinical endpoints and survival were similar between FMR and DMR patients.

The Real World Expanded Multi-center Study of the MitraClip System Continued Access study (REALISM) was a prospective, multicenter, continued access registry to collect data on the "real-world" use of the MitraClip device in both high-risk and non–high-risk surgical patients. Recently, the EVEREST investigators published the aggregate data of REALISM registry with EVEREST-II High Risk Registry in 351 patients. These patients were all considered high risk for surgery (estimated STS >12%). Most patients in this cohort have FMR (70%), and 92% of patients (327 of 351) completed 12 months of follow-up. MitraClip reduced MR to less than 2+ in 86% of patients at discharge (P<.0001). Major adverse events at 30 days were death in 4.8%, myocardial infarction in 1.1%, and stroke in 2.6%; similarly low event rates have been seen in many other series (Fig. 4).[44] At 12 months, 84% of patients had less than 2+ MR (P<.0001). The reverse remodeling indices were measured at 12 months. LVEDV improved from 161 ± 56 mL to 143 ± 53 mL (n = 203; P<.0001) and LVESV improved from 87 ± 47 mL to 79 ± 44 mL (n = 202; P<.0001). NYHA functional class improved from 82% in class III or IV at baseline to 83% in class I or II at 12 months (P<.0001). Annual HF related hospitalization rate reduced from 0.79% before the procedure to 0.41% after the procedure in this cohort and similarly in a DMR subset (Fig. 5).[45]

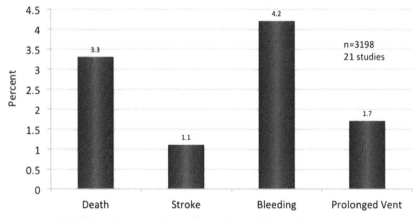

MitraClip 30 Day Outcomes

Fig. 4. A recent review highlights the procedural safety of MitraClip leaflet repair. In a meta-analysis including more than 300 patients from 21 studies, the 30-day outcomes for high-risk patients showed low morbidity and mortality. Vent, ventilation. (Adapted from Philip F, Athappan G, Tuzcu EM, et al. MitraClip for severe symptomatic mitral regurgitation in patients at high surgical risk: a comprehensive systematic review. Catheter Cardiovasc Interv 2014;84(4):581–90; with permission.)

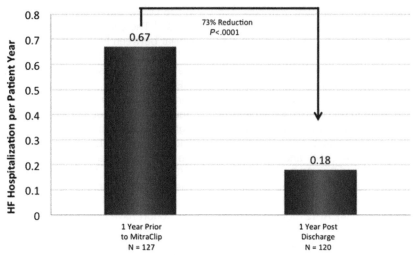

Fig. 5. Heart failure (HF) hospitalizations were reduced by 73% after MitraClip, comparing the year before with the year after treatment. (*Adapted from* Lim DS, Reynolds MR, Feldman T, et al. Improved functional status and quality of life in prohibitive surgical risk patients with degenerative mitral regurgitation following transcatheter mitral valve repair with the mitraclip system. J Am Coll Cardiol 2014;64:182–92; with permission.)

Kaplan-Meier survival estimate at 1 year was 77%.[46] FMR and DMR patient data analysis shows DMR patients were 8 years older, but FMR patients had more comorbidities, including prior myocardial infarction, history of cardiac surgery, and percutaneous coronary intervention. LVEF is also lower in FMR patients. The 30-day mortality was similar between DMR and FMR groups (6.7% vs 4.1%) and there was no difference in 30-day major adverse events. At 12 months, the mortality was 23.8% in DMR and 22.4% in FMR patients. The 12-month major adverse events were similar between the groups at 1 year. Both groups had similar improvement in LVEDV at 12 months (~19 mL), but improvement in LVESV was numerically higher in FMR patients (9 vs 4 mL).

The aggregate of published data on MitraClip demonstrates that this device can favorably impact reverse remodeling in patients with DMR and FMR and is durable to at least 4 years. More important, the unpublished data from the 5-year follow-up of EVEREST II trial has demonstrated that, despite residual MR in the MitraClip arm, patients had favorable remodeling similar to the surgical arm. Furthermore, despite not performing annulus undersizing by MitraClip device, there has been no mitral annular dilatation up to at least 4 years. These results are similar to the Cardiothoracic Surgical Trial Network study, comparing repair versus replacement in FMR and showing no advantage of repair versus replacement on LVESV index.[36] Currently, there

are 2 ongoing clinical trials investigating the effectiveness of MitraClip on FMR patients after optimal medical therapy and CRT (if indicated). The Clinical Outcomes Assessment of the MitraClip Percutaneous Therapy (COAPT) Trial for High Surgical Risk (www.clinicaltrials.gov, identifier NCT01626079) is designed to study the safety and effectiveness of the MitraClip device in HF patients who have FMR. The importance of this trial is that it is the first study to show whether reducing MR has any impact on mortality or other clinical outcomes. The Randomized Study of the MitraClip Device in Heart Failure Patients With Clinically Significant Functional Mitral Regurgitation (RESHAPE) trial (www.clinicaltrials.gov, identifier NCT01772108) is a similar trial being conducted in Europe.

Percu-Pro Cardiosolutions Mitral Spacer

The Cardiosolutions Percu-Pro system (Cardiosolutions Inc, Stoughton, MA) is a percutaneously delivered, balloon-shaped "Mitra-Spacer." The spacer occupies the regurgitant mitral orifice, and anchors to the LV apex (see **Fig. 4**). The spacer has the ability to "self-center" within the regurgitant orifice. There is no available published literature.

Mitral Peak Medical

Mitral Peak Medical (Palo Alto, CA) is designed based on a posterior "neoleaflet." The anterior leaflet occupies one-third of the annular circumference, but controls the majority of flow in diastole and vortex formation in the LV apex. The posterior leaflet has less importance for the overall function of mitral valve coaptation and changes during systole and diastole. The final goal of any mitral valve correction procedure is to restore coaptation of the mitral valve. On the other hand, a majority of the pathology of MR involves the posterior leaflet, so replacing the posterior leaflet may suffice, rather than intervening on the remaining apparatus. This device can be inserted surgically or percutaneously via a transseptal puncture. The shape of the device is designed to replicate the physiologic normal functional anatomy of the posterior leaflet. This device is designed for primary and secondary MR. There is no published clinical experiences.

Chordal Implantation

Synthetic chords can be implanted via a transapical or transseptal approach and are anchored between the LV myocardium and the leaflet. By adjusting the length of the chord, the MR can be reduced or abolished. Currently, there are 3 different systems in the preclinical or clinical stage: the transapically delivered MitraFlex (TransCardiac Therapeutics), NeoChord (Neochord, Inc, Minnetonka, MN) devices, and the transapical-transseptal route of the Babic device.

The NeoChord DS1000 system is a transapically inserted tool that can capture a flail leaflet segment and pierce it with a needle to attach a standard polytetrafluoroethylene artificial chord, which is then anchored to the apical entry site with a pledgeted suture.

There is a single, phase I clinical study with NeoChord and the other 2 devices have not had any clinical studies. The Transapical Artificial Chordae Tendinae (TACT) trial[47] enrolled 30 patients at 7 centers in Europe for this device. Major adverse events included 1 death owing to postcardiotomy syndrome and associated sepsis and 1 minor stroke. Acute procedural success (placement of ≥1 neo-chord and reduction of MR from 3+ or 4+ to ≤2+) was achieved in 26 patients (86.7%). Four patients did not receive repair with the device at the discretion of the surgeon. At 30 days, 17 patients maintained an MR grade of 2+ or greater. Four patients developed recurrent MR and were successfully treated with open MV repair during 30-day follow-up. The success rate of the first 15 cases was 5 (33%), but the success rate in the next 14 cases improved to 12 (86%), underlining the importance of experience with a new device and technology. This technology is mainly designed for DMR with posterior leaflet prolapse.

VENTRICULAR RESHAPING

Several technologies use intracardiac or extracardiac devices that attenuate or reverse remodeling of the LV. By reducing the anteroposterior diameter, the mediolateral distance also decreases in size. Furthermore, papillary muscles will also be closer in systole and improve both the overall function of the LV and coaptation of the mitral leaflets. These devices are designed for FMR. There are 3 major innovations in this category, namely Coapsys (Myocor, Maple Grove, MN), Mardil-BACE (Mardil, Inc, Morrisville, NC), and Parachute (CardioKinetix, Palo Alto, CA).

Coapsys

This device has 2 extracardiac epicardial pads connected by a flexible tether running through transventricular subvalvular space and anchored on the other side of epicardial surface. The chord can be shortened to reduce the MR during the operation. In the Randomized Evaluation of a Surgical Treatment for Off-Pump Repair of the Mitral Valve (RESTORE-MV) Trial,[48] 165 patients were randomly assigned to undergo CABG with or without Coapsys ventricular reshaping. Patients treated with the device had greater reductions in LV end-diastolic diameter, and lesser mortality at 2 years, compared with the conventional annuloplasty control arm. A percutaneous approach was developed. Despite the positive results of the trial, this device is no longer manufactured.

INDIRECT ANNULOPLASTY
Carillon

Because the great cardiac vein and coronary sinus are close to mitral annulus, some of the first attempts to reduce MR without surgery did so by placement of devices in the coronary sinus. Most devices in this category are no longer in development, but clinical trials of the Carillon Mitral Contour System (Cardiac Dimension, Inc, Kirkland, WA) have been completed successfully (**Fig. 6**). The device consists of self-expandable nitinol semihelical distal and proximal anchors connected by a nitinol bridge that are placed in the great cardiac vein and proximal coronary sinus. Tension generated by the system results in cinching of the posterior mitral annulus tissue anteriorly. The device is placed percutaneously via the right internal jugular vein approach and can be easily retrieved if MR reduction is not favorable or coronary artery compromise develops. The device underwent several design iterations to prevent slippage during implantation and reinforcement

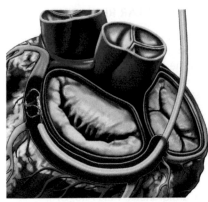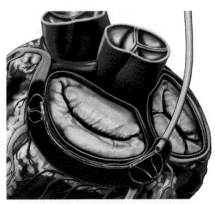

Fig. 6. Coronary sinus annuloplasty. The Cardiac Dimensions Carillon device. The guide catheter is introduced through jugular venous access. The device is delivered in the distal coronary sinus and the distal anchor is released (*left*), and then the guide catheter is pulled back to release the proximal anchor in the coronary sinus ostium. The right panel shows the wireform, made of nitinol wire, after release in the coronary sinus. Cinching pf the mitral annulus results in compression of the septal–lateral dimension and thus the regurgitant orifice. (*From* Feldman T, Young A. Percutaneous approaches to valve repair for mitral regurgitation. J Am Coll Cardiol 2014;63:2057–68. Artwork by Craig Skaggs; with permission.)

of the device at its ends to prevent late wire-form fracture.

The CARILLON Mitral Annuloplasty Device European Union Study (AMADEUS) trial was the first investigation of a percutaneous coronary sinus based intervention to reduce FMR.[49] The AMADEUS trial enrolled 48 symptomatic FMR patients owing to dilated cardiomyopathy, with at least moderate FMR, and an LVEF of less than 40%. Device implantation was successful in 30 patients. The primary safety endpoint was a composite of death, myocardial infarction, or device-related complication at 30 days. FMR grade, NYHA functional indices, Kansas City Cardiomyopathy Questionnaire, and 6-minute walk test were assessed at baseline, 1 month, and 6 months. Of the 48 patients in the trial, 6 (13%) experienced a major adverse event within 30 days; 1 of these 6 patients died, with the remaining events consisting of either clinically silent myocardial infarction or coronary sinus dissection and/or perforation. These early findings of coronary sinus injury led to changes in procedural technique that reduced dramatically the occurrence of this adverse event. There was a 32% reduction in MR grade at 6 months by a composite of 4 echocardiographic parameters that maintained up to 6 months. Despite improvement of quality of life and functional indices, there was no significant change in LV remodeling based on LV size and/or LVEF at 6 months.

The Transcatheter Implantation of Carillon Mitral Annuloplasty Device (TITAN) trial was a prospective nonrandomized trial in which 53 patients with symptomatic FMR were enrolled for CARILLON device therapy.[50] Thirty-six patients (68%)

underwent successful device implantation, whereas 17 devices were not implanted because of insufficient MR reduction (n = 9) or transient coronary compromise (n = 8) in patients. Successful device therapy showed significant reduction in MR grade, favorable LV remodeling, and improved quality of life when compared with the control group of subjects who did not receive implants. There were 9 wire-form device fractures seen in this trial, with no advents attributable to this finding. In only one of the patients with device fracture was a reduction in FMR observed.

DIRECT ANNULOPLASTY

These technologies implant in the mitral annulus. Access to the annulus can be either through transseptal puncture or retrograde through the aortic valve and LV. These devices are implanted onto the annulus and subsequently used to directly reduce the annulus circumference.

Mitralign

The Mitralign Percutaneous Annuloplasty System (Mitralign, Tewksbury, MA) is based on surgical suture plication of the annulus. In this procedure, a deflectable transaortic catheter is advanced to the LV and used to deliver pledgeted anchors through the posterior annulus (**Fig. 7**).[51] These anchors can be pulled together resulting in a segmental posterior annuloplasty to shorten the annulus up to 17 mm. In 15 patients treated in a phase I trial, the 1-year results demonstrated at least 1+ MR reduction that was associated with improved NYHA function class and

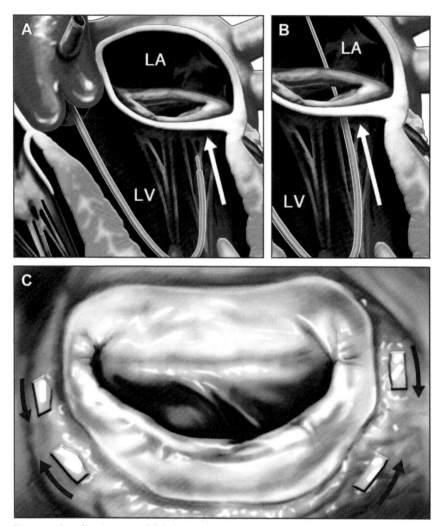

Fig. 7. Mitralign annular plication: Panel (*A*) shows the retrograde guide catheter in the left ventricle (LV), with the distal catheter tip under the mitral annulus, behind the posterior leaflet (*arrow*). (*B*) A wire has been passed from the LV through the annulus and into the left atrium (LA) in panel B. (*C*) Two pairs of wires are used to place pledgets near both commissures, shown from the left atrial side in panel C. The pledgets are drawn together (*arrows*) to decrease the mitral annular circumference. (*From* Feldman T, Young A. Percutaneous approaches to valve repair for mitral regurgitation. J Am Coll Cardiol 2014;63:2057–68. Artwork by Craig Skaggs; with permission.)

reduction in tenting area and depth.[52] A CE-approval trail has completed enrollment and awaits follow-up.

Guided Delivery System Accucinch

The Accucinch system (Guided Delivery Systems, Santa Clara, CA) is based on suture annuloplasty (**Fig. 8**). A retrograde femoral arterial approach to gain access to the LV aspect of the mitral annulus is required. A catheter is placed under the posterior mitral leaflet next to the anterior trigone, adjacent to the annular tissue beneath the valve. Using this catheter, up to 20 anchors can be placed from the anterior to posterior commissures along the

posterior mitral annulus. These anchors are connected by a suture that can plicate the annulus to reduce the mitral annular circumference and MR.

Cardioband

The Cardioband (Valtech, Or Yehuda, Israel) utilizes transseptal percutaneous placement of a series of small corkscrew anchors on the atrial side of the left atrium by transesophageal echocardiogram. The anchors are connected by a Dacron sleeve that can be subsequently tensioned and reduce the mitral annular circumference (**Fig. 9**). This device closely recapitulates surgical

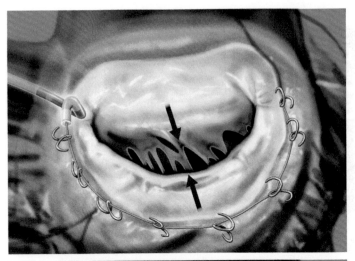

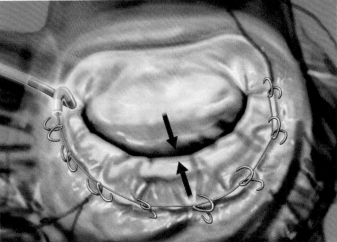

Fig. 8. Direct annuloplasty. The Guided Delivery Systems Accucinch device is delivered through retrograde catheterization of the left ventricle (*top*). The arrows highlight the separation of the leaflet edges, which define the regurgitant orifice. Anchors are placed in the posterior mitral annulus and connected with a "drawstring" to cinch the annular circumference. When the cord is tightened, the basilar myocardium and annulus draw the mitral leaflets together to decrease the regurgitant orifice (*bottom*). (*From* Feldman T, Young A. Percutaneous approaches to valve repair for mitral regurgitation. J Am Coll Cardiol 2014;63: 2057–68. Artwork by Craig Skaggs; with permission.)

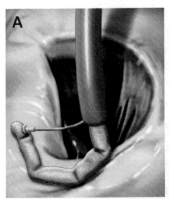

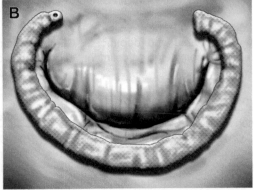

Fig. 9. Valtech CardioBand. (*A*) Transseptal guide catheter delivering the annuloplasty ring in segments. Each segment is sequentially anchored into the annulus. (*B*) Final annuloplasty ring encircling the posterior leaflet. (*From* Feldman T, Young A. Percutaneous approaches to valve repair for mitral regurgitation. J Am Coll Cardiol 2014;63:2057–68. Artwork by Craig Skaggs; with permission.)

annuloplasty with an incomplete ring. The preclinical studies in a swine model has resulted excellent outcomes in short term and for up to 90 days.[53] Early results in patients are promising and a CE approval trial is underway.

Percutaneous Mitral Valve Replacement

Since the introduction of transcutaneous aortic valve replacement, there has been an exponential growth of interest in transcutaneous approach to other valvular diseases. Transcatheter mitral valve replacement (TMVR) may have the potential to become an alternative to treat severe MR in high surgical risk patients.[54]

There are a number of off-label uses of Melody valve and Edwards Sapien and Sapien XT devices in publications using these valves for degenerated surgical bioprostheses in the mitral position, referred to as "mitral valve-in-valve" implants.[55,56] In addition, there are emerging case reports of Edwards Sapien XT valves in severe calcific mitral stenosis patients.[57,58] Despite some success and relatively favorable outcomes of these series, the fundamental problem remains in patients with native mitral valve with FMR or DMR. One of the many key obstacles in designing TMVR valves is the anchorage of the bioprosthesis to the mitral annulus. Fortunately, there are a growing number of TMVR options available, most of which are in the preclinical phase or early human experience. The preclinical studies on TMVR have been successful with different approaches, including transaortic, transapical, and transseptal. There are few reports of first in human TMVR cases at the moment. A rapidly growing number of valve designs are emerging. These procedures have been done initially in high-risk patients, and although technically successful, the clinical outcomes have been mixed owing to severity of illness of these earliest patients.

SUMMARY

Percutaneous treatment of MR is a promising alternative for patients with FMR who do not respond to optimal medical therapy and CRT. The MitraClip has become widely used and in nonrandomized series results in clinical improvement, favorable LV remodeling, and reduced hospitalizations for HF. Several other repair approaches are developing steadily. However, unlike DMR in which medical therapy has little role, there is growing evidence that optimal medical therapy can markedly improve FMR and these percutaneous therapies may not be immediately required at diagnosis of severe FMR. On the other hand, the challenges for all of these novel devices are to demonstrate safety and superior efficacy in comparison to medical management strategies. TMVR is emerging as a feasible therapy, with experience in a small number of cases, but requires significant additional clinical trials to define its place in treating HF related to MR.

REFERENCES

1. Bonow RO, Carabello BA, Chatterjee K, et al. ACC/AHA 2006 guidelines for the management of patients with valvular heart disease: a report of the American College of Cardiology/American Heart Association Task Force on Practice Guidelines (Writing Committee to Develop Guidelines for the Management of Patients With Valvular Heart Disease). American College of Cardiology Web Site. Circulation 2006;114:450–527. Available at: http://www.acc.org/clinical/guidelines/valvular/index.pdf.
2. Nkomo VT, Gardin JM, Skelton TN, et al. Burden of valvular heart diseases: a population-based study. Lancet 2006;368:1005–11.
3. de Marchena E, Badiye A, Robalino G, et al. Respective prevalence of the different Carpentier classes of mitral regurgitation: a stepping stone for future therapeutic research and development. J Card Surg 2011;26(4):385–92.
4. Lamas GA, Mitchell GF, Flaker GC, et al. Clinical significance of mitral regurgitation after acute myocardial infarction. Circulation 1997;96:827–33.
5. Rossi A, Dini FL, Faggiano P, et al. Independent prognostic value of functional mitral regurgitation in patients with heart failure. A quantitative analysis of 1256 patients with ischaemic and non-ischaemic dilated cardiomyopathy. Heart 2011;97(20):1675–80.
6. Baskett RJ, Exner DV, Hirsch GM, et al. Mitral insufficiency and morbidity and mortality in left ventricular dysfunction. Can J Cardiol 2007;23(10):797–800.
7. Grigioni F, Enriquez-Sarano M, Zehr KJ, et al. Ischemic mitral regurgitation: long term outcome and prognostic implications with quantitative Doppler assessment. Circulation 2001;103(13):1759–64.
8. Koelling TM, Aaronson KD, Cody RJ, et al. Prognostic significance of mitral regurgitation and tricuspid regurgitation in patients with left ventricular systolic dysfunction. Am Heart J 2002;144(3):524–9.
9. Lancellotti P, Gerard PL, Pierard LA. Long-term outcome of patients with heart failure and dynamic functional mitral regurgitation. Eur Heart J 2005;26(15):1528–32.
10. Levine RA, Hung J. Ischemic mitral regurgitation, the dynamic lesion: clues to the cure. J Am Coll Cardiol 2003;42(11):1929–32.
11. Beaudoin J, Handschumacher MD, Zeng X, et al. Mitral valve enlargement in chronic aortic

regurgitation as a compensatory mechanism to prevent functional mitral regurgitation in the dilated left ventricle. J Am Coll Cardiol 2013;61(17):1809–16.

12. Ducas RA, White CW, Wassef AW, et al. Functional mitral regurgitation: current understanding and approach to management. Can J Cardiol 2014; 30(2):173–80.

13. Gaasch WH, Meyer TE. Left ventricular response to mitral regurgitation: implications for management. Circulation 2008;118(22):2298–303.

14. Levine RA, Handschumacher MD, Sanfilippo AJ, et al. Three-dimensional echocardiographic reconstruction of the mitral valve, with implications for the diagnosis of mitral valve prolapse. Circulation 1989;80(3):589–98.

15. Dal-Bianco JP, Levine RA. Anatomy of the mitral valve apparatus: role of 2D and 3D echocardiography. Cardiol Clin 2013;31(2):151–64.

16. Lancellotti P, Stainier PY, Lebois F, et al. Effect of dynamic left ventricular dyssynchrony on dynamic mitral regurgitation in patients with heart failure due to coronary artery disease. Am J Cardiol 2005; 96(9):1304–7.

17. van Bommel RJ, Marsan NA, Delgado V, et al. Cardiac resynchronization therapy as a therapeutic option in patients with moderate-severe functional mitral regurgitation and high operative risk. Circulation 2011;124(8):912–9.

18. Madaric J, Vanderheyden M, Van Laethem C, et al. Early and late effects of cardiac resynchronization therapy on exercise-induced mitral regurgitation: relationship with left ventricular dyssynchrony, remodelling and cardiopulmonary performance. Eur Heart J 2007;28(17):2134–41.

19. Yiu SF, Enriquez-Sarano M, Tribouilloy C, et al. Determinants of the degree of functional mitral regurgitation in patients with systolic left ventricular dysfunction: a quantitative clinical study. Circulation 2000;102(12):1400–6.

20. He S, Fontaine AA, Schwammenthal E, et al. Integrated mechanism for functional mitral regurgitation: leaflet restriction versus coapting force: in vitro studies. Circulation 1997;96(6):1826–34.

21. Messas E, Guerrero JL, Handschumacher MD, et al. Paradoxic decrease in ischemic mitral regurgitation with papillary muscle dysfunction: insights from three-dimensional and contrast echocardiography with strain rate measurement. Circulation 2001; 104(16):1952–7.

22. Chinitz JS, Chen D, Goyal P, et al. Mitral apparatus assessment by delayed enhancement CMR: relative impact of infarct distribution on mitral regurgitation. JACC Cardiovasc Imaging 2013; 6(2):220–34.

23. Chaput M, Handschumacher MD, Tournoux F, et al. Mitral leaflet adaptation to ventricular remodeling: occurrence and adequacy in patients with functional mitral regurgitation. Circulation 2008; 118(8):845–52.

24. Seneviratne B, Moore GA, West PD. Effect of captopril on functional mitral regurgitation in dilated heart failure: a randomised double blind placebo controlled trial. Br Heart J 1994;72(1):63–8.

25. Capomolla S, Febo O, Gnemmi M, et al. Betablockade therapy in chronic heart failure: diastolic function and mitral regurgitation improvement by carvedilol. Am Heart J 2000;139(4):596–608.

26. St John Sutton MG, Plappert T, Abraham WT, et al, Multicenter InSync Randomized Clinical Evaluation (MIRACLE) Study Group. Effect of cardiac resynchronization therapy on left ventricular size and function in chronic heart failure. Circulation 2003; 107(15):1985–90.

27. Breithardt OA, Sinha AM, Schwammenthal E, et al. Acute effects of cardiac resynchronization therapy on functional mitral regurgitation in advanced systolic heart failure. J Am Coll Cardiol 2003;41(5): 765–70.

28. Abraham WT, Fisher WG, Smith AL, et al, MIRACLE Study Group. Multicenter InSync Randomized Clinical Evaluation. Cardiac resynchronization in chronic heart failure. N Engl J Med 2002;346(24):1845–53.

29. Cleland JG, Daubert JC, Erdmann E, et al, Cardiac Resynchronization-Heart Failure (CARE-HF) Study Investigators. The effect of cardiac resynchronization on morbidity and mortality in heart failure. N Engl J Med 2005;352(15):1539–49.

30. Cleland J, Freemantle N, Ghio S, et al. Predicting the long-term effects of cardiac resynchronization therapy on mortality from baseline variables and the early response a report from the CARE-HF (Cardiac Resynchronization in Heart Failure) Trial. J Am Coll Cardiol 2008;52(6):438–45.

31. O'Gara PT. Randomized trials in moderate ischemic mitral regurgitation: many questions, limited answers. Circulation 2012;126(21):2452–5.

32. Fattouch K, Guccione F, Sampognaro R, et al. POINT: Efficacy of adding mitral valve restrictive annuloplasty to coronary artery bypass grafting in patients with moderate ischemic mitral valve regurgitation: a randomized trial. J Thorac Cardiovasc Surg 2009;138(2):278–85.

33. Chan KM, Punjabi PP, Flather M, et al, RIME Investigators. Coronary artery bypass surgery with or without mitral valve annuloplasty in moderate functional ischemic mitral regurgitation: final results of the Randomized Ischemic Mitral Evaluation (RIME) trial. Circulation 2012;126(21): 2502–10.

34. Nishimura RA, Otto CM, Bonow RO, et al, ACC/AHA Task Force Members. 2014 AHA/ACC guideline for the management of patients with valvular heart disease: executive summary: a report of the American College of Cardiology/American Heart Association

Task Force on Practice Guidelines. Circulation 2014; 129(23):2440–92.

35. Deja MA, Grayburn PA, Sun B, et al. Influence of mitral regurgitation repair on survival in the surgical treatment for ischemic heart failure trial. Circulation 2012;125(21):2639–48.

36. Acker MA, Parides MK, Perrault LP, et al, for the Cardiothoracic Surgical Trials Network (CTSN). Mitral-valve repair versus replacement for severe ischemic mitral regurgitation. N Engl J Med 2014; 370:23–32.

37. Feldman T. Young A: Transcatheter mitral valve repair. EuroIntervention Valve Supplement 2013;9: S118–23.

38. Fucci C, Sandrelli L, Pardini A, et al. Improved results with mitral valve repair using new surgical techniques. Eur J Cardiothorac Surg 1995;9(11): 621–6.

39. Maisano F, Viganò G, Blasio A, et al. Surgical isolated edge-to-edge mitral valve repair without annuloplasty: clinical proof of the principle for an endovascular approach. EuroIntervention 2006; 2(2):181–6.

40. Feldman T, Foster E, Glower D, et al, for the EVEREST II Investigators. Percutaneous repair or surgery for mitral regurgitation. N Engl J Med 2011;364: 1395–406.

41. Ladich E, Michaels MB, Jones RM, et al, Endovascular Valve Edge-to-Edge Repair Study (EVEREST) Investigators. Pathological healing response of explanted MitraClip devices. Circulation 2011; 123(13):1418–27.

42. Mauri L, Glower DG, Apruzzese P, et al, for the EVEREST II Investigators. Four-year results of a randomized controlled trial of percutaneous repair versus surgery for mitral regurgitation. J Am Coll Cardiol 2013;62:317–28.

43. Whitlow P, Feldman T, Pedersen W, et al, The EVEREST II High Risk Study. Acute and 12 month results with catheter based mitral valve leaflet repair. J Am Coll Cardiol 2012;59:130–9.

44. Philip F, Athappan G, Tuzcu EM, et al. MitraClip for severe symptomatic mitral regurgitation in patients at high surgical risk: a comprehensive systematic review. Catheter Cardiovasc Interv 2014;84(4): 581–90.

45. Lim DS, Reynolds MR, Feldman T, et al. Improved functional status and quality of life in prohibitive surgical risk patients with degenerative mitral regurgitation following transcatheter mitral valve repair with the mitraclip system. J Am Coll Cardiol 2014;64: 182–92.

46. Glower D, Kar S, Lim DS, et al. Percutaneous Mitra-Clip device therapy for mitral regurgitation in 351 patients - high risk subset of the EVEREST II Study. J Am Coll Cardiol 2014;64:172–81.

47. Seeburger J, Rinaldi M, Nielsen SL, et al. Off-pump transapical implantation of artificial neo-chordae to correct mitral regurgitation: the TACT Trial (Transapical Artificial Chordae Tendinae) proof of concept. J Am Coll Cardiol 2014;63(9):914–9.

48. Grossi EA, Patel N, Woo YJ, et al. Outcomes of the RESTOR-MV Trial (randomized evaluation of a surgical treatment for off-pump repair of the mitral valve). J Am Coll Cardiol 2010;56:1984–93.

49. Schofer J, Siminiak T, Haude M, et al. Percutaneous mitral annuloplasty for functional mitral regurgitation: results of the AMADEUS trial. Circulation 2009;120: 326–33.

50. Siminiak T, Wu JC, Haude M, et al. Treatment of functional mitral regurgitation by percutaneous annuloplasty-results of the TITAN Trial. Eur J Heart Fail 2012;14(8):931–8.

51. Siminiak T, Dankowski R, Baszko A, et al. Percutaneous direct mitral annuloplasty using the Mitralign Bident system: description of the method and a case report. Kardiol Pol 2013;71(12):1287–92.

52. Nickenig G. Presentation at TransCatheter Therapeutics 26th Annual Scientific Symposium. Washington, DC, September 13–17, 2014.

53. Maisano F, Vanermen H, Seeburger J, et al. Direct access transcatheter mitral annuloplasty with a sutureless and adjustable device: preclinical experience. Eur J Cardiothorac Surg 2012;42(3):524–9.

54. De Backer O, Piazza N, Banai S, et al. Percutaneous transcatheter mitral valve replacement: an overview of devices in preclinical and early clinical evaluation. Circ Cardiovasc Interv 2014;7(3):400–9.

55. Cheung A, Webb JG, Barbanti M, et al. 5-year experience with transcatheter transapical mitral valve-in-valve implantation for bioprosthetic valve dysfunction. J Am Coll Cardiol 2013;61:1759–66.

56. Cullen MW, Cabalka AK, Alli OO, et al. Transvenous, antegrade Melody valve-in-valve implantation for bioprosthetic mitral and tricuspid valve dysfunction: a case series in children and adults. JACC Cardiovasc Interv 2013;6:598–605.

57. Sinning JM, Mellert F, Schiller W, et al. Transcatheter mitral valve replacement using a balloon-expandable prosthesis in a patient with calcified native mitral valve stenosis. Eur Heart J 2013;34:2609.

58. Guerrero M, Greenbaum A, O'Neill W. First in human percutaneous implantation of a balloon expandable transcatheter heart valve in a severely stenosed native mitral valve. Catheter Cardiovasc Interv 2014;83(7):E287–91.

Percutaneous Left Ventricular Restoration

Mobolaji Ige, MD, Sadeer G. Al-Kindi, MD, Guilherme Attizzani, MD, Marco Costa, MD, Guilherme H. Oliveira, MD*

KEYWORDS

• Left ventricular remodeling • Ventricular partitioning device • Implantation technique • Heart failure

KEY POINTS

- Previous attempts with surgical ventricular restoration were faced with difficulties.
- Parachute is the first percutaneous left ventricular restoration device.
- Studies have proven the feasibility and safety of the Parachute device.
- The ongoing randomized trial is testing the efficacy of Parachute in patients with heart failure.

INTRODUCTION

Heart failure (HF) is one of the leading causes of morbidity and mortality and has become an overwhelming burden on the health care industry in the United States and worldwide.[1] Because left ventricular (LV) geometry is a major prognosticator of HF outcomes,[2–4] the bedrock of HF management, particularly following myocardial infarction (MI), has been to arrest the progressive distortion of LV geometry, otherwise called LV remodeling. An obstructive lesion of the left anterior descending artery may result in a large anterior MI with hypokinesis or akinesis of the LV apical region, which invariably results in progressive LV remodeling and clinical HF. The interventions aimed at reversing the course of LV remodeling are referred to as LV restoration or reverse remodeling therapies. With a limited wherewithal of neurohormonal manipulation at preventing or arresting the progression of LV remodeling, introduction of device-based therapies has generated predicable clinical interest. The idea of a ventricular partitioning device (VPD) was first conceived by Drs Branislav Radovencevic and Serjan Nikolic in 1999 and was first implanted surgically in calf models.[5] To date, the VPD known as Parachute (Cardiokinetix, Menlo Park, CA) is the first and only percutaneously implantable device aimed at restoration of normal LV geometry in humans. Since its conception, this technology has undergone extensive animal and human testing, with proved feasibility and safety, and is currently being studied in a pivotal randomized clinical trial.

This article discusses ventricular remodeling and therapies attempted in the past, details the components of the VPD, describes the implanting technique, and reviews the most current experience of this device in humans.

LEFT VENTRICULAR REMODELING AND RESTORATION

Ventricular remodeling is a histologically mediated process provoked by an inciting event (eg, MI), which leads to altered LV geometry, having been identified as a major prognostic factor for mortality in patients with HF.[2] Remodeling is associated with upregulation of an array of neuroendocrine, paracrine, and autocrine factors particularly those

Funding: No funding was received for this article.

Conflict of Interest: M. Ige, S. Al-Kindi, G. Attizzani, and G.H. Oliveira have no conflict of interest to disclose; M. Costa consults for Cardiokinetix.

Advanced Heart Failure and Transplant Center, Harrington Heart & Vascular Institute, University Hospitals Case Medical Center, Department of Medicine, Case Western Reserve University, 11100 Euclid Avenue, Cleveland, OH 44106, USA

* Corresponding author. Case Western Reserve University School of Medicine; Advanced Heart Failure and Transplantation Center, Harrington Heart & Vascular institute, University Hospitals Case Medical Center, Department of Medicine, 11100 Euclid Avenue, Room: Lakeside, 3012, Cleveland, OH 44106.

E-mail address: guilherme.oliveira@uhhospitals.org

Heart Failure Clin 11 (2015) 261–273
http://dx.doi.org/10.1016/j.hfc.2014.12.005
1551-7136/15/$ – see front matter

involving the renin-angiotensin-aldosterone axis and the adrenergic nervous system.[6–8] Therefore, medical HF therapies have targeted LV remodeling by suppression of the renin-angiotensin system and blockade of the β-adrenergic systems.[9–12] This pathologic mechanism is mediated through myocyte hypertrophy, apoptosis, and infiltration of the myocardium by interstitial collagen.[13] In the early phase of LV remodeling, MI induces fibrotic repair of the area of necrosis, which results in scarring, elongation, and narrowing of this region.[2] As a result, LV volume increases in what is invariably an adaptive mechanism aimed at preserving stroke volume and cardiac output. In the later phase of the remodeling process, there is preponderance of myocyte hypertrophy in the noninfarcted area causing increase in wall mass and further dilatation of LV cavity, thereby rendering the LV more spherical in shape.[14] These geometric alterations result in deterioration of LV function and perpetuate a vicious cycle leading to further LV dilatation and sphericity.[15] In part, the reduction of LV function in the hypertrophied noninfarcted myocardium can also be explained by reduced myocardial stretch during diastole resulting in concomitant diminished systolic contraction as proposed by Frank and Starling.[16] Of note, the authors of the Valsartan in Acute Myocardial Infarction echocardiographic study[17] identified three types of LV remodeling based on assessment of LV mass index and relative wall thickness: (1) concentric remodeling (normal LV mass index; increased relative wall thickness), (2) eccentric hypertrophy (increased LV mass index; normal relative wall thickness), and (3) concentric hypertrophy (increased LV mass index; increased relative wall thickness). Because each of these is associated with increasingly worse outcomes, determination of the specific pattern of LV remodeling also confers prognostic information.[17] The apex of the LV is a particularly susceptible region to remodeling because of its greater curvature and thinner structure.[18] Isolation of an aneurysmal apex decreases LV volume, reduces wall stress, and improves hemodynamics as predicted by Laplace law.[19]

Previously, surgical techniques of LV restoration, known generically as surgical ventricular restoration (SVR), have been attempted. Although met with mixed early results, the largest setback to SVR has been the negative result of the Surgical Treatment for Ischemic Heart Failure trial.[20] This trial, heavily criticized for its methodology and implementation,[21] failed to show mortality benefits in patients who underwent SVR in addition to coronary artery bypass grafting (CABG) compared with those who had CABG alone. Despite notable limitations decried by critics of this trial, SVR has fallen into disfavor and is no longer a commonly performed procedure in clinical HF practice. However, the recent advent of Parachute, a VPD that offers a percutaneous alternative to SVR, has now resparked interest in mechanical LV restoration. Although still investigational, Parachute data have thus far been promising enough to raise careful optimism that this VPD may represent a major breakthrough in LV restoration strategies.

Historically, earlier devices designed to achieve reverse remodeling have been introduced and tested. The Acorn Corcap (Acorn Cardiovascular, Inc, St. Paul, MN) is a flexible, compliant, polyester textile mesh that is surgically implanted around the dilated ventricles to slow down the dilation and promote reverse remodeling. The Acorn trial blindly randomized 300 patients to Corcap or medical treatment.[22] The trial showed improvement in New York Heart Association (NYHA) functional class, quality of life measures, and reduction in LV volumes but it failed to show any reduction in mortality. Paracor HeartNet (Paracor Medical, Cupertino, CA) is another attempt for pericardial straining. It involved a distensible ventricular restraint that is surgically implanted without the need for cardiopulmonary bypass. Although this device showed improvement in symptoms (6-minute walk test) and LV remodeling parameters, it failed to achieve primary end points of survival benefit or improvement in peak oxygen consumption.[23] Myocor Coapsys (Maple Grove, MN) involves tensioning cords that aim at treating ischemic mitral regurgitation in patients with ischemic cardiomyopathy. The trial randomized patients with ischemic cardiomyopathy to CABG alone or combined CABG/Coapsys implantation.[24] The trial showed improvement in survival compared with the CABG-only group.[24] **Table 1** summarizes these devices in comparison with the Parachute experience.

PARACHUTE-PERCUTANEOUS VENTRICULAR PARTITIONING DEVICE

Parachute was primarily designed as a VPD to percutaneously isolate the infarcted, aneurysmal apex of the LV and restore LV geometry from within (**Fig. 1**). It is made up of three main components: (1) an access system, (2) a delivery system, and (3) the VPD (**Fig. 2**). The access system consists of a 14F or 16F guide catheter and a dilator, providing access to the LV apex. The delivery system is composed of a torque shaft contained in the central lumen of a delivery catheter, which has a screw at its distal end that occupies the VPD. Through this means, the collapsed VPD is deployed into the LV apex. The lumen of the

Table 1
Summary of the previous experience with ventricular restoration devices

Device	Main Features	Outcomes	Current Stage
Acorn Corcap	Pericardial strain Surgically implanted	Improvement in NYHA, MLHF Reverse modeling No survival benefit	Not FDA approved
Paracor HeartNet	Elastic ventricular restraint Surgically implanted No cardiopulmonary bypass	Improvement in 6MWT, MLHF, echocardiographic indices, NYHA functional class No improvement in peak Vo_2 No survival benefit	Not FDA approved
Myocor Coapsys	Ventricular tensioning chords Treats functional mitral regurgitation Surgically implanted	Survival benefit Decreased adverse events	Currently developing transcatheter system (iCoapsys)
Cardiokinetix Parachute	First catheter-based device Targeting anterior-apical scars	Improvement in NYHA functional class Trend toward improvement in quality of life, 6MWT	Randomized controlled trial in progress (PARACHUTE IV)

Abbreviations: 6MWT, six-minute walk test; FDA, food and drug administration; MLHF, minnesota living with heart failure.

torque shaft in turn contains a balloon that is located proximal to the distal engagement screw, which when inflated, expands the VPD causing the device struts to engage the ventricular wall.

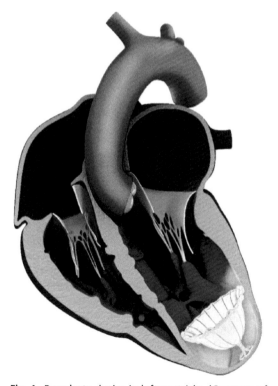

Fig. 1. Parachute device in left ventricle. (*Courtesy of* CardioKinetix, Menlo Park, CA; with permission.)

The VPD itself consists of an umbrella-shaped nitinol frame covered by an expanded polytetrafluoroethylene occlusive membrane and a radiopaque, atraumatic (pebax polymer) foot at the tip of the device, which serves as a contact point with the LV apex and also facilitates proper visualization of the device. The nitinol frame of the VPD has 16 struts, the tip of each ending in a 2-mm anchor. When the device is expanded, these anchors engage the myocardium and in the process stabilize the device, preventing potential dislodgement and migration of the VPD, and the occlusive membrane presents a barrier that separates and seals off the akinetic chamber on the distal side of the device. There are eight available sizes of the VPD (65, 75, 85, and 95 mm, each in regular and short foot). The appropriate device size depends on the LV end-diastolic cavity and it is advocated that Parachute diameter exceeds the largest LV diameter by 30% to 60% to allow for adequate adherence to the ventricular wall.[25]

ANATOMIC CRITERIA FOR VENTRICULAR PARTITIONING DEVICE PLACEMENT AND THE ROLE OF MULTIMODAL IMAGING

Multimodality imaging is paramount in the selection of Parachute candidates to ensure that strict anatomic specifications are met. Anatomic criteria used thus far are (1) ejection fraction (EF) less than 40% with akinetic apex or aneurysm, (2) LV

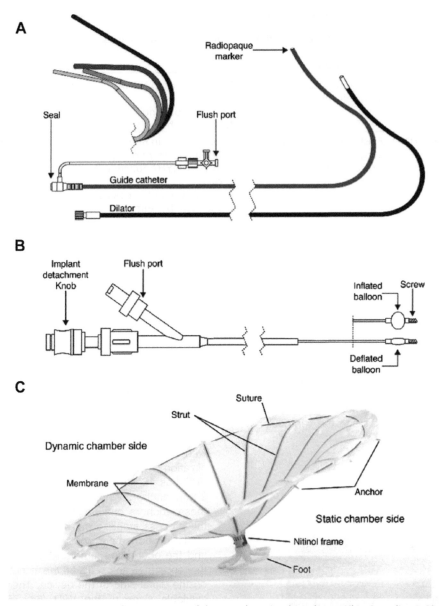

A

Radiopaque marker

Seal

Flush port

Guide catheter

Dilator

B

Implant detachment Knob

Flush port

Inflated balloon   Screw

Deflated balloon

C

Suture

Strut

Dynamic chamber side

Membrane

Anchor

Static chamber side

Nitinol frame

Foot

Fig. 2. (A–C) Catheter apparatus and components of the Parachute implant. (*From* Silva G, Melica B, Pires de Morais G, et al. Percutaneous implantation of a ventricular partitioning device for treatment of ischemic heart failure: initial experience of a center. Rev Port Cardiol 2012;31(12):795–801; with permission.)

diameter 55 to 70 mm, (3) LV wall thickness greater than 3.5 mm, (4) apex diameter 4 × 5 cm, and (5) normal trabeculation and papillary muscle.[25]

In Parachute trials, a multistage screening format was adopted with transthoracic two-dimensional echocardiography as a screening test, followed by three-dimensional cardiac computed tomography (CT) with contrast as a confirmatory test. This stepwise system offers the advantages of minimizing radiation exposure and improving cost effectiveness by using echocardiography to exclude patients that would not meet criteria.

Echocardiography is a well-established, noninvasive imaging modality that serves as the initial screening tool of LV function and geometry.[26,27] It is free of radiation and can be safely performed in most patients, including the critically ill. For Parachute trial purposes, echocardiography is sensitive enough to identify potential candidates for a VPD and specific enough to exclude those that clearly do not qualify. In the PARACHUTE trials, echocardiographic inclusion criteria were (1) LVEF less than 40%, (2) LV dilatation (LV end-diastolic diameter >56 mm, LV end-systolic diameter >38 mm), (3) anteroapical regional wall motion abnormalities (akinesia or dyskinesia), and (4) LV apical dimensions 4.0 cm × 5.0 cm.

However, limitations intrinsic to this method prevent its use as the only imaging modality. In addition to heavy operator dependence, variable imaging quality, limited reproducibility, and wide intraobserver and interobserver variability,[26] it is unable to provide LV anatomic assessment accurate enough for VPD deployment. LV volumes and structure assessed by echo can be unreliable for such reasons as poor selection of imaging planes, volumetric assessment using geometric assumptions, obscurity of the endocardial borders, and beat-to-beat variability of LV size and function, among others. The advent and increasing availability of real-time three-dimensional echocardiography with superior exactness and reproducibility has the potential to limit most of the drawbacks identified with two-dimensional echocardiography and may become incorporated into the screening process of VPD implantation in the future.

Because of the limitations of echocardiography, three-dimensional CT is used at the second stage of the evaluation process, and used to exclude patients with unsuitable anatomy and for implantation planning purposes. Compared with two-dimensional echocardiography, it offers better and more reproducible determination of LV size, wall thickness,[28] and assessment of ventricular trabeculae and bands. It also quantifies endocardial calcium deposit vital for device implantation. The importance of CT validation was shown in a study in which echocardiography identified 28 patients for VPD, only nine (32%) of whom met anatomic criteria by CT.[29]

Unsuitable Left Ventricular Anatomy by Computed Tomography for Parachute Deployment

An LV cavity that is too large precludes satisfactory strut anchorage, whereas incomplete expansion of the device results from inappropriately small LV cavity. Also, the risk of myocardial perforation with device implantation depends on the LV wall thickness, which takes into account the size of the tip of each strut anchor (typically 2 mm), hence the reason why LV wall thickness is greater than 3.5 mm. Excessive calcification of the endocardium seen on CT and the presence of intraventricular bands impedes adequate strut anchorage and device stabilization, whereas deeply embedded papillary muscles can result in predisposition to severe mitral regurgitation following device placement. The VPD has not been determined to provide any clinical or hemodynamic benefit in a globally dilated LV or EF greater than 40%.

Even though cardiac MRI is considered the gold standard for noninvasive assessments of LV function and volumes, its role is limited in the available VPD trials. This is probably the result of most eligible patients being treated with implantable devices at some point during the course of their disease making MRI contraindicated (Fig. 3).

THE IMPLANTATION TECHNIQUE

Following informed consent, the procedure takes place in the cardiac catheterization laboratory under local anesthesia and conscious sedation. With aseptic technique, a 14F or 16F guide catheter is introduced via the femoral artery to access the LV. Following placement of a preshaped delivery catheter near the LV apex, the device is then advanced through the sheath under fluoroscopy guidance until the foot is exposed. Positioning can further be verified with transthoracic echocardiogram. With the retraction of the delivery catheter, the device is then deployed and expansion is expedited by inflating the low-pressure contrast-filled balloon until the anchors are fully stretched to abut the LV wall, creating a barrier to separate the dyskinetic or aneurysmal portion of the LV on the distal side of the implant. Finally, contrast LV angiography is used to confirm correct positioning before the device is released (Fig. 4). The VPD can then be detached by rotating the knob located proximally on the delivery catheter. At this point, the catheters can then be removed together with the femoral access sheath when appropriate. Manual compression or a closure device system is essential in closing the access site and maintaining hemostasis. In most of the human trials, total procedure duration and estimated length of hospital stay averaged 1 hour and 2 days, respectively. As part of the study protocol, all the patients were required to receive 12 months of aspirin, 6 months of clopidogrel, and 3 months of warfarin following device placement. Fig. 5 shows a CT of VPD in the left ventricle at 9-month follow-up.

THE PARACHUTE EXPERIENCE

Nikolic and colleagues[16] first assessed the hemodynamic effects of the VPD in an ovine model by artificially inducing anteroapical MI by placing a coil in the left anterior descending arteries in 10 animals. Five of the animals had VPD implanted 6 weeks post-MI, whereas the other five received no intervention and served as the control group. After 30 weeks postinfarction, the VPD group

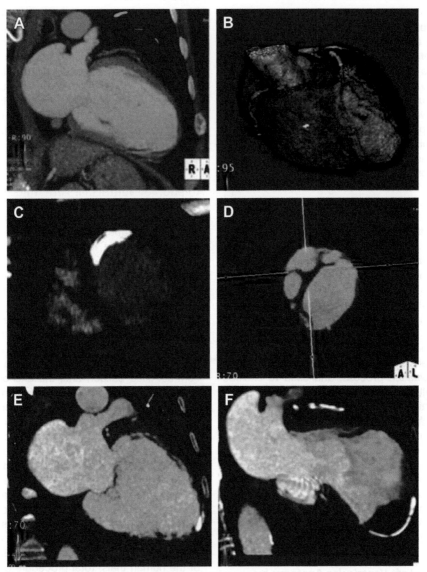

Fig. 3. Preimplantation cardiac CT exclusion criteria. (*A*) LV aneurysm. (*B*) Three-dimensional view of anteroapical LV infarction. (*C*) Presence of excessive calcium. (*D*) Transverse trabeculae. (*E*) Unfavorable LV anatomy. (*F*) Presence of massive thrombus in LV.

showed improved hemodynamic variables compared with the control group: LV end-systolic volume (70.1 ± 9.0 mL vs 102.9 ± 10.3 mL; *P*<.02), EF (46.9 ± 5.2% vs 34.7 ± 6.8%; *P*<.04), and cardiac output (5.2 ± 0.7 L/min vs 5.0 ± 1.8 L/min; *P* = NS). These experimental results indicated potential benefits of the VPD in the human trials to follow.

The Percutaneous Ventricular Restoration in Chronic Heart Failure (PARACHUTE) trial research is comprised of four trials at various stages of conclusion. The PARACHUTE Cohort A and PARACHUTE US feasibility study represented the first-in-human, prospective, single arm, multicenter trial

carried out in the United States and Europe. These were pilot studies of 39 patients between 2005 and 2009 designed to test feasibility and safety of VPD delivery and deployment, and absence of device-related major adverse cardiac events (MACE) at 6 months. MACE was characterized as the presence of cardiac death, emergent cardiac surgery, erosion of the LV by the device, cardiac tamponade, peripheral embolization (including cerebrovascular accident [CVA]), new or worsening HF, migration of the device or embolization, or introduction of a mechanical support device. Secondary objectives included serial assessment of hemodynamic (LV volume measurements, EF and

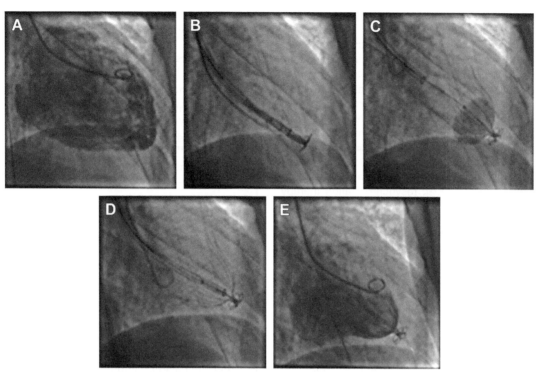

Fig. 4. Angiographic sequence of a Parachute implantation in the left ventricle (LV). (*A*) Pigtail in the LV cavity to perform LV angiography. (*B*) Device placement with foot exposed and in contact with the anteroapical wall. (*C*) Balloon inflation to facilitate self-expansion of the device. (*D*) Device fully expanded but still attached to the delivery system. (*E*) Final positioning after release of the device.

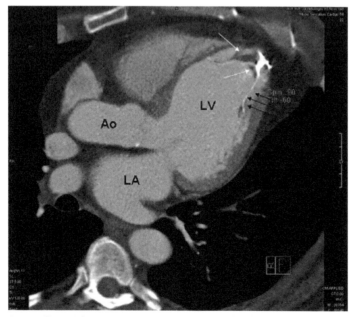

Fig. 5. Postimplantation cardiac CT showing VPD opposed to LV apex at 9 months (*arrows* show thrombi attached to the device on both sides). Ao, aortic; LA, left atrium; LV, left ventricle. (*From* Otasevic P, Sagic D, Antonic Z, et al. First-in-man implantation of left ventricular partitioning device in a patient with chronic heart failure: 12-month follow-up. J Card Fail 2007;13(7):517–20; with permission.)

stroke volumes) and functional changes (6-minute walk distance, NYHA class, and quality of life [QOL]) throughout the duration of the study. Inclusion criteria for enrollment include age greater than 18 years, anteroapical akinesis or dyskinesis caused by MI, EF less than 40%, and NYHA classes II-IV on stable doses of evidenced based HF medical therapy for at least 3 months before enrollment in the trial. Allowance was made for adjustment of medication doses during the study. Exclusion criteria included ischemic heart disease revascularized within the last 60 days, revascularization and/or cardiac resynchronization therapy within the last 60 days, and severe valvular heart disease, **Box 1**.

Of the 39 patients initially enrolled, five were found to have incompatible LV anatomy identified by cardiac CT and did not have VPD implanted. Unsuitability of these patients previously screened by two-dimensional echocardiogram was found to be mainly because of inaccurate estimation of the LV volume (caused by suboptimal two-dimensional echocardiogram windows), and severe apical deformity not identified on two-dimensional echocardiogram leading to inadequate contact of the footplate with the apex. Four of the "nonimplants" were found in the European arm. This then led to the incorporation of cardiac CT scan as part of the enrollment screening process in the US protocol. As a result, the inclusion criteria were modified based on CT screening.

Of the 34 (87%) patients implanted, three patients had device explantation in the immediate postprocedure period because of unrelated sepsis, incomplete device expansion, and excessive endocardial calcification making the implantation success rate 79% and 91% of enrolled and implanted patients, respectively.

Mazzaferri and colleagues[30] was first to publish the 24-month outcomes of this study. In the first 6 months post-Parachute device implant, five (15%) of the implanted patients had data and safety monitoring board–determined MACE events. Two of these patients had worsening HF (device related), whereas two died and one had a heart transplant (non–device related). Therefore, the primary end point of successful delivery and deployment of the Parachute in the absence of device-related MACE was met in 29 (74%) of the enrolled patients. There were no CVAs noted within the first 12 months of follow-up. However, one ischemic stroke was noted at 24 months follow-up. Notably, the data were inconclusive on the occurrence of bleeding complications, worsening arrhythmias, and device-related thrombus formation because these were not prespecified as study objectives. Assessment of changes in

---

Box 1
Major inclusion criteria for PARACHUTE IV trial

1. The patient is ≥18 years of age and ≤79 years of age.

2. The patient has a BMI <40.

3. The patient has symptomatic ischemic heart failure (NYHA class III or "ambulatory" class IV) after an MI in the LAD territory that occurred at least 60 days before enrollment.

4. The patient is not hospitalized at the time of enrollment.

5. The patient is receiving appropriate medical treatment for heart failure according to the ACC/AHA 2009 Guideline Update for the Diagnosis and Management of Chronic Heart Failure in the Adult during the 3 months before enrollment.

6. The patient or the patient's legal representative has been informed of the nature of the study, agrees to its provisions, and has provided written informed consent as approved by the IRB of the respective clinical site.

7. The patient and the treating physician agree that the patient will return for all required postprocedure follow-up visits.

Inclusion criteria based on imaging

1. The patient has LVEF ≥15% and ≤35% assessed by TTE.

2. The patient has LV post-MI structural heart dysfunction represented by LV wall motion abnormality assessed by TTE.

3. The patient's left ventricle must have appropriate anatomy (size and morphology) for implant placement using cardiac computed tomography scan and confirmed by left ventriculogram.

Abbreviations: ACC/AHA, American College of Cardiology/American Heart Association; BMI, body mass index; IRB, institutional review board; LAD, left anterior descending; LVEF, left ventricular ejection fraction; MI, myocardial infarction; NYHA, New York Heart Association; TTE, transthoracic echocardiogram.

From Costa MA, Pencina M, Nikolic S, et al. The PARACHUTE IV trial design and rationale: percutaneous ventricular restoration using the Parachute device in patients with ischemic heart failure and dilated left ventricles. Am Heart J 2013;165(4):533; with permission.

---

hemodynamics and functional status represented secondary end points of the study. There was a significant reduction noted in the LV end-systolic volume and end-diastolic volume at 12-month follow-up compared with baseline, whereas there were no significant changes noted in the EF and stroke volume index. Interestingly, subjects reported significant decreases in NYHA class but only a nonsignificant trend toward enhanced QOL and 6-minute walk distance.

The 3-year outcomes were recently published by Costa and colleagues.[31] Only 23 (74%) patients still had the device implanted at 36 months. Two LV assist devices, one transplant, and two noncardiac deaths (caused by malignancy and CVA) occurred between the 12- and 36-month period. Improvement in the LV indices was reportedly maintained in the remainder of the patients, in whom NYHA class symptoms were improved or sustained in 85% and worse in 15% of patients. The 3-year cumulative incidence of HF hospitalizations and mortality were 33% and 13.9%, respectively, whereas four patients had CVA between the 12- and 36-month period. Hemodynamically, significant reductions in LV end-diastolic volume index were maintained at 36 months, whereas reductions in LV end-systolic volume index tailed off to a nonsignificant trend over the same time period. This finding indicates that, unlike optimal medical or cardiac resynchronization therapies, reduction in LV volumes by Parachute occurs in the immediate aftermath of device placement with no further reduction noted over time. **Table 2** and **Fig. 6** summarize the most recent published results of the PARACHUTE trial.

The PARACHUTE III trial is designed as a dual arm nonrandomized trial (Parachute vs optimal medical therapy) enrolling up 100 patients in 20 European centers. PARACHUTE IV trial[32] is the only randomized (1:1, Parachute vs optimal medical therapy) trial currently ongoing in 65 US centers with the aim of enlisting up to 500 patients with NYHA III-IV, dyskinetic or aneurysmal LV apex, and EF between 15% and 35% with a primary objective of establishing the safety and efficacy of the Parachute with a follow-up period of 5 years. Outcomes of these trials are yet to be published.

Several smaller, single-arm, nonrandomized studies of Parachute have also been reported. Silva and colleagues[18] published the in-hospital outcomes of five patients who were implanted in a Portuguese center. In addition to significant

Table 2
Most recent available data from US feasibility and EU safety surveillance data

	US Feasibility and CE Mark Approval Data	EU Safety Surveillance
Number of patients (intention-to-treat analysis)	34	100
Procedure success	91%	97%
Clinical end points		
Mortality at 1 y	6.5%	9.5%
Mortality and heart failure hospitalization at 1 y	16.1%	26.0%
Functional		
NYHA baseline, class	2.6	2.5
NYHA change at 1 y	−0.9 (P<.0001)	−0.5 (P<.0001)
% NYHA improved at 1 y	71%	43%
% NYHA maintained at 1 y	19%	37%
6MWT baseline (m)	357	372
6MWT change at 1 y	+16.1 (P = .20)	+24.7 (P<.01)
% 6MWT improved at 1 y	39%	46%
% 6MWT maintained at 1 y	19%	30%
Hemodynamics and geometry		
LVESVi baseline, mm/M^2	93.2	84
LVESVi change at 1 y	−16.2 (P<.001)	−13.5 (P<.0001)
LVEDP baseline, mm Hg	18.2	23.8
LVEDP change at 6 mo	−5.3 (P = .02)	Not measured
LAVi baseline, mm/M^2	Not measured	42.5
LAVi change at 1 y	Not measured	−4.2 (P = .05)

Abbreviations: 6MWT, six-minute walk test; LAVi, left atrial volume index; LVEDP, left ventricular end-diastolic pressure; LVESVi, left ventricular end-systolic volume index; NYHA, New York Heart Association functional class.

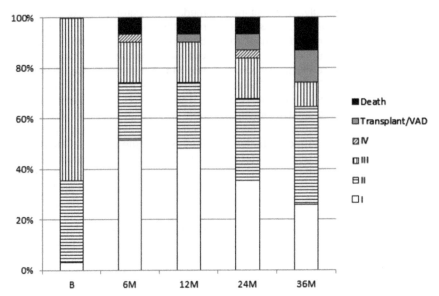

Fig. 6. Clinical outcomes of treated subjects (N = 31) according to New York Heart Association class (I-IV). (*From* Costa MA, Mazzaferri EL Jr, Sievert H, et al. Percutaneous ventricular restoration using the Parachute device in patients with ischemic heart failure: 3-year outcomes of the PARACHUTE first-in-human study. Circ Heart Fail 2014;7(5):752–8; with permission.)

reductions in LV volumes as noted in the first-in-human (FIH) trial, renal function and cardiac biomarkers also remained at baseline levels, the latter implying that no myocardial damage occurred during the implantation. Another study by Sagic and colleagues[33] in which 15 patients were implanted reported similar findings. Bozdag-Turan and coworkers[25] instead highlighted the importance of adequate patient screening in improving patient outcomes. They emphasized the usefulness of two-dimensional echocardiography in identifying the predetermined LV volumes, whereas three-dimensional cardiac CT was essential for determining the architecture, geometry, and trabeculation of the LV.[29] Therefore out of the 50 patients initially screened for their study, only eight patients had device implantation following screening with echo and cardiac CT. Unlike the previous quoted studies including the FIH trial, this study also reported a significant increase in LVEF, N-terminal fragment of the prohormone B-type natriuretic peptide, and QOL at 3-month follow-up. They reported similar significant decreases in LV volumes and improvement of NYHA class as the other studies. Ladich and colleagues[34] examined the histologic features of seven Parachute devices that were explanted either at autopsy or during transplant with average implant duration of 408 days (15–1533 days). The explanted devices all had organized thrombus with subsequent development of neoendocardial thickening at the free edge of the device and the

adjacent endocardium. Notably, the two implants that had duration of greater than 300 days both had fractures of the struts and foot, and one had tearing of the expanded polytetrafluoroethylene, which may be a significant indicator of long-term durability of the presently available Parachute devices. **Table 2** shows the most recent data from US feasibility and EU safety data. **Fig. 6** shows the functional status of patients implanted with VPD at baseline through 36 months of follow-up.

POTENTIAL COMPLICATIONS AND CONCERNS

Although the procedural success is more than 90%, potential postimplantation complications have been reported. Device implantation may exclude a myocardial region from where a subsequent ventricular tachycardia may develop. Lauschke and colleagues[35] reported a case of ventricular tachycardia in a patient with a Parachute device with the substrate being behind the Parachute with failed epicardial ablation. This suggests that patients should be evaluated for VT ablation before device implantation.

The Parachute device acts as a foreign body, and thus concerns for bacterial seeding and endocarditis are substantial. The infection risk should be assessed before device implantation. In addition, the Parachute induces thrombus formation and thus embolization may occur. A study of seven explanted devices showed that four devices had thrombus formation, five devices had fibrous

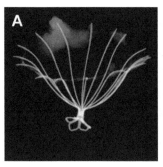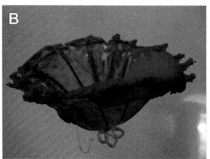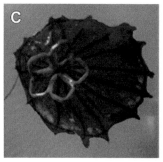

Fig. 7. Explanted device after 15 days. (*A*) Radiograph of the Parachute device. (*B, C*) Device-attached thrombi. (*Courtesy of* CardioKinetix, Menlo Park, CA; with permission.)

tissue formation, and one had pannus formation.[34] **Fig. 7** illustrates these findings.

Another concern is possible implantation of LV assist devices in those patients where the in-flow cannula is attached to the LV apex and is thus covered with the Parachute device. Apical removal of the device is possibly feasible given its elastic nature,[36] and this has been reported in two patients.[31]

SUMMARY

In the face of persistent unacceptably high morbidity and mortality of HF despite guideline-directed medical therapy, the advent of a percutaneous VPD capable of restoring LV geometry is cause for enthusiasm. Parachute has been designed to serve as an adjunct to medical therapy in restoring LV size and function. As a percutaneous intervention, it also offers the advantage of a less invasive intervention compared with SVR and is performed under local anesthesia and conscious sedation. Parachute was constructed in a way that its conical shape provides a more predictable and reproducible restoration compared with SVR where results are more surgeon dependent.[32] It also avoids the possibility of suture-related myocardial scarring, which can ultimately be a nidus for ventricular arrhythmias.

Experience with Parachute has not shown it to interfere with placement of other devices, such as pacemakers, defibrillators, or percutaneous valve solutions essential in the management of patients with HF. Furthermore, the device can be explanted through apical core at the time of implantation of an LV assist device. Even though available outcomes reported only nonsignificant increase in LVEF, it is feasible that newer-generation VPDs may be comprised of elastic recoil capabilities that may potentially augment LV systolic function.[36] Segregation of the scarred anteroapical wall with the VPD theoretically may

also improve diastolic compliance. This can be verified with paired echocardiographic data pre and post device placement and by assessing for other more muted changes in myocardial functions. In fact, it has been postulated that early isolation of infarcted myocardium in the immediate aftermath of anterior MI may prevent LV remodeling and could serve as a potential basis of future prospective studies with increased experience with the VPD.[36]

Amid the euphoria of this novel invention, it should be noted that the data reported so far are fraught with limitations. The FIH trial and other studies are unblinded, uncontrolled, with small numbers of subjects and quite indulgent end points that mainly serve as pilot studies. Placebo effect, especially with the reporting of functional and surrogate end points, cannot yet be ruled out. It should also be noted that the 39 patients that participated in the FIH trial were enrolled over a period greater than 2 years. This implies that the stringent screening criteria may make this device extraneous to a wider patient population.

So far, experience with Parachute is still very limited. As noted in our recent report, reduction in LV volumes attained at 12 months post device placement was not sustained at 36 months, even though the left ventricular end-diastolic volume was still significantly reduced compared with baseline. Similarly, significant reductions in left ventricular end-systolic volume at 12 and 24 months were not present at 36 months. This may imply that Parachute has short-lived early efficacy and may only serve as a bridge to more definitive therapy, such as mechanical support and heart transplantation. This is also corroborated by defects in mechanical integrity of explanted Parachute devices with intraventricular duration of greater than 300 days as reported by Ladich and colleagues.[34]

It is hoped that the results of the ongoing PARACHUTE IV trial will provide better answers to these questions and establish this device as a major innovation in the treatment of advanced ischemic cardiomyopathy. Until then, Parachute remains an appealing innovation, the feasibility and safety of which are expected to improve along with more operator experience and newer iterations of the device.

REFERENCES

1. Ambrosy AP, Fonarow GC, Butler J, et al. The global health and economic burden of hospitalizations for heart failure: lessons learned from hospitalized heart failure registries. J Am Coll Cardiol 2014;63(12): 1123–33.
2. Konstam MA, Kramer DG, Patel AR, et al. Left ventricular remodeling in heart failure: current concepts in clinical significance and assessment. JACC Cardiovasc Imaging 2011;4(1):98–108.
3. White HD, Norris RM, Brown MA, et al. Left ventricular end-systolic volume as the major determinant of survival after recovery from myocardial infarction. Circulation 1987;76(1):44–51.
4. Yamaguchi A, Ino T, Adachi H, et al. Left ventricular volume predicts postoperative course in patients with ischemic cardiomyopathy. Ann Thorac Surg 1998;65(2):434–8.
5. Sharkey H, Nikolic S, Khairkhahan A, et al. Left ventricular apex occluder. Description of a ventricular partitioning device. EuroIntervention 2006;2(1):125–7.
6. Remme WJ. Therapeutic strategies and neurohormonal control in heart failure. Eur Heart J 1994; 15(Suppl D):129–38.
7. Francis GS. Neurohormonal control of heart failure. Cleve Clin J Med 2011;78(Suppl 1):S75–9.
8. Young JB. Heart failure, ventricular remodelling and the renin-angiotensin system: insights from recently completed clinical trials. Eur Heart J 1993; 14(Suppl C):14–7.
9. Pitt B, Remme W, Zannad F, et al. Eplerenone, a selective aldosterone blocker, in patients with left ventricular dysfunction after myocardial infarction. N Engl J Med 2003;348(14):1309–21.
10. Udelson JE, Feldman AM, Greenberg B, et al. Randomized, double-blind, multicenter, placebo-controlled study evaluating the effect of aldosterone antagonism with eplerenone on ventricular remodeling in patients with mild-to-moderate heart failure and left ventricular systolic dysfunction. Circ Heart Fail 2010;3(3):347–53.
11. Colucci WS, Kolias TJ, Adams KF, et al. Metoprolol reverses left ventricular remodeling in patients with asymptomatic systolic dysfunction: the REversal of VEntricular Remodeling with Toprol-XL (REVERT) trial. Circulation 2007;116(1):49–56.
12. Kelesidis I, Varughese CJ, Hourani P, et al. Effects of beta-adrenergic blockade on left ventricular

13. Cohn JN, Ferrari R, Sharpe N. Cardiac remodeling–concepts and clinical implications: a consensus paper from an international forum on cardiac remodeling. Behalf of an International Forum on Cardiac Remodeling. J Am Coll Cardiol 2000;35(3): 569–82.
14. Sutton MG, Sharpe N. Left ventricular remodeling after myocardial infarction: pathophysiology and therapy. Circulation 2000;101(25):2981–8.
15. Douglas PS, Morrow R, Ioli A, et al. Left ventricular shape, afterload and survival in idiopathic dilated cardiomyopathy. J Am Coll Cardiol 1989;13(2): 311–5.
16. Nikolic SD, Khairkhahan A, Ryu M, et al. Percutaneous implantation of an intraventricular device for the treatment of heart failure: experimental results and proof of concept. J Card Fail 2009;15(9):790–7.
17. Aguilar D, Solomon SD, Kober L, et al. Newly diagnosed and previously known diabetes mellitus and 1-year outcomes of acute myocardial infarction: the VALsartan In Acute myocardial iNfarcTion (VALIANT) trial. Circulation 2004;110(12):1572–8.
18. Silva G, Melica B, Pires de Morais G, et al. Percutaneous implantation of a ventricular partitioning device for treatment of ischemic heart failure: initial experience of a center. Rev Port Cardiol 2012; 31(12):795–801.
19. Di Donato M, Sabatier M, Toso A, et al. Regional myocardial performance of non-ischaemic zones remote from anterior wall left ventricular aneurysm. Effects of aneurysmectomy. Eur Heart J 1995; 16(9):1285–92.
20. Velazquez EJ, Lee KL, Deja MA, et al. Coronary-artery bypass surgery in patients with left ventricular dysfunction. N Engl J Med 2011;364(17):1607–16.
21. Shroyer AL, Collins JF, Grover FL. Evaluating clinical applicability: the STICH trial's findings. J Am Coll Cardiol 2010;56(6):508–9.
22. Mann DL, Acker MA, Jessup M, et al. Clinical evaluation of the CorCap cardiac support device in patients with dilated cardiomyopathy. Ann Thorac Surg 2007;84(4):1226–35.
23. Costanzo MR, Ivanhoe RJ, Kao A, et al. Prospective evaluation of elastic restraint to lessen the effects of heart failure (PEERLESS-HF) trial. J Card Fail 2012; 18(6):446–58.
24. Grossi EA, Patel N, Woo YJ, et al. Outcomes of the RESTOR-MV Trial (Randomized Evaluation of a Surgical Treatment for Off-Pump Repair of the Mitral Valve). J Am Coll Cardiol 2010;56(24):1984–93.
25. Bozdag-Turan I, Bermaoui B, Paranskaya L, et al. Challenges in patient selection for the Parachute device implantation. Catheter Cardiovasc Interv 2013; 82(5):E718–25.

26. Gottdiener JS, Bednarz J, Devereux R, et al. American Society of Echocardiography recommendations for use of echocardiography in clinical trials. J Am Soc Echocardiogr 2004;17(10):1086–119.

27. Oh JK, Pellikka PA, Panza JA, et al. Core lab analysis of baseline echocardiographic studies in the STICH trial and recommendation for use of echocardiography in future clinical trials. J Am Soc Echocardiogr 2012;25(3):327–36.

28. Schwarz F, Takx R, Schoepf UJ, et al. Reproducibility of left and right ventricular mass measurements with cardiac CT. J Cardiovasc Comput Tomogr 2011; 5(5):317–24.

29. Bozdag-Turan I, Bermaoui B, Turan RG, et al. Parachute implant: CT morphological criteria of our center to identify the suitable patient. Cardiovasc Ther 2014;32(1):26–31.

30. Mazzaferri EL Jr, Gradinac S, Sagic D, et al. Percutaneous left ventricular partitioning in patients with chronic heart failure and a prior anterior myocardial infarction: results of the PercutAneous Ventricular RestorAtion in Chronic Heart failUre PaTiEnts Trial. Am Heart J 2012;163(5):812–20.e1.

31. Costa MA, Mazzaferri EL Jr, Sievert H, et al. Percutaneous ventricular restoration using the Parachute(r) device in patients with ischemic heart failure: three-year outcomes of the PARACHUTE first-in-human study. Circ Heart Fail 2014;7:752–8.

32. Costa MA, Pencina M, Nikolic S, et al. The PARACHUTE IV trial design and rationale: percutaneous ventricular restoration using the Parachute device in patients with ischemic heart failure and dilated left ventricles. Am Heart J 2013;165(4):531–6.

33. Sagic D, Otasevic P, Sievert H, et al. Percutaneous implantation of the left ventricular partitioning device for chronic heart failure: a pilot study with 1-year follow-up. Eur J Heart Fail 2010;12(6):600–6.

34. Ladich E, Otsuka F, Virmani R. A pathologic study of explanted Parachute devices from seven heart failure patients following percutaneous ventricular restoration. Catheter Cardiovasc Interv 2013;83(4): 619–30.

35. Lauschke J, Schneider R, Bansch D. Ventricular tachycardia ablation in a patient with a Parachute device: a decent word of warning. Europace 2014; 16(2):207.

36. Oliveira GH, Al-Kindi SG, Bezerra HG, et al. Left ventricular restoration devices. J Cardiovasc Transl Res 2014;7(3):282–91.

Stem Cell Therapy for Heart Failure

 CrossMark

Amit N. Patel, MD, MS*, Francisco Silva, MS, Amalia A. Winters, BSc

KEYWORDS

• Stem cell • Delivery • Heart failure • Clinical trials

KEY POINTS

- During the past decade, studies in animals and humans have suggested that cell therapy has positive effects for the treatment of heart failure.
- This clinical effect may be mediated by angiogenesis and reduction in fibrosis rather than by regeneration of myocytes.
- Increased microvasculature and decreased scar also likely lead to improved cardiac function in the failing heart.
- The effects of cell therapy are not limited to one type of cell or delivery technique.
- Well-designed, large-scale, randomized clinical trials with objective end points will help to fully realize the therapeutic potential of cell-based therapy for treating heart failure.

STEM CELL THERAPY FOR HEART FAILURE

Heart failure (HF) is the inability of the heart to pump sufficient blood to meet the body's oxygen demands. It is classified as ischemic (cause by atherosclerosis, decreased perfusion, or myocardial infarction) or nonischemic (caused by viral infection or congenital or idiopathic disease). Regardless of the cause, congestive HF is the final common pathway, marked by cardiomyocyte death, inflammation, and scar formation resulting in loss of contractility. Despite significant therapeutic advances, the prognosis for patients hospitalized with HF remains poor, with a 5-year mortality of approximately 50%. Additionally, HF creates a heavy burden on health care resources.

HF therapies improve symptoms and can prolong life, but are unable to replace scar tissue or awaken hibernating myocardium via angiogenesis. Currently, cell-based technology is emerging as a novel therapy with the potential to dramatically transform the treatment of HF through inducing myocardial repair and regeneration.

Efficient delivery of cells to the target site is critical for effective clinical outcomes. Cell therapy may be delivered to the heart through several routes: direct injection into the myocardium via endocardial or epicardial approaches, coronary artery infusion, intravenous infusion, epicardial patch, or retrograde coronary sinus infusion.

This article discusses the use and delivery techniques of various stem cell-based therapeutics for the treatment of HF, along with advances, challenges, and future directions.

EPIDEMIOLOGY, PATHOPHYSIOLOGY, AND TREATMENT OF HEART FAILURE

HF is a common, lethal, and expensive disorder. It is one of the most common causes of hospitalization in industrialized countries, and the incidence is increasing with concomitant increases of morbidity, mortality, and consumption of health care resources. Although ischemic and nonischemic heart disease contribute to a final common pathway marked by a cycle of inflammatory

University of Utah School of Medicine, 30 North 1900 East 3c127 SOM, Salt Lake City, UT 84132, USA
* Corresponding author. University of Utah School of Medicine, 30 North 1900 East 3c127 SOM, Salt Lake City, UT 84132.
E-mail address: amit.patel@hsc.utah.edu

Heart Failure Clin 11 (2015) 275–286
http://dx.doi.org/10.1016/j.hfc.2014.12.006
1551-7136/15/$ – see front matter © 2015 Elsevier Inc. All rights reserved.

mediator release, cardiomyocyte death, and scar formation, leading to HF, development of novel therapies requires an understanding of the different pathophysiology of these causes.[1–3]

Pathophysiology of Ischemic Heart Failure

Ischemic HF is the end result of insufficient blood flow to the myocardium caused by occlusive disease of the coronary arteries. Atherosclerosis narrows the arterial lumen and leads to decreased myocardial oxygen delivery, with both chronic and acute effects. Narrowed, calcified coronary arteries cannot accommodate the increased blood flow required in the setting of increased oxygen demand (eg, exercise). A myocardial infarction occurs when myocardium distal to the arterial blockage receives no blood flow and subsequently dies. Infarcted myocardium is replaced by fibrotic tissue that does not have the same contractile properties as healthy heart muscle, resulting in a heart that functions abnormally. The fraction of myocardium replaced with fibrosis is a predictor of all-cause mortality and adverse cardiovascular events in patients with HF.[4] If the areas of ischemia are large enough, valvular integrity and contractile function can be compromised and HF can develop. Current treatments focus on improving blood flow through these major arteries using angioplasty or stenting, or providing a new source of blood flow to an ischemic region, such as through coronary artery bypass grafting.

Pathophysiology of Nonischemic Heart Failure

Nonischemic HF is a disease characterized by microvascular dysfunction. The major coronary arteries remain patent, but the disease is marked by decreased capillary density, increased microvascular resistance, and insufficient vasodilation of the small myocardial vessels in response to increased oxygen demand. Patients demonstrate reduced myocardial blood flow even at rest.[5] This "blunted perfusion reserve" in the setting of normal coronary arteries is the main feature of nonischemic HF.[6] Microvascular dysfunction sets the stage for recurrent, frequent episodes of myocardial ischemia. This condition ultimately leads to ventricular wall thinning and global cardiac dysfunction marked by pump failure and arrhythmias.[7] The degree of microcirculatory dysfunction is an independent predictor of mortality. It is important to note that coronary microvascular dysfunction is not an effect of myocardial damage but rather is the cause of the ischemic substrate that results in progressive myocardial injury and HF. In nonischemic HF, the pattern of myocardial injury is more diffuse than in ischemic disease. This global dysfunction means that treatments for nonischemic HF are limited to inotropic medications or ventricular-assist devices (neither of which stop or reverse HF), or cardiac transplantation. An intervention targeted at improving microvascular function in nonischemic cardiomyopathy may improve outcomes in HF or prevent patients from progressing to failure.

CELL OPTIONS FOR THE TREATMENT FOR HEART FAILURE

This article discusses the source of stem cells and routes of delivery along with their safety and efficacy for the treatment of HF. Clinical trials that have been registered with ClinicalTrials.gov are mentioned, along with their assigned numbers.

Skeletal Myoblasts

Skeletal myoblasts are progenitor cells derived from skeletal muscle. They were the first cells to be tested in both preclinical and clinical studies for HF.[8–11] Although early clinical studies reported engraftment and significant improvement in cardiac function, subsequent clinical studies, including a 97-patient phase II randomized, placebo-controlled, double-blind trial, failed to reproduce these results.[9] In several patients, ventricular tachyarrhythmias were noted after cell transplantation. With poor clinical outcomes and the potential for increased adverse events, skeletal myoblasts have a limited role in cell-based therapy for HF.

Peripheral Blood Cells

Peripheral blood–selected CD34+ cells have been used in the treatment of patients with ischemic HF with promising results.[12] The issues related to using granulocyte colony-stimulating factors for peripheral blood mobilization, apheresis, and the costs associated with CD34+ selection have limited the use of this cell product. The long-term benefits of using blood-selected cells in patients with acute myocardial infarction have been shown to be less favorable compared with using bone marrow cells.[13] This finding has further limited the use of peripheral blood for treating ischemic heart disease. However, this technique still has potential benefit, which is currently being evaluated (ClinicalTrials.gov identifier: NCT01350310).[14] The mechanism of possible benefit for peripheral blood CD34+ cells in patients with nonischemic versus ischemic HF has not been identified.

Bone Marrow Mononuclear Cells

Bone marrow mononuclear cells (BMMNCs) are a heterogeneous cell population composed of several cell types derived from bone marrow. Early preclinical clinical studies have reported that transplanted cells undergo transdifferentiation into cardiomyocytes and supporting vasculature, resulting in improved left ventricular function.[15–18] Although initially encouraging, subsequent studies have failed to demonstrate any meaningful degree of transdifferentiation.[19] Additionally, BMMNCs stimulate angiogenesis, which improves microcirculation, but do not stimulate vasculogenesis.[16] Perin and colleagues[20] demonstrated in the National Institute of Health–sponsored FOCUS-HF (Autologous Stem Cells for Cardiac Angiogenesis) trial that a small potential benefit in the left ventricular ejection is seen in patients with ischemic HF but viable myocardium treated with endocardial BMMNCs (ClinicalTrials.gov identifier: NCT00824005). A recent trial (PreSERVE-AMI (AMR001 Versus Placebo Post ST Segment Elevation Myocardial Infarction); ClinicalTrials.gov identifier: NCT01495364) used intracoronary bone marrow–selected CD34+ cell delivery in patients with post–myocardial infarction LV dysfunction, demonstrating that a minimum dose of 20×10^6 cells were required to show potential benefit. The purification of BMMNCs from bone marrow can be performed easily using density gradient centrifugation, and now can be performed at bedside using commercial cell processing systems. Despite the simplicity of processing bone marrow, a large discrepancy exists in the outcomes of clinical trials based on the variety of purification or concentrating methods.[21] Several meta-analyses suggest that the use of BMMNCs in ischemic cardiomyopathy is safe and feasible, but significant positive clinical outcomes are limited.[22–24]

Autologous Cultured Bone Marrow Cells

As a result of the many issues related to rapid processing of autologous bone marrow, culture processes were developed to address issues with BMMNCs, specifically donor age and comorbidities. Ixmyelocel-T is a product derived from a small sample of autologous bone marrow that is cultured for 12 days. The culture process results in an enhanced product of mesenchymal cells and M2 macrophages, which have the potential for angiogenesis and remodeling of fibrosis.[25] The ixmyelocel-T product was used in the phase IIa IMPACT-DCM trial (Use of Ixmyelocel-T (Formerly Cardiac Repair Cell [CRC] Treatment) in Patients With Heart Failure Due to Dilated Cardiomyopathy), which demonstrated benefit in only patients with ischemic HF (ClinicalTrials.gov identifier: NCT00765518).[26] A follow-up trial, (IDCM)-ixCELL DCM (An Efficacy, Safety and Tolerability Study of

Ixmyelocel-T Administered Via Transendocardial Catheter-based Injections to Subjects With Heart Failure Due to Ischemic Dilated Cardiomyopathy), is enrolling only patients with ischemic dilated cardiomyopathy (ClinicalTrials.gov identifier: NCT01670981). Similarly, the C-CURE (C-Cure Clinical Trial) program harvested a small amount of autologous bone marrow, which was cultured for several weeks in a cardiopoetic cocktail of growth factors (ClinicalTrials.gov identifier: NCT00810238).[27] This trial also demonstrated benefits in patients with ischemic HF and is currently enrolling in CHART-2 (Congestive Heart Failure Cardiopoietic Regenerative Therapy), a global phase III study (ClinicalTrials.gov identifier: NCT01768702).[28]

Bone Marrow Mesenchymal Stem Cells

The use of bone marrow mesenchymal stem cells (MSCs) for the treatment of HF has great potential because they can be easily harvested and cultured.[29] They also have immune-modulating and anti-inflammatory properties, making them immune-privileged. MSCs typically express CD105, CD73, and CD90, but lack hematopoietic markers (CD45, CD34, and CD14/CD11b).[30] Preclinical studies using MSCs in both ischemic and nonischemic cardiomyopathy have shown signs of angiogenesis, including reduced fibrosis, and improved cardiac function.[31–33] A clinical study by Hare and colleagues[31] compared 3 doses of autologous or allogeneic MSCs (20, 100, and 200 x 10^6 cells) in patients with ischemic cardiomyopathy and showed that all doses resulted in improved patient functional capacity, quality of life, and ventricular remodeling.[32] MSCs were also shown to function better than BMMNCs. MSCs have the potential to be used as an allogeneic cell source, which leads to a very stable and reliable cell source.[31] Phase III trials are currently underway in patients with HF, using endocardial delivery of allogeneic bone marrow MSCs in the DREAM-HF trial (The purpose of this Study is to evaluate the efficacy and safety of a Allogeneic Mesenchymal Precursor Cells (CEP-41750) for the treatment of chronic heart failure) (ClinicalTrials.gov identifier: NCT02032004).

Adipose-Derived Stem Cells

Adipose-derived stem cells (ADSCs) also are a form of MSCs but are more abundant than bone marrow MSCs. They have also been used in several trials for the treatment of HF.[34] The PRECISE trial (A Randomized Clinical Trial of adiPose-deRived stEm & Regenerative Cells In the Treatment of Patients With Non revaScularizable ischEmic Myocardium) used autologous ADSCs in patients with HF demonstrating a modest potential benefit (ClinicalTrials.gov identifier: NCT00426868).[35] However, ADSCs are more difficult to process and have been used strictly in an autologous manner, unlike bone marrow MSCs. Some preclinical models of allogeneic use of ADSCs have shown benefit in cardiac models, which also resulted in allogeneic immune responses.[36]

Umbilical/Placental/Endometrial Mesenchymal Stem Cells

Several mesenchymal cells have been isolated from pregnancy and gynecologic organs that have potential benefit in HF models. They are all derived and used in an allogeneic manner. Limited information is available, but many of these cells are being used in preclinical or early clinical trials.[37–40]

Cardiac Stem Cells

Recent studies have shown that the postnatal heart undergoes a continuous turnover of its cellular components. As a result, several cardiac-derived stem cell (CSC) populations have been identified and isolated.[41] Preclinical models using various CSC populations have demonstrated their therapeutic potential.[42] The encouraging results of these early preclinical studies established the translatability of intracoronary CSC transplantation. Cardiac Stem Cell Infusion in Patients With Ischemic Cardiomyopathy (SCIPIO) is the first clinical trial using CSCs (ClinicalTrials.gov identifier: NCT00474461).[43] Results from the trial showed improvement in global and regional left ventricular function and a reduction in infarct size compared with use of conventional treatment. In a similar approach, autologous 3-dimensional CSCs (cardiospheres) have also demonstrated a benefit in a preclinical model and have been translated into clinical trials.[44] The CADUCEUS trial (CArdiosphere-Derived aUtologous Stem CElls to Reverse ventricUlar dySfunction) also demonstrated a benefit in scar reduction using autologous cardiosphere-derived cells (ClinicalTrials.gov identifier: NCT00893360).[45] Based on these data, Tseliou and colleagues[46] have demonstrated that these cells can be made allogeneic from donor hearts. Currently a phase II trial (ALLSTAR (Allogeneic Heart Stem Cells to Achieve Myocardial Regeneration); ClinicalTrials.gov identifier: NCT01458405) is using allogeneic CSCs in patients with myocardial ischemia and decreased left ventricular function. A phase I trial using allogeneic CSCs is being conducted in patients with nonischemic HF (DYNAMIC (Dilated cardiomYopathy iNtervention With Allogeneic MyocardIally-regenerative Cells); ClinicalTrials.gov identifier: NCT02293603).

Embryonic and Induced Pluripotent Stem Cells

Both embryonic and induced pluripotent stem cells have demonstrated the potential for engraftment in prehuman models of HF.[47,48] Sheets of cells have also been used in prehuman models showing functional engraftment, but translation to humans has also been difficult because of the scalability of manufacturing large sheets of cells.[49] Many scientists believe that even with the great potential of both cells types, translation may be premature.[50] However, based on their preclinical data, Menasche's group in Paris have obtained European Union (EU) approval to start a first-in-man study (ESCORT (Transplantation of Human Embryonic Stem Cell-derived Progenitors in Severe Heart Failure); ClinicalTrials.gov identifier: NCT02057900) using embryonic-derived sheets of cardiac progenitor cells in patients with HF.[51]

MECHANISMS OF ACTION OF CELL THERAPY IN HEART FAILURE

The exact mechanism of action of cell therapy in HF is unknown. Although early research suggested that delivered cells transformed into new heart muscle, subsequent research by many investigators, including Mirotsou and colleagues,[52] indicates that transplanted cells do not remain in the heart for more than a few days. Therefore, the benefit is likely related to the release of paracrine factors into the injured myocardium that mediate neovascularization and remodeling. The other proposed mechanisms of engraftment, cell fusion, and endogenous cell recruitment have not been verified clinically.[53]

DELIVERY METHODS FOR CELL THERAPY IN HEART FAILURE

Many routes for delivering cell therapy to the heart are available, including intramyocardial via an endocardial or epicardial approach, epicardial patch, intracoronary, intravenous, and retrograde through the coronary sinus.[54–56]

Intramyocardial

Intramyocardial delivery, which includes epicardial and endocardial approaches, consists of direct injection of cells into the heart muscle. The epicardial approach is very accurate and reproducible but is invasive, because it is typically performed under direct vision either during a median sternotomy, video-assisted thoracoscopic surgery, or pericardioscopy.[57–61] This method is best suited for combined procedures in patients who are undergoing surgery, such as the delivery of cell therapy during coronary artery bypass grafting, valve surgery, ventricular assist device implantation or transmyocardial laser revascularization.[57–61] The endocardial approach is much less invasive, and allows one to achieve direct delivery of cells to target peri-infarct regions, but has the potential for cell loss during delivery.[54] This method can also result in myocardial injury, inflammation, and scarring, all of which disrupt the conduction pathways and can contribute to arrhythmias. One risk associated with endomyocardial injection is the perforation of a thinned or damaged ventricle. Endomyocardial delivery of cells also results in localized islets of cells rather than a homogeneous distribution, and access to regions of the heart other than the left ventricle remains difficult. To optimize the targeting of desired regions and minimize potential damage, many intramyocardial protocols use electromechanical mapping catheters (NOGA, Biologics Delivery Systems, Irwindale, CA, USA), which allow real-time evaluation of myocardial viability before cell therapy injection.[62] However, safety and precision are gained at the expense of availability; NOGA mapping is an expensive technique and requires significant supervised clinical experience to develop proficiency.[63] Another catheter for endocardial delivery is the BioCardia Helical Infusion Catheter (HIC-BioCardia Inc, San Carlos, CA, USA). It has the ability to stay engaged in myocardium to enable reproducible delivery. With this catheter, there is no 3-dimensional mapping or viability, and therefore preoperative viability and wall thickness measurements are required. Therefore, intramyocardial injection may be useful when targeting discrete segments of myocardium, such as peri-infarct regions, but it may be less effective in more global HF, particularly in the setting of nonischemic cardiomyopathy.[64,65] Another endocardial delivery catheter in clinical trials is the C-Cath (Cardio3 Biosciences, Mont-Saint-Guibert, Belgium), which has a curved end needle to minimize the risk of perforation.[66] Despite the advantages and disadvantages of epicardial and endocardial delivery methods, endocardial has become the most used technique for cell therapy in current HF trials.

Intracoronary

Intracoronary delivery consists of infusing cells antegrade (in the direction of arterial flow) into the coronary arteries. This technique can be performed invasively, during a combined open heart surgical procedure, or percutaneously through catheter access via a peripheral artery to the left side of the heart. Cell therapy delivered via the intracoronary route is used most often as an adjunct in patients with acute myocardial infarction in an attempt to promote angiogenesis and rescue heart muscle served by compromised vasculature and maybe amenable to repeat dosing.[67,68]

Intracoronary infusion relies on cell migration through the endothelial layer of the artery, and homing of cells to damaged tissue. However, atherosclerotic or occluded vessels prevent infused cells from reaching the myocardium. Furthermore, although delivery of cell therapy via the coronary arteries may result in new blood vessel development, the increase in growth signals may also result in accelerated atherosclerosis of the targeted arteries. This double-edged sword of angiogenesis versus accelerated atherogenesis has been termed the *Janus phenomenon*[69] and has been seen in the setting of accelerated stenosis within coronary stents after intracoronary infusion of peripheral blood stem cells and bone marrow–derived stem cells.[69,70] Additionally, delivery of large cells or particularly viscous cell suspensions via the antegrade coronary route also poses the risk of artery occlusion or embolization. Occlusion of the coronaries results in transient ischemia; therefore, infusion of cell therapy via this route is limited in terms of infusion time, particularly if balloon occlusion is used to minimize proximal antegrade flow. Repeated instrumentation of, or balloon inflation within, the coronary arteries risks dislodging plaque or causing endothelial damage that serves as a nidus for plaque formation. The muscular wall of the arteries (compared with thinner-walled veins) presents a further distance through which delivered cells must migrate to reach the target myocardium. Although this approach has generally been considered safe, several papers highlight unique risks of the procedure.

As mentioned previously, accelerated atherosclerosis or restenosis has occurred in patients receiving intracoronary infusions of both peripheral blood–derived and bone marrow–derived stem cells.[69–71] Another risk of this infusion route is dissection of the coronary artery. In the TOPCARE-CHD trial (Transplantation Of Progenitor Cells And Recovery Of Left Ventricular Function In Patients With Nonischemic Dilatative Cardiomyopathy), for example, this complication was seen in 3 of 69 patients.[67] All underwent immediate stenting across the dissection and no further complication occurred in their clinical course. In progressive ischemic disease, the heart may collateralize to compensate for decreased flow. Nonischemic disease, however, is more a disease of the microcirculation, and without such collateralization, patients may be much less tolerant of balloon occlusion of their coronary arteries. A pilot trial of cell therapy for dilated cardiomyopathy had to be halted because of this complication in several patients.[72] Given the issues related to intracoronary delivery, other routes of delivery have been evaluated. Comparison of endocardial versus intracoronary delivery of cells in patients with nonischemic dilated cardiomyopathy showed improved outcomes in the endocardial group.[73] As a result of these issues, intracoronary delivery of cell therapy for HF is not currently being used except in cardiac stem cell clinical trials.

Intravenous

Intravenous infusions of cell therapy via the peripheral vein is the least invasive method but also the least reliable. Preclinical studies demonstrate low retention rates in the heart and significant cell trapping in the lungs. The intravenous route relies entirely on the homing of stem cells to the site of injury, and without means to augment or facilitate localization, sufficient cells are unlikely to be delivered to injured myocardium to demonstrate a clinical effect.[73] Using labeled stem cells in a porcine model of myocardial infarction, Forest and colleagues[74] found that intravenously injected cells were not detectable in the heart at 24 hours and instead localized to the lung; this was in contrast to cells delivered via the intracoronary route, which demonstrated signal in both the heart and lungs at 24 hours. In a randomized controlled trial of allogeneic, culture-expanded MSCs that were delivered intravenously (Prochymal, Osiris Therapeutics Inc, Columbia, MD, USA) to patients after acute myocardial infarction, no clinically significant differences were seen between groups in terms of cardiovascular parameters.[75] Because of these findings, intravenous cell therapy is not currently used for clinical trials.

Retrograde

The coronary sinus drains deoxygenated blood from the heart via cardiac veins into the right atrium. Because it lies on the right side of the circulation, the coronary sinus can be accessed transvenously via the femoral, jugular, or antecubital veins. This method of access is less invasive and presents a lower risk than the left-sided arterial access required for antegrade intracoronary delivery. The retrograde route is well suited to

"no-option" patients with significant coronary disease or thin myocardial walls, and allows for the safe and repeated delivery of cell therapy.[76–79] Temporary occlusion of the coronary sinus and cardiac veins does not lead to clinically significant ischemia; therefore, longer infusion and dwell times may be used than with antegrade coronary delivery. Retrograde coronary sinus infusion of cell therapy achieves uniform distribution of cells, avoids the islet-like clustering and arrhythmias associated with intramyocardial delivery, and allows distribution to ischemic zones that cannot be accessed via the antegrade route because of diseased coronary arteries.[80]

Many patients with HF also have coronary sinus leads implanted for biventricular pacing. The presence of these leads was thought to be a contraindication to early coronary sinus delivery of cells; however, with highly compliant balloons that can allow adequate sealing around the lead during cell infusion, this issue has safely been addressed. Human experience with retrograde delivery of cell therapy for chronic myocardial ischemia has been shown to be safe, feasible, and effective, leading to trials in patients with HF.[81] This method of delivery can be used in patients with ischemic and nonischemic HF. Several clinical trials are currently using retrograde coronary sinus delivery of cells for HF.

Epicardial Patches

To address issues related to cell retention and engraftment, which have plagued the field of cell therapy, cell sheets have been engineered. Despite the potential advantages of cell sheets demonstrated in preclinical models, they are highly invasive because they require a sternotomy or thoracotomy for implantation.[32] Currently, the use of embryonic-derived sheets of cardiac progenitor cells in patients with HF is approved in the EU (ESCORT; ClinicalTrials.gov identifier: NCT02057900).[51]

CLINICAL TRIALS AND END POINTS

Several trials have used the various cell types and delivery approaches described earlier in patients with HF (**Table 1**). Other than skeletal myoblasts, all other clinically used cell types have demonstrated safety and a modest clinical benefit. The issue with these modest benefits is determining which end points are required for these approaches to be considered successful in a clinical HF trial that will be accepted by the cardiology and reimbursement community.[82] Most trials have used ejection fraction along with 6-minute walk time, maximum oxygen consumption, brain

Table 1
Cell therapy clinical trials in heart failure

Trial Name/Investigator	ClinicalTrials.gov Identifier	Cell Type	End Point	Patients	Delivery Route	HF Cause
MARVEL[11]	00526253	Skeletal muscle	Safety + QOL	170	Endocardial	Ischemic
FOCUS-HF[20]	00824005	BMMNC vs placebo	LVESV	92	Endomyocardial	Ischemic
Pokushalov et al[85]	00841958	BMMNC	LVEF	109	Endomyocardial	Ischemic
REGEN-IHD	00747708	Intracoronary BMMNC + G-CSF vs endomyocardial BMMNC + G-CSF vs G-CSF vs placebo	LVEF	148	Intracoronary/ Endomyocardial	Ischemic
DANCELL-CHF[68]	00235417	Repeated BMMNC	LVEF	35	Intracoronary	Ischemic
REVIVE-1	01299324	BMMNC vs medical therapy	Safety + SAE	60	Retrograde	Ischemic
PreSERVE-AMI	01495364	BMMNC vs placebo	Safety + SAE	160	Intracoronary	Ischemic
BAMI	01569178	BMMNC vs placebo	All-cause mortality	3000	Intracoronary	Ischemic
REPEAT	01693042	Single vs repeated (2 times) BMC infusions	Mortality + morbidity	676	Intracoronary	Ischemic
Patel et al[57]	00130377	BMMNC/CD34+ vs placebo	LVEF	50	Epicardial	Ischemic
Patila et al[86]	00418418	BMMNC vs placebo	LVEF	104	Epicardial	Ischemic
PERFECT[87]	00950274	Bone marrow CD133+ vs placebo	LVEF	142	Epicardial	Ischemic
PRECISE[35]	00426868	ADSC vs placebo	SAE + infarct size	27	Endomyocardial	Ischemic
Parcero et al	01502514	ADSC	Safety + QOL	10	Endomyocardial/ Intravenous	Ischemic
Yan et al	01946048	Allogeneic USCs	Safety + LVEF	10	Endomyocardial	Ischemic
CHART-1	01768702	Cultured bone marrow -cardiopoetic	Time to SAE	240	Endocardial	Ischemic
TAC-HFT[32]	00768066	MSCs (100 or 200 million) vs BMCs (100 or 200 million) vs placebo	SAE + LVEF	67	Endomyocardial	Ischemic
Anastasiadis et al	01753440	Allogeneic MSCs	LVEF	30	Epicardial	Ischemic
ixCELL DCM[26]	01670981	Cultured bone marrow	Time to SAE	108	Endomyocardial	Ischemic

(continued on next page)

Table 1
(continued)

Trial Name/Investigator	ClinicalTrials.gov Identifier	Cell Type	End Point	Patients	Delivery Route	HF Cause
PROMETHEUS[88]	00587990	Low- vs high-dose MSCs vs placebo	SAE	7	Endomyocardial	Ischemic
MSC-HF[89]	00644410	MSCs vs placebo	LVEF	60	Endomyocardial	Ischemic
SCIPIO[43]	00474461	Cultured cardiac progenitors	SAE	33	Intracoronary	Ischemic
Perin et al	00555828	25 vs 75 vs 150 million allogeneic MSCs vs placebo	Safety + LVEF	60	Endomyocardial	Both
IMPACT-DCM[26]	01020968	Cultured bone marrow	Safety + SAE	60	Endomyocardial/Epicardial	Both
DREAM-HF	02032004	Allogeneic MSCs	Time to SAE	1730	Endomyocardial	Both
POSEIDON-DCM[31]	01392625	MSCs vs allogeneic MSCs	Safety + SAE	36	Endocardial	Nonischemic
Suzrez et al	00629096	BMMNC	LVEF	28	Intracoronary	Nonischemic
Ribeiro et al	00349271	BMMNC	LVEF	234	Intracoronary	Nonischemic
Vrtovec et al[14]	01350310	G-CSF/blood/CD34+	LVEF	60	Intracoronary/ Endomyocardial	Nonischemic
DYNAMIC	02293603	Allogeneic cardiac progenitor cells	Safety + SAE	42	Intracoronary	Nonischemic
TOPCARE-DCM	00284713	BMMNC	LVEF	30	Intracoronary	Nonischemic
Martino et al	00612911	BMMNC	LVEF	24	Intracoronary	Nonischemic

All cells are autologous unless stated otherwise.
Abbreviations: ADSC, adipose-derived stem cell; BMMNC, bone marrow mononuclear cell; G-CSF, granulocyte colony-stimulating factor; LVEF, left ventricular ejection fraction; LVESV, left ventricular end-systolic volume; MSC, mesenchymal stem cell; NCT, National Clinical Trial; QOL, quality of life; SAE, serious adverse event; USC, umbilical mesenchymal cell.

natriuretic peptide, or myocardial perfusion as clinical end points. However, these are not hard end points, such as mortality, readmission, reintervention, defibrillator event, left ventricular assist device placement, or recurrent HF symptoms, which have been used in other HF trials and are accepted end points.[83] The CUPID trial (A Phase 2b, Double-Blind, Placebo-Controlled, Multinational, Multicenter, Randomized Study Evaluating the Safety and Efficacy of Intracoronary Administration of MYDICAR® (AAV1/SERCA2a) in Subjects With Heart Failure) for gene therapy in patients with HF has used time to recurrent HF symptoms along with composite end points to determine success (ClinicalTrials.gov identifier: NCT01643330).[84] Thus, several methodologies are available that can be used to determine success. However, because no approved cell therapy exists for HF, each group has set its own parameters for clinical success, working with opinion leaders in the field of HF and with the FDA.

SUMMARY

During the past decade, studies in animals and humans have suggested that cell therapy has positive effects for the treatment of HF. This clinical effect may be mediated by angiogenesis and reduction in fibrosis rather than by regeneration of myocytes. Increased microvasculature and decreased scar also likely lead to improved cardiac function in the failing heart. The effects of cell therapy are not limited to one type of cell or delivery technique. Well-designed, large-scale, randomized clinical trials with objective end points will help to fully realize the therapeutic potential of cell-based therapy for treating HF.

REFERENCES

1. Roger VL. The heart failure epidemic. Int J Environ Res Public Health 2010;7:1807–30.
2. Giamouzis G, Kalogeropoulos A, Georgiopoulou V, et al. Hospitalization epidemic in patients with heart failure: risk factors, risk prediction, knowledge gaps, and future directions. J Card Fail 2011;17:54–75.
3. Pocock SJ, Wang D, Pfeffer MA, et al. Predictors of mortality and morbidity in patients with chronic heart failure. Eur Heart J 2006;27:65–75.
4. Aoki T, Fukumoto Y, Sugimura K, et al. Prognostic impact of myocardial interstitial fibrosis in non-ischemic heart failure. Comparison between preserved and reduced ejection fraction heart failure. Circ J 2011;75:2605–13.
5. Neglia D, L'Abbate A. Coronary microvascular dysfunction and idiopathic dilated cardiomyopathy. Pharmacol Rep 2005;57(Suppl):151–5.
6. Knaapen P, Germans T, Camici PG, et al. Determinants of coronary microvascular dysfunction in symptomatic hypertrophic cardiomyopathy. Am J Physiol Heart Circ Physiol 2008;294:H986–93.
7. Cecchi F, Sgalambro A, Baldi M, et al. Microvascular dysfunction, myocardial ischemia, and progression to heart failure in patients with hypertrophic cardiomyopathy. J Cardiovasc Transl Res 2009;2:452–61.
8. Fukushima S, Coppen SR, Lee J, et al. Choice of cell-delivery route for skeletal myoblast transplantation for treating post-infarction chronic heart failure in rat. PLoS One 2008;3:e3071.
9. Menasche P, Alfieri O, Janssens S, et al. The Myoblast Autologous Grafting in Ischemic Cardiomyopathy (MAGIC) trial: first randomized placebo-controlled study of myoblast transplantation. Circulation 2008;117:1189–200.
10. Guarita-Souza LC, Francisco JC, Simeoni R, et al. Benefit of stem cells and skeletal myoblast cells in dilated cardiomyopathies. World J Cardiol 2011;3: 93–7.
11. Povsic TJ, O'Connor CM, Henry T, et al. A double-blind, randomized, controlled, multicenter study to assess the safety and cardiovascular effects of skeletal myoblast implantation by catheter delivery in patients with chronic heart failure after myocardial infarction. Am Heart J 2011;162(4):654–62.e1. http://dx.doi.org/10.1016/j.ahj.2011.07.020.
12. Poglajen G, Sever M, Cukjati M, et al. Effects of transendocardial CD34+ cell transplantation in patients with ischemic cardiomyopathy. Circ Cardiovasc Interv 2014;7(4):552–9.
13. Delewi R, van der Laan AM, Robbers LF, et al. Long term outcome after mononuclear bone marrow or peripheral blood cells infusion after myocardial infarction. Heart 2014 [pii:heartjnl-2014-305892]. [Epub ahead of print].
14. Vrtovec B, Poglajen G, Lezaic L, et al. Comparison of transendocardial and intracoronary CD34+ cell transplantation in patients with nonischemic dilated cardiomyopathy. Circulation 2013;128(11 Suppl 1): S42–9.
15. Orlic D, Kajstura J, Chimenti S, et al. Bone marrow cells regenerate infarcted myocardium. Nature 2001;410:701–5.
16. Zhang N, Li J, Luo R, et al. Bone marrow mesenchymal stem cells induce angiogenesis and attenuate the remodeling of diabetic cardiomyopathy. Exp Clin Endocrinol Diabetes 2008;116: 104–11.
17. Duong Van Huyen JP, Smadja DM, Bruneval P, et al. Bone marrow-derived mononuclear cell therapy induces distal angiogenesis after local injection in critical leg ischemia. Mod Pathol 2008;21:837–46.
18. Hamano K, Nishida M, Hirata K, et al. Local implantation of autologous bone marrow cells for therapeutic angiogenesis in patients with ischemic heart

disease: clinical trial and preliminary results. Jpn Circ J 2001;65:845–7.

19. Murry CE, Soonpaa MH, Reinecke H, et al. Haematopoietic stem cells do not transdifferentiate into cardiac myocytes in myocardial infarcts. Nature 2004; 428:664–8.

20. Perin EC, Silva GV, Henry TD, et al. A randomized study of transendocardial injection of autologous bone marrow mononuclear cells and cell function analysis in ischemic heart failure (FOCUS-HF). Am Heart J 2011;161:1078–87.e3.

21. Seeger FH, Tonn T, Krzossok N, et al. Cell isolation procedures matter: a comparison of different isolation protocols of bone marrow mononuclear cells used for cell therapy in patients with acute myocardial infarction. Eur Heart J 2007;28:766–72.

22. Abdel-Latif A, Bolli R, Tleyjeh IM, et al. Adult bone marrow-derived cells for cardiac repair: a systematic review and meta-analysis. Arch Intern Med 2007;167:989–97.

23. Matar AA, Chong JJ. Stem cell therapy for cardiac dysfunction. Springerplus 2014;3:440. http://dx.doi.org/10.1186/2193-1801-3-440.

24. Xiao C, Zhou S, Liu Y, et al. Efficacy and safety of bone marrow cell transplantation for chronic ischemic heart disease: a meta-analysis. Med Sci Monit 2014;20:1768–77.

25. Ledford KJ, Zeigler F, Bartel RL. Ixmyelocel-T, an expanded multicellular therapy, contains a unique population of M2-like macrophages. Stem Cell Res Ther 2013;4(6):134.

26. Henry TD, Traverse JH, Hammon BL, et al. Safety and efficacy of ixmyelocel-T: an expanded, autologous multi-cellular therapy, in dilated cardiomyopathy. Circ Res 2014;115(8):730–7.

27. Behfar A, Yamada S, Crespo-Diaz R, et al. Guided cardiopoiesis enhances therapeutic benefit of bone marrow human mesenchymal stem cells in chronic myocardial infarction. J Am Coll Cardiol 2010;56(9):721–34.

28. Bartunek J, Behfar A, Dolatabadi D, et al. Cardiopoietic stem cell therapy in heart failure: the C-CURE (Cardiopoietic stem Cell therapy in heart failURE) multicenter randomized trial with lineage-specified biologics. J Am Coll Cardiol 2013;61(23): 2329–38.

29. Narita T, Suzuki K. Bone marrow-derived mesenchymal stem cells for the treatment of heart failure. Heart Fail Rev 2015;20:53–68.

30. Lv FJ, Tuan RS, Cheung KM, et al. Concise review: the surface markers and identity of human mesenchymal stem cells. Stem Cells 2014;32(6): 1408–19.

31. Hare JM, Fishman JE, Gerstenblith G, et al. Comparison of allogeneic vs. autologous bone marrow-derived mesenchymal stem cells delivered by transendocardial injection in patients with ischemic cardiomyopathy: the POSEIDON randomized trial. JAMA 2012;308:2369–79.

32. Heldman AW, DiFede DL, Fishman JE, et al. Transendocardial mesenchymal stem cells and mononuclear bone marrow cells for ischemic cardiomyopathy: the TAC-HFT randomized trial. JAMA 2014;311(1):62–73.

33. Tano N, Narita T, Kaneko M, et al. Epicardial placement of mesenchymal stromal cell-sheets for the treatment of ischemic cardiomyopathy; in vivo proof-of-concept study. Mol Ther 2014;22(10): 1864–71.

34. Chen L, Qin F, Ge M, et al. Application of adipose-derived stem cells in heart disease. J Cardiovasc Transl Res 2014;7(7):651–63.

35. Perin EC, Sanz-Ruiz R, Sánchez PL, et al. Adipose-derived regenerative cells in patients with ischemic cardiomyopathy: the PRECISE Trial. Am Heart J 2014;168(1):88–95.e2.

36. Rigol M, Solanes N, Roura S, et al. Allogeneic adipose stem cell therapy in acute myocardial infarction. Eur J Clin Invest 2014;44(1):83–92.

37. Bockeria L, Bogin V, Bockeria O, et al. Endometrial regenerative cells for treatment of heart failure: a new stem cell enters the clinic. J Transl Med 2013; 11:56.

38. Passipieri JA, Kasai-Brunswick TH, Suhett G, et al. Improvement of cardiac function by placenta-derived mesenchymal stem cells does not require permanent engraftment and is independent of the insulin signaling pathway. Stem Cell Res Ther 2014;5(4):102.

39. Latifpour M, Nematollahi-Mahani SN, Deilamy M, et al. Improvement in cardiac function following transplantation of human umbilical cord matrix-derived mesenchymal cells. Cardiology 2011; 120(1):9–18.

40. Roura S, Gálvez-Montón C, Bayes-Genis A. Umbilical cord blood-derived mesenchymal stem cells: new therapeutic weapons for idiopathic dilated cardiomyopathy? Int J Cardiol 2014;177(3):809–18 [pii: S0167-5273(14) 01848-8].

41. Laugwitz KL, Moretti A, Lam J, et al. Postnatal isl1+ cardioblasts enter fully differentiated cardiomyocyte lineages. Nature 2005;433(7026):647–53.

42. Tang XL, Rokosh G, Sanganalmath SK, et al. Intracoronary administration of cardiac progenitor cells alleviates left ventricular dysfunction in rats with a 30-day-old infarction. Circulation 2010;121(2):293–305.

43. Chugh AR, Beache GM, Loughran JH, et al. Administration of cardiac stem cells in patients with ischemic cardiomyopathy: the SCIPIO trial: surgical aspects and interim analysis of myocardial function and viability by magnetic resonance. Circulation 2012;126(11 Suppl 1):S54–64.

44. Malliaras K, Zhang Y, Seinfeld J, et al. Cardiomyocyte proliferation and progenitor cell recruitment underlie therapeutic regeneration after myocardial

infarction in the adult mouse heart. EMBO Mol Med 2013;5(2):191–209.

45. Malliaras K, Makkar RR, Smith RR, et al. Intracoronary cardiosphere-derived cells after myocardial infarction: evidence of therapeutic regeneration in the final 1-year results of the CADUCEUS trial (CArdiosphere-Derived aUtologous stem CElls to reverse ventricUlar dySfunction). J Am Coll Cardiol 2014; 63(2):110–22.

46. Tseliou E, Pollan S, Malliaras K, et al. Allogeneic cardiospheres safely boost cardiac function and attenuate adverse remodeling after myocardial infarction in immunologically mismatched rat strains. J Am Coll Cardiol 2013;61(10):1108–19.

47. Chong JJ, Yang X, Don CW, et al. Human embryonic-stem-cell-derived cardiomyocytes regenerate non-human primate hearts. Nature 2014;510(7504):273–7.

48. Christoforou N, Liau B, Chakraborty S, et al. Induced pluripotent stem cell-derived cardiac progenitors differentiate to cardiomyocytes and form biosynthetic tissues. PLoS One 2013;8(6):e65963.

49. Masumoto H, Ikuno T, Takeda M, et al. Human iPS cell-engineered cardiac tissue sheets with cardiomyocytes and vascular cells for cardiac regeneration. Sci Rep 2014;4:6716.

50. Anderson ME, Goldhaber J, Houser SR, et al. Embryonic stem cell-derived cardiac myocytes are not ready for human trials. Circ Res 2014;115(3):335–8.

51. Menasché P, Vanneaux V, Fabreguettes JR, et al. Towards a clinical use of human embryonic stem cell-derived cardiac progenitors: a translational experience. Eur Heart J 2014 [pii:ehu192].

52. Mirotsou M, Jayawardena TM, Schmeckpeper J, et al. Paracrine mechanisms of stem cell reparative and regenerative actions in the heart. J Mol Cell Cardiol 2011;50(2):280–9.

53. Chou SH, Lin SZ, Kuo WW, et al. Mesenchymal stem cell insights: prospects in cardiovascular therapy. Cell Transplant 2014;23(4–5):513–29.

54. Hastings CL, Roche ET, Ruiz-Hernandez E, et al. Drug and cell delivery for cardiac regeneration. Adv Drug Deliv Rev 2014. http://dx.doi.org/10.1016/j.addr.2014.08.0062014 [pii:S0169–S0409X(14)00180-X].

55. Dib N, Khawaja H, Varner S, et al. Cell therapy for cardiovascular disease: a comparison of methods of delivery. J Cardiovasc Transl Res 2011;4:177–81.

56. Dib N, Menasche P, Bartunek JJ, et al. Recommendations for successful training on methods of delivery of biologics for cardiac regeneration: a report of the International Society for Cardiovascular Translational Research. JACC Cardiovasc Interv 2010;3: 265–75.

57. Patel AN, Geffner L, Vina RF, et al. Surgical treatment for congestive heart failure with autologous adult stem cell transplantation: a prospective randomized study. J Thorac Cardiovasc Surg 2005; 130:1631–8.

58. Thompson RB, Parsa CJ, van den Bos EJ, et al. Video-assisted thoracoscopic transplantation of myoblasts into the heart. Ann Thorac Surg 2004; 78(1):303–7.

59. Donndorf P, Kaminski A, Steinhoff G, et al. Transvalvular intramyocardial bone marrow stem cell transplantation in combination with videoscopic mitral valve repair. Interact Cardiovasc Thorac Surg 2010;11(6):806–8.

60. Reyes G, Allen KB, Alvarez P, et al. Mid term results after bone marrow laser revascularization for treating refractory angina. BMC Cardiovasc Disord 2010;10:42.

61. Ascheim DD, Gelijns AC, Goldstein D, et al. Mesenchymal precursor cells as adjunctive therapy in recipients of contemporary left ventricular assist devices. Circulation 2014;129(22):2287–96.

62. Perin EC, Silva GV. Autologous cell-based therapy for ischemic heart disease: clinical evidence, proposed mechanisms of action, and current limitations. Catheter Cardiovasc Interv 2009;73:281–8.

63. Perin EC, Silva GV, Willerson JT. Training on the use of transendocardial delivery of biologics for cardiac regeneration. JACC Cardiovasc Interv 2010;3:991.

64. Kumar A, Haralampus CA, Hughes M, et al. Assessment of safety, accuracy, and human CD34+ cell retention after intramyocardial injections with a helical needle catheter in a porcine model. Catheter Cardiovasc Interv 2013;81(6):970–7.

65. Suncion VY, Ghersin E, Fishman JE, et al. Does transendocardial injection of mesenchymal stem cells improve myocardial function locally or globally?: An analysis from the percutaneous stem cell injection delivery effects on neomyogenesis (POSEIDON) randomized trial. Circ Res 2014; 114(8):1292–301.

66. Behfar A, Latere JP, Bartunek J, et al. Optimized delivery system achieves enhanced endomyocardial stem cell retention. Circ Cardiovasc Interv 2013; 6(6):710–8.

67. Fischer-Rasokat U, Assmus B, Seeger FH, et al. A pilot trial to assess potential effects of selective intracoronary bone marrow-derived progenitor cell infusion in patients with nonischemic dilated cardiomyopathy: final 1-year results of the transplantation of progenitor cells and functional regeneration enhancement pilot trial in patients with nonischemic dilated cardiomyopathy. Circ Heart Fail 2009;2(5): 417–23.

68. Diederichsen AC, Moller JE, Thayssen P, et al. Effect of repeated intracoronary injection of bone marrow cells in patients with ischaemic heart failure the Danish stem cell study– congestive heart failure trial (DanCell-CHF). Eur J Heart Fail 2008;10:661–7.

69. Epstein SE, Stabile E, Timothy K, et al. Janus phenomenon: the interrelated tradeoffs inherent in

therapies designed to enhance collateral formation and those designed to inhibit angiogenesis. Circulation 2004;109:2826–31.

70. Kang HJ, Kim HS, Zhang SY, et al. Effects of intracoronary infusion of peripheral blood stem-cells mobilised with granulocyte-colony stimulating factor on left ventricular systolic function and restenosis after coronary stenting in myocardial infarction: the MAGIC cell randomised clinical trial. Lancet 2004; 363:751–6.

71. Mansour S, Vanderheyden M, De Bruyne B, et al. Intracoronary delivery of hematopoietic bone marrow stem cells and luminal loss of the infarct-related artery in patients with recent myocardial infarction. J Am Coll Cardiol 2006;47:1727–30.

72. Widimsky P, Penicka M. Complications after intracoronary stem cell transplantation in idiopathic dilated cardiomyopathy. Int J Cardiol 2006;111: 178–9.

73. Thompson CA. Transvascular cellular cardiomyoplasty. Int J Cardiol 2004;95(Suppl 1):S47–9.

74. Forest VF, Tirouvanziam AM, Perigaud C, et al. Cell distribution after intracoronary bone marrow stem cell delivery in damaged and undamaged myocardium: implications for clinical trials. Stem Cell Res Ther 2010;1:4.

75. Hare JM, Traverse JH, Henry TD, et al. A randomized, double-blind, placebo-controlled, dose-escalation study of intravenous adult human mesenchymal stem cells (prochymal) after acute myocardial infarction. J Am Coll Cardiol 2009;54: 2277–86.

76. Siminiak T, Lipiecki J. Trans-coronary-venous interventions. Circ Cardiovasc Interv 2008;1:134–42.

77. Mohl W, Mina S, Milasinovic D, et al. The legacy of coronary sinus interventions: endogenous cardioprotection and regeneration beyond stem cell research. J Thorac Cardiovasc Surg 2008;136: 1131–5.

78. Giordano FJ. Retrograde coronary perfusion: a superior route to deliver therapeutics to the heart? J Am Coll Cardiol 2003;42:1129–31.

79. Yokoyama S, Fukuda N, Li Y, et al. A strategy of retrograde injection of bone marrow mononuclear cells into the myocardium for the treatment of ischemic heart disease. J Mol Cell Cardiol 2006; 40:24–34.

80. Muller WA. Mechanisms of transendothelial migration of leukocytes. Circ Res 2009;105:223–30.

81. Tuma J, Fernández-Viña R, Carrasco A, et al. Safety and feasibility of percutaneous retrograde coronary sinus delivery of autologous bone marrow mononuclear cell transplantation in patients with chronic refractory angina. J Transl Med 2011;9:183.

82. Malliaras K, Marbán E. Moving beyond surrogate endpoints in cell therapy trials for heart disease. Stem Cells Transl Med 2014;3(1):2–6.

83. Zannad F, Garcia AA, Anker SD, et al. Clinical outcome endpoints in heart failure trials: a European Society of Cardiology Heart Failure Association consensus document. Eur J Heart Fail 2013; 15(10):1082–94.

84. Zsebo K, Yaroshinsky A, Rudy JJ, et al. Long-term effects of AAV1/SERCA2a gene transfer in patients with severe heart failure: analysis of recurrent cardiovascular events and mortality. Circ Res 2014; 114(1):101–8.

85. Pokushalov E, Romanov A, Chernyavsky A, et al. Efficiency of intramyocardial injections of autologous bone marrow mononuclear cells in patients with ischemic heart failure: a randomized study. J Cardiovasc Transl Res 2010;3(2):160–8.

86. Pätilä T, Lehtinen M, Vento A, et al. Autologous bone marrow mononuclear cell transplantation in ischemic heart failure: a prospective, controlled, randomized, double-blind study of cell transplantation combined with coronary bypass. J Heart Lung Transplant 2014;33(6):567–74.

87. Donndorf P, Kaminski A, Tiedemann G, et al. Validating intramyocardial bone marrow stem cell therapy in combination with coronary artery bypass grafting, the PERFECT Phase III randomized multicenter trial: study protocol for a randomized controlled trial. Trials 2012;13:99.

88. Karantalis V, DiFede DL, Gerstenblith G, et al. Autologous mesenchymal stem cells produce concordant improvements in regional function, tissue perfusion, and fibrotic burden when administered to patients undergoing coronary artery bypass grafting: The Prospective Randomized Study of Mesenchymal Stem Cell Therapy in Patients Undergoing Cardiac Surgery (PROMETHEUS) trial. Circ Res 2014;114(8):1302–10.

89. Mathiasen AB, Jørgensen E, Qayyum AA, et al. Rationale and design of the first randomized, doubleblind, placebo-controlled trial of intramyocardial injection of autologous bone-marrow derived Mesenchymal Stromal Cells in chronic ischemic Heart Failure (MSC-HF Trial). Am Heart J 2012; 164(3):285–91.

Cardiac Resynchronization Therapy: Past, Present, and Future

Neal A. Chatterjee, MD[a], Jagmeet P. Singh, MD, DPhil[b],*

KEYWORDS

- Cardiac resynchronization therapy • Heart failure • Electrical dyssynchrony • Biventricular pacing

KEY POINTS

- Cardiac resynchronization therapy (CRT) has revolutionized the care of patients with heart failure and electrical dyssynchrony.
- CRT fundamentally modifies the natural history of the pathologic ventricle, improves patient symptoms and functional capacity, and incrementally improves survival beyond optimized medical therapy.
- Ongoing studies will identify expanding populations who may benefit from CRT and further identify novel pacing approaches and technologies that augment the efficacy of resynchronization.
- Consensus efforts toward defining the response to CRT, earlier identification of those at risk for nonresponse, and enhancing implantation rates in those meeting contemporary guideline indications will only improve the delivery and effectiveness of CRT in our patients.

Videos of unipolar isochrones assessed via noncontact mapping, cardiac computed tomography kinematics to reflect mechanical activation pattern, and modalities of coronary vein assessment accompany this article at http://www.heartfailure.theclinics.com/

INTRODUCTION

Cardiac resynchronization therapy (CRT), or biventricular pacing, has become a standard therapeutic modality for patients with symptomatic heart failure (HF), depressed left ventricular (LV) function, and electrical dyssynchrony.[1,2] Resynchronization of the failing ventricle leads to improvement in mechanical pumping efficiency, reduction in mitral regurgitation, and optimization of ventricular filling. Over time, CRT facilitates favorable remodeling of the ventricle, characterized by reductions in LV volumes and improvement in ejection fraction, which in turn translates to significant improvement in quality of life, functional capacity, and survival.[3–7] In the nearly 20 years of clinical implementation,[8] the deployment of CRT has catalyzed cooperation and integration of multiple fields of cardiology, including HF, electrophysiology, and cardiovascular imaging.[9]

Despite the overall success of CRT in improving morbidity and mortality in selected patients with HF, a significant minority demonstrates nonresponse. This review describes the electrical and physiologic rationale for biventricular pacing therapy, summarizes landmark clinical trials assessing CRT efficacy, highlights strategies to optimize the response to CRT, and frames future

[a] Cardiology Division, Department of Medicine, Massachusetts General Hospital, Harvard Medical School, 55 Fruit Street, Boston, MA 02114, USA; [b] Harvard Medical School, Cardiology Division, Electrophysiology Laboratory, Cardiac Arrhythmia Service, Department of Medicine, Massachusetts General Hospital, Harvard Medical School, 55 Fruit Street, Boston, MA 02114, USA
* Corresponding author.
E-mail address: JSINGH@mgh.harvard.edu

Heart Failure Clin 11 (2015) 287–303
http://dx.doi.org/10.1016/j.hfc.2014.12.007
1551-7136/15/$ – see front matter © 2015 Elsevier Inc. All rights reserved.

challenges in the use, delivery, and care of patients undergoing CRT.

ELECTRICAL DYSSYNCHRONY AND THE FAILING HEART: IMPACT OF CARDIAC RESYNCHRONIZATION THERAPY

The coordinated electrical activation of the heart is a critical determinant of coordinated mechanical contraction, myocardial relaxation, and mechanical efficiency.[10] Approximately half of all patients with LV systolic dysfunction (LVSD) demonstrate evidence of electrical conduction delay.[11–13] Although primary abnormalities of the electrical conduction system yield dyssynchronous ventricular activation that diminishes cardiac function,[14] pathobiologic changes underlying cardiomyopathy (eg, myocyte hypertrophy, inflammation, fibrosis, electrical remodeling[15]) as well as additional myocardial characteristics (eg, scar, ischemia) can also affect the ventricular conduction system.

Late-activated segments of myocardium (eg, the lateral wall in patients with left bundle branch block [LBBB]) demonstrate unique metabolic, transcriptional, and electrical signatures of dyssynchrony[16] characterized, for example, by pathologic changes in mitochondrial function,[17,18] abnormalities of calcium handling,[19,20] and alteration in action potential duration.[19] Asynchronous ventricular activation is associated with a localized increase in myocardial work, heterogeneity of myocardial blood flow, increased oxygen consumption, and reduced mechanical pumping efficiency as late-activated segments are passively stretched early in systole and early activated segments are relaxing and stretched at the time of late segment activation (**Fig. 1**).[20–23] To the extent that biventricular pacing reverses underlying electrical dyssynchrony, CRT restores coordinated mechanical contraction with related improvements in cardiac function. These mechanical improvements are mirrored by normalization of subcellular dysfunction ranging from improved calcium handling, upregulation of cell

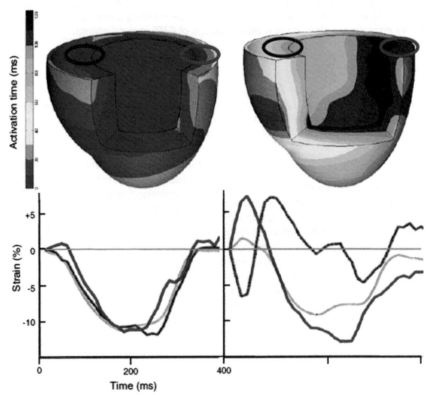

Fig. 1. Electrical and mechanical dyssynchrony in LBBB. Colorimetric representation of electrical activation (*upper panels*) and mechanical strain (*lower panels*) in a normal (*left panels*) versus LBBB (*right panels*) canine heart. Compared with the normal heart, in the LBBB heart there is early electrical activation of the septum (*right upper panel, blue circle*) correlating to early mechanical shortening of the septum (*right lower panel*). In addition, there is relatively delayed electrical activation of the lateral LV wall (*right upper panel, red circle*), which is mechanically stretched during early systole (*right lower panel, red tracing*) with subsequent shortening in late systole. (*Adapted from* Prinzen FW, Vernooy K, De Boeck BW, et al. Mechano-energetics of the asynchronous and resynchronized heart. Heart Fail Rev 2011;16:216; with permission.)

surface β-receptor expression, shortening of the action potential duration, and mitochondrial energetics.[16,19,24] In contrast to other HF therapies that enhance systolic function (eg, inotropes), CRT improves cardiac function without an associated increase in myocardium oxygen consumption (ie, CRT improves myocardial energetic efficiency).[10,25]

LANDMARK TRIALS IN CARDIAC RESYNCHRONIZATION THERAPY
Severe Heart Failure

The first large-scale comparison of CRT efficacy was the MUSTIC (Multisite Stimulation in Cardiomyopathy) trial in which 67 patients with New York Heart Association (NYHA) class III HF in sinus rhythm and electrical dyssynchrony (QRS >150 milliseconds) underwent single-blind randomized controlled crossover with 3 months of inactive versus biventricular pacing.[26] CRT was associated with significant improvement in 6-minute walk distance (6MWD), quality-of-life scores, and peak oxygen consumption (pVO$_2$) as well as a significant reduction in HF hospitalizations. The first double-blind randomized controlled comparison of CRT occurred in the MIRACLE (Multicenter In-Sync Randomized Clinical Evaluation) trial, which compared optimal medical therapy (OMT) with OMT plus CRT in 453 patients with severe HF (NYHA III/IV), LVSD (LV ejection fraction [LVEF] ≤35%), and electrical dyssynchrony (QRS ≥130 milliseconds).[3] CRT demonstrated improvement in functional capacity and symptoms (6MWD, NYHA class, quality of life) as well as reversal of pathologic remodeling (LVEF improvement, LV diastolic dimension reduction, mitral regurgitation reduction) at 6-month follow-up. There was a 40% reduction in the composite end point of death or HF hospitalization driven by a significant reduction in HF hospitalization. In a similar comparison of CRT pacing (CRT-P) + OMT versus OMT, the CARE-HF (Cardiac Resynchronization on Morbidity and Mortality in Heart Failure) trial demonstrated improvements in quality of life, LV reverse remodeling, and reduction in HF hospitalization in patients with severe HF (NYHA III/IV), systolic dysfunction (LVEF ≤35%), and electrical dyssynchrony (QRS >120 milliseconds).[5] Unlike previous trials, patients with borderline electrical dyssynchrony (QRS 120–150 milliseconds) were additionally required to demonstrate evidence of mechanical dyssynchrony. Over longer-term follow-up (30 months) in CARE-HF, CRT-P was associated with a 40% reduction in the composite endpoint of death and HF hospitalization as well as a 36% reduction in all-cause mortality.[27]

Coincident with the initial demonstration of CRT efficacy was the proliferation of evidence supporting the efficacy of implantable cardioverter-defibrillator (ICD) therapy in the primary prevention of sudden death in patients with systolic HF.[28–30] The COMPANION (Comparison of Medical Therapy, Pacing and Defibrillation in Heart Failure) trial was the largest study to compare the efficacy of OMT with that of CRT-P and CRT with ICD (CRT-D).[4] In a 1:2:2 ratio, the trial randomized 1520 patients with advanced LVSD (LVEF ≤35%, NYHA III/IV) and wide QRS (>120 milliseconds) to OMT, CRT-P, or CRT-D. Compared with OMT, both CRT-P and CRT-D significantly reduced the risk of death or HF hospitalization by approximately 20%. Similarly, both CRT-P and CRT-D reduced the hazard of all-cause mortality (24% and 36%, respectively), although the reduction in mortality was only of borderline significance for CRT-P. Comparison between CRT-P and CRT-D was not prespecified in COMPANION; to date, there remains no direct comparison of CRT-D and CRT-P therapy.

Mild Heart Failure

Initial support for the efficacy of CRT in patients with less severe HF was framed by the CONTAK-CD (Cardiac Resynchronization Therapy for the Treatment of Heart Failure Patients with Intraventricular Conduction Delay and Malignant Ventricular Tachyarrhythmias)[31] and MIRACLE ICD-II[32] trials, which included patients with NYHA II symptoms and showed favorable reverse remodeling in the subgroup of patients with mild HF. The efficacy of CRT in patients with mildly symptomatic HF was subsequently demonstrated in a series of large-scale randomized comparisons (REVERSE [Resynchronization Reverse Remodeling in Systolic Left Ventricular Dysfunction], MADIT-CRT [Multicenter Automatic Defibrillator Implantation Trial with Cardiac Resynchronization Therapy], RAFT [Resynchronization/Defibrillation for Ambulatory Heart Failure Trial]).[6,7,33]

In the REVERSE study, 610 patients with LVSD (LVEF <40%), electrical dyssynchrony (QRS ≥120 milliseconds), and mild HF (NYHA II or NYHA I with previous HF symptoms) were randomized to biventricular therapy.[33] Although CRT did not reduce the primary end point (composite of HF hospitalization, worsening NYHA class, quality-of-life score), CRT was associated with significant LV reverse remodeling (reductions in LV volume, improvement in LVEF) as well as a 50% reduction in HF hospitalization over the 1-year follow-up. The subsequently reported MADIT-CRT trial randomized 1820 patients with minimally or mildly symptomatic HF (NYHA II or NYHA I with an ischemic cause of HF), systolic dysfunction (LVEF <30%) and electrical dyssynchrony (QRS >130 milliseconds) to either CRT-D or ICD.[6] Over more than 2 years of follow-up, CRT was associated with a 34% reduction in the composite end point of death or incident symptomatic HF, driven primarily by a significant reduction in HF events. More recently, the RAFT study randomized 1798 patients to either CRT-D or ICD and examined a primary composite outcome of death or HF over 3.3 years of follow-up.[7] Subjects were required to have mild to moderately symptomatic HF (NYHA II/III), LVEF of 30% or less, and QRS greater than 120 milliseconds (or paced QRS >200 milliseconds). In all patients, CRT was associated with significant reduction in the primary outcome of death/HF hospitalization (25% risk reduction), which was driven both by reductions in HF hospitalization (30% risk reduction) as well as mortality (25% risk reduction; absolute incidence: 26.1% vs 20.8%, $P = .003$). In summary, in patients with mildly symptomatic HF, CRT is associated with substantial LV reverse remodeling and a 30% to 50% risk reduction in HF hospitalization. The RAFT study was the only study of those in mild HF to demonstrate a significant reduction in all-cause mortality, likely reflecting the relative incidence of mortality in RAFT (NYAH II/III patients; placebo group mortality: 21%) compared with trials inclusive of NYHA I patients (MADIT-CRT, REVERSE) in which the mortality was significantly lower (placebo group mortality: 2%–7%) and the follow-up time was shorter.

Narrow QRS and Mechanical Dyssynchrony: Futility of Cardiac Resynchronization Therapy

Following the successful demonstration of LV reverse remodeling and significant reduction of HF morbidity and mortality in patients with LVSD and wide QRS, there was interest in examining the efficacy of CRT in patients with narrow QRS.[34] In particular, given the potential imprecision of the surface QRS to identify asynchronous ventricular contraction, several smaller studies identified the presence of mechanical dyssynchrony in patients with relatively narrow QRS as a predictor of response to CRT.[34,35] The efficacy of CRT in patients with narrow QRS was subsequently examined in a series of larger randomized comparisons (RethinQ [Cardiac Resynchronization Therapy in Patients with Heart Failure and Narrow QRS], LESSER-EARTH [Evaluation of Resynchronization Therapy for Heart Failure], ECHO-CRT [Echocardiography Guided Cardiac Resynchronization Therapy]), all of which showed

no benefit and some of which were terminated prematurely given possible harm.[36–38] The RethinQ study enrolled 250 patients with advanced HF (NYHA III), systolic dysfunction (LVEF ≤35%), and standard indication for ICD. Patients had a QRS less than 130 milliseconds with echocardiographic evidence of mechanical dyssynchrony as assessed by tissue Doppler imaging (TDI).[36] At the 6-month follow-up, there was no difference in the primary end point of pVO$_2$ or LV reverse remodeling associated with CRT therapy. In LESSER-EARTH, patients with symptomatic HF, LVEF of 35% or less, and a narrow QRS (<120 milliseconds) were randomized to CRT-on versus CRT-off.[38] The trial was terminated early because of demonstrable futility and a trend to increased HF hospitalization associated with CRT. Following the neutral result of RethinQ and LESSER-EARTH, some suggested that more definitive assessment of CRT in narrow QRS would require use of hard clinical end points (as opposed to surrogates, such as oxygen consumption) and more rigorously defined metrics of mechanical dyssynchrony. In particular, the tissue Doppler–based criterion for dyssynchrony used in RethinQ was questioned as the optimal method for assessment given its inability to distinguish between passive myocardial motion versus active contraction as well as limitations of resolution. Alternative methods of dyssynchrony assessment, including speckle tracking, which directly measures strain along longitudinal, circumferential, and radial axes, had been shown to predict the response to CRT in smaller studies (**Fig. 2**).[39,40] These data framed the design of the recently reported ECHO-CRT study, which assessed the efficacy of CRT in patients with moderate to severe HF (NYHA III/IV), LVSD, and narrow QRS (QRS <130 milliseconds) with evidence of mechanical dyssynchrony as defined by TDI or by means of speckle-tracking radial strain delay.[37] Similar to LESSER-EARTH, the study was terminated early on account of futility with respect to the primary end point (composite of death/HF) as well as a significant increase in mortality associated with CRT therapy (11.0% vs 6.4%) over 20 months before study closure.

The failure of contemporary echocardiographic dyssynchrony parameters to predict the CRT response in patients with narrow QRS was similarly identified in patients meeting the standard indications for CRT.[41] In the prospective, nonrandomized PROSPECT (Predictors of Response to CRT) study, 498 patients with standard indications for CRT (including QRS ≥130 milliseconds) underwent baseline echocardiographic assessment including multiple metrics of mechanical dyssynchrony. Using a rigorous composite

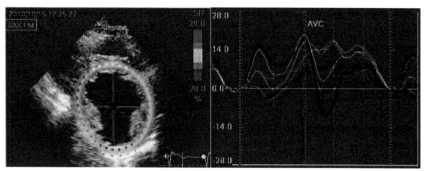

Fig. 2. Speckle-tracking strain imaging. Shown in the left panel are representative 2-dimensional strain images. The right panel demonstrates temporal strain curves of LV myocardial segments relative to aortic valve closure (AVC). The time differences in peak systolic strain between segments are assessed in the determination of mechanical dyssynchrony. (*Adapted from* Singh JP, Gras D. Biventricular pacing: current trends and future strategies. Eur Heart J 2012;33:307; with permission.)

outcome of clinical and echocardiographic response, no single echocardiographic parameter predicted either clinical or echocardiographic response to CRT. The failure of standard echocardiographic parameters to identify the CRT response may reflect the heterogeneous factors that contribute to mechanical dyssynchrony beyond electrical dyssynchrony, including abnormalities of myocardial perfusion, viability, and relaxation, all of which may not be directly addressed by biventricular pacing. Furthermore, the impact of LV lead location and device programming may further add to the heterogeneity of response, thereby further impacting the predictive role of a baseline echocardiographic measure of dyssynchrony. Whether or not imaging modalities (eg, 3-dimensional [3D] ultrasound, computed tomography [CT], or MRI)[42–44] that can integrate measures of dyssynchrony with the presence of scar and coronary venous anatomy offer incremental value in patient selection remains to be determined in larger prospective analyses (Video 1). Early work is promising; for example, a recent single-center study of 75 patients used MRI-based determination of dyssynchrony (global and circumferential strain) coupled with scar localization to identify patients at significant risk of nonresponse.[42]

Chronic Right Ventricular Pacing

Right ventricular (RV) apical pacing is associated with asynchronous activation of the left ventricle. Chronic RV apical pacing has been associated an increased risk of HF hospitalization, atrial fibrillation (AF), and incident LVSD.[45–47] Although patients with chronic RV pacing have been historically underrepresented in landmark CRT trials, given the implications of chronic RV apical pacing

in patients with systolic HF, the current North American guidelines recommend biventricular pacing therapy in patients with LVEF of 35% or less who are undergoing a new or replacement device with anticipated requirement for significant (>40%) ventricular pacing.[2] The more recently reported BLOCK-HF (Biventricular vs Right Ventricular Pacing in Heart Failure Patients with Atrioventricular Block) study enrolled 691 patients with standard indications for pacing caused by atrio-ventricular (A-V) pacing, LVEF of 50% or less, and HF (NYHA I-III).[48] Approximately one-third of patients met the criteria for ICD implantation. Biventricular pacing was associated with a significant (26%) reduction in a composite end point of death and HF, driven primarily by a reduction in HF hospitalization. This benefit accrued to both patients with mildly versus significantly depressed LVEF. In contrast, the recently completed BIOPACE (Biventricular Pacing for Atrioventricular Block to Prevent Cardiac Desynchronization) study failed to show the benefit of biventricular pacing over RV pacing in patients with a preserved LVEF.[49]

DEFINING RESPONSE: CLINICAL VERSUS ECHOCARDIOGRAPHIC RESPONSE

With the expanding indication and use of CRT to treat patients with HF, there has been increasing focus on maximizing the response to biventricular pacing. With this focus has come significant heterogeneity in the definition of response, which has included metrics of ventricular reverse remodeling, improvement in functional capacity or symptoms, and reduction in clinical end points, such as HF hospitalization or mortality.[50] Some have even argued that the spectrum of response and nonresponse is to be expected following any therapy, and the application of a nonresponse metric is inappropriately applied to device therapy.[51] In the most elegant and comprehensive analysis to date, Fornwalt and colleagues[52] applied 17 echocardiographic and clinical criteria for a CRT response to the PROSPECT study population. The investigators used a method of analysis known as κ-coefficient to assess the difference between the actual agreement between 2 response criteria compared with the expected agreement caused by chance alone. Among the echocardiographic response criteria agreement was poor (mean κ = 0.35), whereas among the clinical response criteria response agreement was only moderate (mean κ = 0.44). Of striking note, agreement between the echocardiographic and clinical criteria was poor (mean κ = 0.05), suggesting that the agreement was nearly no better than chance alone. Others have shown that short-term LV reverse remodeling, but not clinical improvement, predicts long-term survival in CRT.[53] There are additionally a subset of patients who demonstrate so-called super-response following CRT as defined by significant improvement in LVEF (>10%–15%) or reductions in LV volumes (>20%–30% reduction).[54,55] In this population, there is a more clear relationship with improved long-term clinical outcomes (mortality/HF hospitalization) as shown in the MADIT-CRT population.[54] To date, there remains no standardized definition to response to CRT, though the authors would favor a composite of short-term echocardiographic reverse remodeling as well as longer-term clinical outcomes, including survival and HF hospitalization.

MAXIMIZING RESPONSE

Notwithstanding the heterogeneous definitions of nonresponse, approximately one-third of patients will demonstrate a lack of echocardiographic reverse remodeling or poor clinical outcome following CRT. Given the substantial morbidity and mortality associated with HF and the significant associated health care costs,[56] there has been increasing focus on maximizing the response to CRT. The authors review the role for optimal patient selection, procedural strategies at the time of lead implantation, as well as optimizing postimplant care in patients undergoing CRT.

Patient Selection: QRS Duration, Morphology and Beyond

To date, wide QRS duration has been used as the gold standard identification of patients in whom ventricular asynchrony could be ameliorated by LV pacing. During CRT, the RV and LV leads generate 2 ventricular wave fronts and the benefit of CRT turns on the effective fusion of these wave fronts, synchronizing the contraction of the ventricles. For example, in patients with LBBB, seminal work from Auricchio and colleagues[57] demonstrated that the LV activation wave front initiates anteriorly and then courses inferiorly toward the apex (around a proposed functional line of block) before propagating to the basal posterior/posterolateral segment of the LV (Video 2). Given that this pattern of electrical activation is associated with delayed mechanical activation of the posterior basal lateral wall, targeting this region for LV pacing has been the intuitive approach standardly used in CRT. In contrast to LBBB, patients with a right bundle branch block (RBBB) or nonspecific intraventricular conduction delay (IVCD) do not share similar activation patterns and may, therefore, not benefit as much from CRT.[58] Of important note, there is substantial heterogeneity of activation wave fronts within bundle branch type that may be further modified by substrate phenotype, including myocardial scar and inflammation. For example, a significant minority of patients with LBBB demonstrates normal or near-normal LV endocardial activation times, and prolongation of QRS duration may be related to prolonged intramural activation time or the underlying myopathic process.[59] Alternatively, some patients with RBBB or IVCD (particularly those with very wide QRS >150 milliseconds) demonstrate prolonged LV activation times that may respond to biventricular pacing.[58,60]

Understanding the electrical pathophysiology and rationale for CRT frames the most recent North American guidelines for CRT therapy restricting a class I recommendation only for patients with LBBB and a QRS of 150 milliseconds or greater.[2] Meta-analysis of several landmark trials (COMPANION, CARE-HF, REVERSE, MADIT-CRT, RAFT) suggested that significant reduction of composite clinical events was present only in patients with a baseline QRS of 150 milliseconds or greater (40% risk reduction, P<.001) but not those with a QRS less than 150 milliseconds (5% risk reduction, P = .49).[61] A continuous (as opposed to dichotomized) approach to analysis identified a continuous relationship and benefit between lengthening the QRS duration and echocardiographic remodeling[62] as well as clinical outcome,[63] although these relationships were identified only in patients with an LBBB (Fig. 3). Indeed, recent meta-analyses suggest that the clinical benefit of CRT may only accrue to patients with LBBB and not to those with IVCD or RBBB.[64] For example, in patients with LBBB undergoing CRT, there was a significant

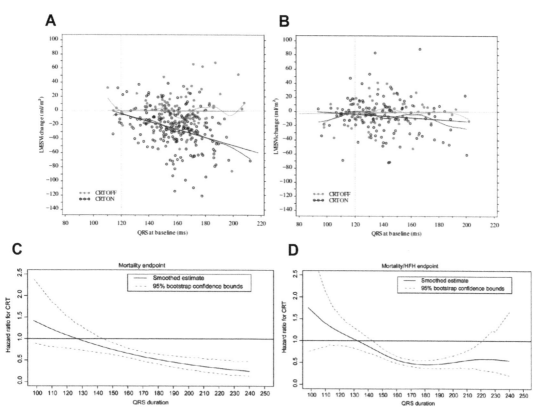

Fig. 3. QRS duration and CRT response. (*A*, *B*): Shown is the continuous relationship between QRS duration and absolute change in LV systolic volume index (LVESVi) with CRT-ON versus CRT-OFF in patients with LBBB (*A*) and non-LBBB (*B*) for patients in the REVERSE trial. (*C*, *D*): Shown is the relationship between QRS duration and mortality (*C*) and a composite of mortality and HF hospitalization (HFH) (*D*) in meta-analysis of CRT trials. The 95% confidence intervals intersect the line of unity at a QRS duration of ~140 milliseconds for each end point suggesting a benefit in patients with QRS duration wider than 140 milliseconds. (*Adapted from* [*A*, *B*] Cleland JG, Abraham WT, Linde C, et al. An individual patient meta-analysis of five randomized trials assessing the effects of cardiac resynchronization therapy on morbidity and mortality in patients with symptomatic heart failure. Eur Heart J 2013;34:3553; and [*C*, *D*] Gold MR, Thebault C, Linde C, et al. Effect of QRS duration and morphology on cardiac resynchronization therapy outcomes in mild heart failure: results from the Resynchronization Reverses Remodeling in Systolic Left Ventricular Dysfunction (REVERSE) study. Circulation 2012;126:826; with permission.)

40% reduction in composite clinical events, whereas no such benefit was identified in patients with non-LBBB morphology (relative risk: 0.97, P = .75).[64]

In addition to QRS morphology and duration, there are several other baseline clinical features that may influence the response to CRT. In AF, there is loss of A-V synchrony as well as suboptimal effective biventricular capture on account of irregular and high ventricular rates leading to fusion, pseudofusion, or loss of fusion. Given the coincidence of AF and HF, the impact of AF on CRT efficacy is of substantial importance. Previous meta-analyses suggest attenuated efficacy of CRT in patients with AF when compared with those in sinus rhythm.[65,66] A recent subanalysis of patients with AF enrolled in the RAFT trial showed that, although CRT did reduce HF

hospitalization (40% risk reduction), it had no influence on cardiovascular death (hazard ratio: 0.97, 95% confidence intervals: 0.55–1.71, P = .91).[67] In the largest registry to date, Gasparini and colleagues[68] report that atrio-ventricular (A-V) junction ablation at the time of CRT in patients with AF led to improved outcomes, a finding that was similarly suggested in a recent meta-analysis.[69] The role for this approach remains to be assessed in a larger prospective randomized fashion.

In addition to QRS duration and AF, several other factors have been shown to influence the efficacy of CRT, including medical comorbidities (chronic renal insufficiency),[70,71] hemodynamic abnormalities (precapillary pulmonary hypertension),[72] and abnormalities of LV substrate (nonrevascularized coronary artery disease, myocardial scar).[73,74] There has also been a suggestion that women may benefit from CRT more so than men, particularly in patients with LBBB and even at a QRS duration less than 150 milliseconds.[75,76] Whether these factors only attenuate the efficacy of CRT versus obviate the benefit of biventricular pacing remains to be assessed in future prospective studies.

Intraprocedural Strategies: Lead Targeting, Alternative Implantation Approaches

The conventional approach to implantation of the LV lead is via a transvenous approach targeting the lateral or posterolateral location within a second- or third-order branch of the coronary sinus veins (**Fig. 4**, Video 3). This strategy reflects the intuitive and expected pattern of delayed electrical and mechanical activation of the lateral and posterolateral wall, particularly in patients with LBBB. Placement of the LV lead can be challenged by the heterogeneity of coronary sinus venous anatomy.[44,77] The response to CRT is often variable even when the LV lead is placed in this optimal anatomic position,[78] reflecting the complex interaction of myocardial substrate (eg, scar), heterogeneity of ventricular wave front activation even within similar QRS duration or bundle branch morphology, as well as RV pacing-induced shifts in LV activation. Anatomically, placement of the LV lead can be organized along the long and short axes (**Fig. 4**). Placement of the

LV lead in an apical position seems to confer an increased risk of poor clinical outcome compared with nonapical locations likely reflecting the absence of electrical delay at apical locations in patients undergoing CRT (ie, wave front activation of the apex occurs relatively early in ventricular depolarization).[79]

Beyond anatomic targeting, alternative approaches include identification of regions of maximal electrical delay,[80,81] maximal mechanical delay,[21,40,42] or lead positions that maximize hemodynamic improvement.[82] Given that CRT is a form of electrical therapy for patients with abnormalities of electrical conduction, it remains intuitive that targeting the site of latest electrical activation may yield an optimal CRT response. Although the site of latest electrical delay has been identified using various methods, including 3D noncontact endocardial mapping,[83] a more practical strategy has been the use of intracardiac electrograms to measure the delay between the surface QRS and the initial sensed intracardiac signal of the LV lead (QLV).[84] This difference can be further corrected for baseline QRS duration to yield the LV lead electrical delay (LVLED) (**Fig. 5**).[81] Lead placement at sites of increasing QLV is associated with greater rates of LV reverse remodeling and improvement in patient symptoms.[81,84] Recent efforts have also demonstrated the feasibility of newer electroanatomical mapping catheters to define sites of electrical delay (**Fig. 6**).[85]

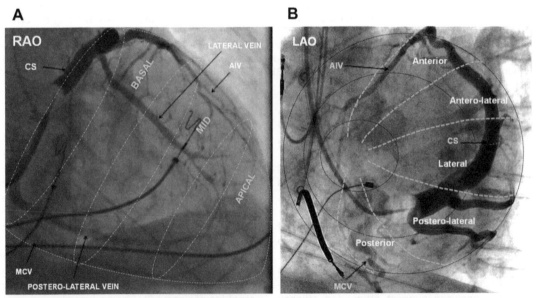

Fig. 4. Angiographic classification of LV lead position. A right anterior oblique (RAO) (*A*) view enables segmentation of the heart along the long axis into basal, midventricular (MID), and apical segments. The left anterior oblique (LAO) (*B*) view enables segmentation of the heart along the short axis into anterior, anterolateral, lateral, posterolateral, and posterior segments. AIV, anterior interventricular vein; CS, coronary sinus; MCV, middle cardiac vein.

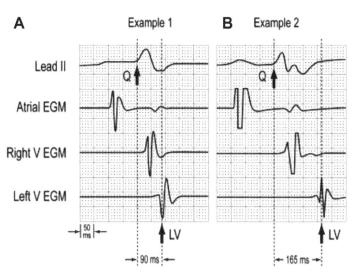

Fig. 5. Two examples of QLV measurements. The calipers are aligned with the onset of QRS and peak of the LV electrogram (EGM). The QLV was calculated as 90 milliseconds for the patient in (A) and 165 milliseconds for the patient in (B). (*Adapted from* Gold MR, Yu Y, Singh JP, et al. The effect of left ventricular electrical delay on A-V optimization for cardiac resynchronization therapy. Heart Rhythm 2013;10:989; with permission.)

Although mechanical dyssynchrony has historically failed to predict CRT response or identify patients with narrow QRS who may benefit from CRT, newer modalities of mechanical dyssynchrony assessment (eg, speckle tracking and cardiac MRI)[40,42] have shown promise. In the STARTER (Speckle Tracking Assisted Resynchronization Therapy for Electrode Region) trial, a lead targeting strategy at sites of latest activation with avoidance of areas of scar was associated with significant reduction in composite outcome.[40] Of note, exact concordance was only achieved in 30% of patients highlighting the limitations of coronary venous anatomy. Whether or not the improved outcome was related to avoidance of scar versus targeted mechanical dyssynchrony is also unknown. LV lead implantation at sites of scar (even in optimal anatomic location) has been associated with poor response to CRT[73]; whether routine use of imaging to guide lead targeting

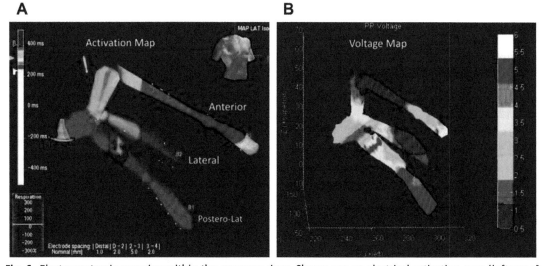

Fig. 6. Electroanatomic mapping within the coronary sinus. Shown are an electrical activation map (*left panel*) and voltage map (*right panel*) within branches of the coronary sinus (NavX catheter system, St. Jude Medical, St. Paul, MN). The area of most delayed activation is present in the lateral and posterolateral branches (*left panel*, *blue*). Furthermore, voltage mapping demonstrates an area of scar in the posterolateral segment (*right panel*, *red*) suggesting that the optimal LV lead location is the lateral midventricular region. Postero-Lat, posterolateral. (*Adapted from* Ryu K, D'Avila A, Heist EK, et al. Simultaneous electrical and mechanical mapping using 3D cardiac mapping system: novel approach for optimal cardiac resynchronization therapy. J Cardiovasc Electrophysiol 2010;21:221; with permission.)

(eg, cardiac MRI) is of benefit remains to be seen. Finally, recent work has shown that conventional anatomically guided LV lead targeting is rarely associated with optimal hemodynamic improvement at the time of implant.[78] Although the degree of acute hemodynamic improvement has been associated with greater LV reverse remodeling,[82] whether or not this approach is superior to anatomic, electrical, or mechanical targeting strategies remains to be determined.

Strategies to overcome potential limitations in lead targeting include the use of multisite pacing, surgical implantation of epicardial leads, and endocardial pacing. Multisite pacing (MSP) offers the possibility of generating multiple wave fronts whose fusion may further improve resynchronization over standard lead configurations.[86] MSP was historically achieved via implantation of multiple leads (eg, 2 LV leads)[86,87] although more recent technology has developed multipolar leads capable of delivering LV stimulation at multiple sites.[88] MSP has been shown to yield more substantial reverse remodeling in select patients with AF and slow ventricular rate,[89] and more recent data using quadripolar pacing leads have demonstrated superior improvement in acute hemodynamics (eg, rate of pressure change) and short-term ventricular reverse remodeling.[88,90] Ongoing studies are examining the incremental benefit of quadripolar lead technology (MultiPoint Pacing IDE Study; NCT01786993)[91] and specifically in those demonstrating nonresponse (More Response on CRT with MultiPoint Pacing study; NCT02006069).[92] In circumstances whereby an optimal lead location cannot be achieved via transvenous approach, surgical epicardial lead placement is feasible, though technical challenges include optimizing lead fixation strategies as well as minimizing the risk of laceration or damage of the adjacent arterial coronary tree.[93] Given the limitations of the transvenous route, alternative pacing approaches, such as endocardial pacing, have the potential to significantly impact CRT.[78,94] Endocardial pacing may offer more physiologic depolarization of the ventricles, which extends from the endocardium to the epicardium in the nonpathologic ventricle. Several techniques for endocardial pacing have been proposed, including transapical, transaortic, as well as transseptal. In the recently presented ALSYNC (Alternate Site Cardiac Resynchronization) study, the safety and efficacy of LV endocardial pacing was assessed in 138 patients in whom LV lead placement was not technically possible or who demonstrated CRT nonresponse. In this select population, LV endocardial pacing was associated with clinical and echocardiographic improvement in nearly two-thirds of patients.[95] Even more recently, the WiSE-CRT (Wireless Stimulation Endocardially for CRT) study demonstrated the feasibility and safety of an endocardial LV pacing system using a leadless ultrasound-based algorithm.[94] The routine use, standard procedural approach, and efficacy of endocardial pacing remain points of active investigation.

Postimplant Care: Device Programming, Optimization, and Monitoring

Care of the patient following implantation of CRT includes optimization of device programming as well as early recognition of patients at risk for nonresponse. Optimizing the A-V delay in patients with ventricular pacemakers has been shown to influence cardiac function and hemodynamics by allowing for optimal ventricular filling and ensuring biventricular pacing before native conduction.[96,97] Optimization algorithms include the use of echocardiography-guided assessment of mitral inflow patterns[98] as well as device algorithms that account for intrinsic A-V intervals, interventricular timing, and LV lead location.[84,99,100] To date, routine echocardiographic and intrinsic device-based optimization of A-V intervals has not been associated with improved clinical outcome in most studies (SmartDelay; Boston Scientific, Marlborough, MA),[84,99,100] although A-V optimization may be of particular benefit to patients who demonstrate nonresponse.[9] In addition to AV optimization, interventricular optimization has also been shown to improve hemodynamic outcomes in patients undergoing CRT.[101,102] Similar to A-V optimization, RV-LV (V-V) optimization algorithms include echocardiography-guided as well as those intrinsic to the device itself and have not shown a clinical benefit when applied routinely eg, SmartAV algorithm.[97,100,101] V-V optimization may be of particular importance to patients with heterogeneous activation patterns (eg, those with LBBB but significant LV scar) and previous work suggests there may incremental benefit of such optimization in ischemic as opposed to nonischemic patients.[103]

Despite the general lack of benefit of routine optimization, 2 recent algorithms based on hemodynamic optimization (SonR sensor; Sorin Group, Milan, Italy)[104,105] and effective fusion of LV pacing and native RV conduction (AdaptivCRT; Medtronic, Minneapolis, MN)[106] have shown promise. In the recently reported CLEAR (Clinical Evaluation on Advanced Resynchronization) study, an accelerometer-based technology implanted in the RV lead (SonR) was used to impute LV contractility to guide optimization of both A-V and V-V intervals.[105] Use of the accelerometer-based algorithm was associated with an improved NYHA class at the short-term follow-up when compared with standard echocardiographic optimization[105]; post hoc analysis suggested a possible mortality benefit in patients undergoing frequent, systematic optimization compared with standard care.[104] The ongoing RESPOND CRT (SonRtip Lead and Automatic AV-VV Optimization Algorithm in the PARADYM RF SonR) study will definitively assess the clinical benefits of this accelerometer-based algorithm in a randomized study (NCT01534234).[107] In addition, the use of a dynamic LV-only pacing algorithm (AdaptivCRT; Medtronic, Minneapolis, MN)[106] that allows for physiologic activation of the RV and avoidance of RV pacing-induced dyssynchrony has also shown a possible clinical benefit.[100,108] Patients randomized to the (AdaptivCRT; Medtronic, Minneapolis, MN) algorithm experienced a 44% reduction in RV pacing when compared with those undergoing standard echocardiography-guided optimization.[106] Increased percentage of LV-only pacing in all patients, as well as the use of the (AdaptivCRT; Medtronic, Minneapolis, MN) algorithm in patients with normal PR interval, were associated with a clinical benefit.[108] There may be a particular benefit of LV-only pacing algorithms in patients demonstrating nonresponse to CRT as suggested recently.[109]

Contemporary CRT devices similarly offer a range of monitoring parameters that are relevant for the longitudinal care of patients with HF.[110] For example, information regarding patient activity, heart rate, autonomic activity, atrial and ventricular ectopic burden, and transthoracic impedance are available in present-day CRT devices and may frame providers' understanding of HF symptoms; identify those at risk of nonresponse; and possibly recognize worsening HF status earlier and, thus, prevent poor clinical outcome and HF hospitalizations.[111,112] Biventricular pacing percentage has been identified as an important determinant of clinical outcomes following CRT. A recent report from the LATITUDE investigators (Boston Scientific, Marlborough, MA) of nearly 37,000 patients suggested biventricular pacing percentages greater than 98% were associated with improved survival relative to lower pacing percentages.[113] Device data including burden of atrial or ventricular ectopy or tachyarrhythmias may facilitate targeted intervention to improve CRT pacing percentage and clinical outcomes.[114]

Caring for CRT patients requires the integrated and synergistic cooperation of several cardiology specialists from electrophysiology, HF, and cardiac imaging. Multidisciplinary care offers a coordinated application of expertise to recognize patients at risk for nonresponse, optimize device programming, as well as expert management of pathologic conditions known to influence outcomes in CRT (eg, management RV dysfunction, pulmonary hypertension).[9] In addition, multidisciplinary infrastructure may also assist in the optimization of medical therapy, adherence, and patient education. Such a multidisciplinary approach was associated with improved clinical outcomes in a recent retrospective report[115]; the efficacy of routine application of such care remains to be assessed in a prospective study.

FUTURE TRENDS, CHALLENGES, AND CONTROVERSIES IN CARDIAC RESYNCHRONIZATION THERAPY

The future of CRT is replete with ongoing investigation and challenges along the spectrum of clinical care, from patient selection to implantation and postprocedure care. The optimal selection of patients for biventricular pacing therapy remains challenging particularly for patients with non-LBBB morphology. For example, more careful preprocedure identification of dyssynchrony or intraprocedural targeting of electrical delay may identify the subset of these patients who are likely to derive a clinical benefit from CRT. This strategy is currently being evaluated in the ENHANCE-CRT study (CRT Implant Strategy Using the Longest Electrical Delay for Non-left Bundle Branch Block Patients; NCT01983293).[116] Recent single-center retrospective work assessing clinical outcome in non-LBBB is supportive; lead targeting to sites of maximal electrical delay (ie, prolonged LVLED) was associated with improved clinical outcome.[117] The expansion of CRT to nonstandard population also remains an area of active investigation. For example, the MADIT-CHIC (MADIT-Chemotherapy Induced Cardiomyopathy; NCT02164721) trial recently began enrollment and will assess the efficacy of CRT-D therapy in patients with chemotherapy-induced cardiomyopathy.[118] As more data accrue, biventricular pacing therapy may also become more prevalent in patients with relatively preserved LVEF and significant pacing. With respect to procedural and implant technology, the benefit of multisite and sequential pacing to reduce nonresponders and enhance response remains a point of active investigation (eg, MORE-CRT MPP study).[86] With the introduction of leadless endocardial pacing technology, the potential for targeting LV endocardial pacing sites remains to be established. Integration of these pacing technologies with advanced imaging (cardiac MRI, CT, speckle tracking) may ultimately offer a tailored pacing approach uniquely responsive to each patient's dyssynchrony signature. Finally, there remain several open questions and opportunities for improvement in postimplant care. With respect to monitoring, continued sharpening of technologies that offer beat-to-beat hemodynamic assessment in patients undergoing CRT may further optimize clinical outcome after implant.[110] In the longer-term, the management ICD replacement in patients who demonstrate a super-response and normalization of LVEF remains uncertain.[119] Recent appropriate-use guidelines suggest that ICD generator replacement may be deferred in patients demonstrating LVEF recovery (>5%) and for whom the index indication for ICD implantation was primary prevention.[120] Given the substantial cost associated with such replacement[121] and the potential morbidity of inappropriate shock therapy in patients with CRT,[122] this remains one of several important questions in the longer-term management of patients undergoing CRT.

SUMMARY

CRT has revolutionized the care of patients with HF and electrical dyssynchrony. CRT fundamentally modifies the natural history of the pathologic ventricle, improves patient symptoms and functional capacity, and incrementally improves survival beyond OMT. Ongoing studies will identify expanding populations who may benefit from CRT and further identify novel pacing approaches and technologies that augment the efficacy of resynchronization. Consensus efforts toward defining response to CRT, earlier identification of those at risk for nonresponse, and enhancing implantation rates in those meeting contemporary guideline indications[123] will only improve the delivery and effectiveness of CRT in our patients.

SUPPLEMENTARY DATA

Supplementary data related to this article can be found online at http://dx.doi.org/10.1016/j.hfc.2014.12.007.

REFERENCES

1. Brignole M, Auricchio A, Baron-Esquivias G, et al. 2013 ESC guidelines on cardiac pacing and cardiac resynchronization therapy: the task force on cardiac pacing and resynchronization therapy of the European Society of Cardiology (ESC). Developed in collaboration with the European Heart Rhythm Association (EHRA). Europace 2013;15:1070–118.

2. Epstein AE, DiMarco JP, Ellenbogen KA, et al. 2012 ACCF/AHA/HRS focused update incorporated into the ACCF/AHA/HRS 2008 guidelines for device-based therapy of cardiac rhythm abnormalities: a report of the American College of Cardiology Foundation/American Heart Association Task Force on Practice Guidelines and the Heart Rhythm Society. J Am Coll Cardiol 2013;61:e6–75.

3. Abraham WT, Fisher WG, Smith AL, et al. Cardiac resynchronization in chronic heart failure. N Engl J Med 2002;346:1845–53.

4. Bristow MR, Saxon LA, Boehmer J, et al. Cardiac-resynchronization therapy with or without an implantable defibrillator in advanced chronic heart failure. N Engl J Med 2004;350:2140–50.

5. Cleland JG, Daubert JC, Erdmann E, et al. The effect of cardiac resynchronization on morbidity and mortality in heart failure. N Engl J Med 2005; 352:1539–49.

6. Moss AJ, Hall WJ, Cannom DS, et al. Cardiac-resynchronization therapy for the prevention of heart-failure events. N Engl J Med 2009;361: 1329–38.

7. Tang AS, Wells GA, Talajic M, et al. Cardiac-resynchronization therapy for mild-to-moderate heart failure. N Engl J Med 2010;363:2385–95.

8. Cazeau S, Ritter P, Bakdach S, et al. Four chamber pacing in dilated cardiomyopathy. Pacing Clin Electrophysiol 1994;17:1974–9.

9. Mullens W, Grimm RA, Verga T, et al. Insights from a cardiac resynchronization optimization clinic as part of a heart failure disease management program. J Am Coll Cardiol 2009;53:765–73.

10. Nelson GS, Berger RD, Fetics BJ, et al. Left ventricular or biventricular pacing improves cardiac function at diminished energy cost in patients with dilated cardiomyopathy and left bundle-branch block. Circulation 2000;102:3053–9.

11. Baldasseroni S, Opasich C, Gorini M, et al. Left bundle-branch block is associated with increased 1-year sudden and total mortality rate in 5517 outpatients with congestive heart failure: a report from the Italian network on congestive heart failure. Am Heart J 2002;143:398–405.

12. Hawkins NM, Wang D, McMurray JJ, et al. Prevalence and prognostic impact of bundle branch block in patients with heart failure: evidence from the CHARM programme. Eur J Heart Fail 2007;9:510–7.

13. Ghio S, Constantin C, Klersy C, et al. Interventricular and intraventricular dyssynchrony are common in heart failure patients, regardless of QRS duration. Eur Heart J 2004;25:571–8.

14. Liu L, Tockman B, Girouard S, et al. Left ventricular resynchronization therapy in a canine model of left bundle branch block. Am J Physiol Heart Circ Physiol 2002;282:H2238–44.

15. Han W, Chartier D, Li D, et al. Ionic remodeling of cardiac Purkinje cells by congestive heart failure. Circulation 2001;104:2095–100.
16. Kirk JA, Kass DA. Electromechanical dyssynchrony and resynchronization of the failing heart. Circ Res 2013;113:765–76.
17. Agnetti G, Kaludercic N, Kane LA, et al. Modulation of mitochondrial proteome and improved mitochondrial function by biventricular pacing of dyssynchronous failing hearts. Circ Cardiovasc Genet 2010;3:78–87.
18. Wang SB, Foster DB, Rucker J, et al. Redox regulation of mitochondrial ATP synthase: implications for cardiac resynchronization therapy. Circ Res 2011;109:750–7.
19. Aiba T, Hesketh GG, Barth AS, et al. Electrophysiological consequences of dyssynchronous heart failure and its restoration by resynchronization therapy. Circulation 2009;119:1220–30.
20. Chakir K, Daya SK, Aiba T, et al. Mechanisms of enhanced beta-adrenergic reserve from cardiac resynchronization therapy. Circulation 2009;119:1231–40.
21. Prinzen FW, Hunter WC, Wyman BT, et al. Mapping of regional myocardial strain and work during ventricular pacing: experimental study using magnetic resonance imaging tagging. J Am Coll Cardiol 1999;33:1735–42.
22. Rosen BD, Fernandes VR, Nasir K, et al. Age, increased left ventricular mass, and lower regional myocardial perfusion are related to greater extent of myocardial dyssynchrony in asymptomatic individuals: the multi-ethnic study of atherosclerosis. Circulation 2009;120:859–66.
23. Vernooy K, Verbeek XA, Peschar M, et al. Left bundle branch block induces ventricular remodelling and functional septal hypoperfusion. Eur Heart J 2005;26:91–8.
24. Prinzen FW, Vernooy K, De Boeck BW, et al. Mechano-energetics of the asynchronous and resynchronized heart. Heart Fail Rev 2011;16:215–24.
25. Ukkonen H, Beanlands RS, Burwash IG, et al. Effect of cardiac resynchronization on myocardial efficiency and regional oxidative metabolism. Circulation 2003;107:28–31.
26. Cazeau S, Leclercq C, Lavergne T, et al. Effects of multisite biventricular pacing in patients with heart failure and intraventricular conduction delay. N Engl J Med 2001;344:873–80.
27. Cleland JG, Freemantle N, Daubert JC, et al. Long-term effect of cardiac resynchronisation in patients reporting mild symptoms of heart failure: a report from the CARE-HF study. Heart 2008;94:278–83.
28. Kadish A, Dyer A, Daubert JP, et al. Prophylactic defibrillator implantation in patients with nonischemic dilated cardiomyopathy. N Engl J Med 2004;350:2151–8.
29. Moss AJ, Zareba W, Hall WJ, et al. Prophylactic implantation of a defibrillator in patients with myocardial infarction and reduced ejection fraction. N Engl J Med 2002;346:877–83.
30. Myerburg RJ, Reddy V, Castellanos A. Indications for implantable cardioverter-defibrillators based on evidence and judgment. J Am Coll Cardiol 2009;54:747–63.
31. Higgins SL, Hummel JD, Niazi IK, et al. Cardiac resynchronization therapy for the treatment of heart failure in patients with intraventricular conduction delay and malignant ventricular tachyarrhythmias. J Am Coll Cardiol 2003;42:1454–9.
32. Abraham WT, Young JB, Leon AR, et al. Effects of cardiac resynchronization on disease progression in patients with left ventricular systolic dysfunction, an indication for an implantable cardioverter-defibrillator, and mildly symptomatic chronic heart failure. Circulation 2004;110:2864–8.
33. Linde C, Abraham WT, Gold MR, et al. Randomized trial of cardiac resynchronization in mildly symptomatic heart failure patients and in asymptomatic patients with left ventricular dysfunction and previous heart failure symptoms. J Am Coll Cardiol 2008;52:1834–43.
34. Yu CM, Chan YS, Zhang Q, et al. Benefits of cardiac resynchronization therapy for heart failure patients with narrow QRS complexes and coexisting systolic asynchrony by echocardiography. J Am Coll Cardiol 2006;48:2251–7.
35. Achilli A, Sassara M, Ficili S, et al. Long-term effectiveness of cardiac resynchronization therapy in patients with refractory heart failure and "narrow" QRS. J Am Coll Cardiol 2003;42:2117–24.
36. Beshai JF, Grimm RA, Nagueh SF, et al. Cardiac-resynchronization therapy in heart failure with narrow QRS complexes. N Engl J Med 2007;357:2461–71.
37. Ruschitzka F, Abraham WT, Singh JP, et al. Cardiac-resynchronization therapy in heart failure with a narrow QRS complex. N Engl J Med 2013;369:1395–405.
38. Thibault B, Harel F, Ducharme A, et al. Cardiac resynchronization therapy in patients with heart failure and a QRS complex <120 milliseconds: the Evaluation of Resynchronization Therapy for Heart Failure (LESSER-EARTH) trial. Circulation 2013;127:873–81.
39. Delgado V, Ypenburg C, van Bommel RJ, et al. Assessment of left ventricular dyssynchrony by speckle tracking strain imaging comparison between longitudinal, circumferential, and radial strain in cardiac resynchronization therapy. J Am Coll Cardiol 2008;51:1944–52.
40. Saba S, Marek J, Schwartzman D, et al. Echocardiography-guided left ventricular lead placement for cardiac resynchronization therapy: results of the

Speckle Tracking Assisted Resynchronization Therapy for Electrode Region trial. Circ Heart Fail 2013;6:427–34.

41. Chung ES, Leon AR, Tavazzi L, et al. Results of the Predictors of Response to CRT (PROSPECT) trial. Circulation 2008;117:2608–16.

42. Bilchick KC, Dimaano V, Wu KC, et al. Cardiac magnetic resonance assessment of dyssynchrony and myocardial scar predicts function class improvement following cardiac resynchronization therapy. JACC Cardiovasc Imaging 2008;1:561–8.

43. Sohal M, Duckett SG, Zhuang X, et al. A prospective evaluation of cardiovascular magnetic resonance measures of dyssynchrony in the prediction of response to cardiac resynchronization therapy. J Cardiovasc Magn Reson 2014; 16:58.

44. Truong QA, Hoffmann U, Singh JP. Potential uses of computed tomography for management of heart failure patients with dyssynchrony. Crit Pathw Cardiol 2008;7:185–90.

45. Leclercq C, Cazeau S, Lellouche D, et al. Upgrading from single chamber right ventricular to biventricular pacing in permanently paced patients with worsening heart failure: the RD-CHF Study. Pacing Clin Electrophysiol 2007;30(Suppl 1):S23–30.

46. Sweeney MO, Hellkamp AS, Ellenbogen KA, et al. Adverse effect of ventricular pacing on heart failure and atrial fibrillation among patients with normal baseline QRS duration in a clinical trial of pacemaker therapy for sinus node dysfunction. Circulation 2003;107:2932–7.

47. Wilkoff BL, Cook JR, Epstein AE, et al. Dual-chamber pacing or ventricular backup pacing in patients with an implantable defibrillator: the Dual Chamber and VVI Implantable Defibrillator (DAVID) Trial. JAMA 2002;288:3115–23.

48. Curtis AB, Worley SJ, Adamson PB, et al. Biventricular pacing for atrioventricular block and systolic dysfunction. N Engl J Med 2013;368:1585–93.

49. Funck RC, Blanc JJ, Mueller HH, et al. Biventricular stimulation to prevent cardiac desynchronization: rationale, design, and endpoints of the 'Biventricular Pacing for Atrioventricular Block to Prevent Cardiac Desynchronization (BioPace)' study. Europace 2006;8:629–35.

50. Kandala J, Altman RK, Park MY, et al. Clinical, laboratory, and pacing predictors of CRT response. J Cardiovasc Transl Res 2012;5:196–212.

51. Leyva F, Nisam S, Auricchio A. 20 years of cardiac resynchronization therapy. J Am Coll Cardiol 2014; 64:1047–58.

52. Fornwalt BK, Sprague WW, BeDell P, et al. Agreement is poor among current criteria used to define response to cardiac resynchronization therapy. Circulation 2010;121:1985–91.

53. Yu CM, Bleeker GB, Fung JW, et al. Left ventricular reverse remodeling but not clinical improvement predicts long-term survival after cardiac resynchronization therapy. Circulation 2005;112:1580–6.

54. Hsu JC, Solomon SD, Bourgoun M, et al. Predictors of super-response to cardiac resynchronization therapy and associated improvement in clinical outcome: the MADIT-CRT (Multicenter Automatic Defibrillator Implantation Trial with Cardiac Resynchronization Therapy) study. J Am Coll Cardiol 2012;59:2366–73.

55. Rickard J, Kumbhani DJ, Popovic Z, et al. Characterization of super-response to cardiac resynchronization therapy. Heart Rhythm 2010;7:885–9.

56. Voigt J, Sasha John M, Taylor A, et al. A reevaluation of the costs of heart failure and its implications for allocation of health resources in the United States. Clin Cardiol 2014;37:312–21.

57. Auricchio A, Fantoni C, Regoli F, et al. Characterization of left ventricular activation in patients with heart failure and left bundle-branch block. Circulation 2004;109:1133–9.

58. Fantoni C, Kawabata M, Massaro R, et al. Right and left ventricular activation sequence in patients with heart failure and right bundle branch block: a detailed analysis using three-dimensional non-fluoroscopic electroanatomic mapping system. J Cardiovasc Electrophysiol 2005;16:112–9 [discussion: 120–1].

59. Rodriguez LM, Timmermans C, Nabar A, et al. Variable patterns of septal activation in patients with left bundle branch block and heart failure. J Cardiovasc Electrophysiol 2003;14:135–41.

60. Richman JL, Wolff L. Left bundle branch block masquerading as right bundle branch block. Am Heart J 1954;47:383–93.

61. Sipahi I, Carrigan TP, Rowland DY, et al. Impact of QRS duration on clinical event reduction with cardiac resynchronization therapy: meta-analysis of randomized controlled trials. Arch Intern Med 2011;171:1454–62.

62. Gold MR, Thebault C, Linde C, et al. Effect of QRS duration and morphology on cardiac resynchronization therapy outcomes in mild heart failure: results from the Resynchronization Reverses Remodeling in Systolic Left Ventricular Dysfunction (REVERSE) study. Circulation 2012; 126:822–9.

63. Cleland JG, Abraham WT, Linde C, et al. An individual patient meta-analysis of five randomized trials assessing the effects of cardiac resynchronization therapy on morbidity and mortality in patients with symptomatic heart failure. Eur Heart J 2013;34:3547–56.

64. Sipahi I, Chou JC, Hyden M, et al. Effect of QRS morphology on clinical event reduction with cardiac resynchronization therapy: meta-analysis of

randomized controlled trials. Am Heart J 2012;163: 260–7.e3.

65. Upadhyay GA, Choudhry NK, Auricchio A, et al. Cardiac resynchronization in patients with atrial fibrillation: a meta-analysis of prospective cohort studies. J Am Coll Cardiol 2008;52:1239–46.

66. Wilton SB, Leung AA, Ghali WA, et al. Outcomes of cardiac resynchronization therapy in patients with versus those without atrial fibrillation: a systematic review and meta-analysis. Heart Rhythm 2011;8: 1088–94.

67. Healey JS, Hohnloser SH, Exner DV, et al. Cardiac resynchronization therapy in patients with permanent atrial fibrillation: results from the Resynchronization for Ambulatory Heart Failure Trial (RAFT). Circ Heart Fail 2012;5:566–70.

68. Gasparini M, Leclercq C, Lunati M, et al. Cardiac resynchronization therapy in patients with atrial fibrillation: the CERTIFY study (Cardiac Resynchronization Therapy in Atrial Fibrillation Patients Multinational Registry). JACC Heart Fail 2013;1:500–7.

69. Yin J, Hu H, Wang Y, et al. Effects of atrioventricular nodal ablation on permanent atrial fibrillation patients with cardiac resynchronization therapy: a systematic review and meta-analysis. Clin Cardiol 2014;37(11):707–15.

70. Fung JW, Szeto CC, Chan JY, et al. Prognostic value of renal function in patients with cardiac resynchronization therapy. Int J Cardiol 2007;122:10–6.

71. Garg N, Thomas G, Jackson G, et al. Cardiac resynchronization therapy in CKD: a systematic review. Clin J Am Soc Nephrol 2013;8:1293–303.

72. Chatterjee NA, Upadhyay GA, Singal G, et al. Pre-capillary pulmonary hypertension and right ventricular dilation predict clinical outcome in cardiac resynchronization therapy. JACC Heart Fail 2014;2:230–7.

73. Adelstein EC, Saba S. Scar burden by myocardial perfusion imaging predicts echocardiographic response to cardiac resynchronization therapy in ischemic cardiomyopathy. Am Heart J 2007;153: 105–12.

74. Bilchick KC, Kuruvilla S, Hamirani YS, et al. Impact of mechanical activation, scar, and electrical timing on cardiac resynchronization therapy response and clinical outcomes. J Am Coll Cardiol 2014;63: 1657–66.

75. Arshad A, Moss AJ, Foster E, et al. Cardiac resynchronization therapy is more effective in women than in men: the MADIT-CRT (Multicenter Automatic Defibrillator Implantation Trial with Cardiac Resynchronization Therapy) trial. J Am Coll Cardiol 2011;57:813–20.

76. Zusterzeel R, Curtis JP, Canos DA, et al. Sex-specific mortality risk by QRS morphology and duration in patients receiving CRT: results from the NCDR. J Am Coll Cardiol 2014;64:887–94.

77. Blendea D, Shah RV, Auricchio A, et al. Variability of coronary venous anatomy in patients undergoing cardiac resynchronization therapy: a high-speed rotational venography study. Heart Rhythm 2007;4:1155–62.

78. Derval N, Steendijk P, Gula LJ, et al. Optimizing hemodynamics in heart failure patients by systematic screening of left ventricular pacing sites: the lateral left ventricular wall and the coronary sinus are rarely the best sites. J Am Coll Cardiol 2010;55: 566–75.

79. Singh JP, Klein HU, Huang DT, et al. Left ventricular lead position and clinical outcome in the Multicenter Automatic Defibrillator Implantation Trial-Cardiac Resynchronization Therapy (MADIT-CRT) trial. Circulation 2011;123:1159–66.

80. Gold MR, Yu Y, Singh JP, et al. The effect of left ventricular electrical delay on AV optimization for cardiac resynchronization therapy. Heart Rhythm 2013;10:988–93.

81. Singh JP, Fan D, Heist EK, et al. Left ventricular lead electrical delay predicts response to cardiac resynchronization therapy. Heart Rhythm 2006;3: 1285–92.

82. Duckett SG, Ginks M, Shetty AK, et al. Invasive acute hemodynamic response to guide left ventricular lead implantation predicts chronic remodeling in patients undergoing cardiac resynchronization therapy. J Am Coll Cardiol 2011;58:1128–36.

83. Faris OP, Evans FJ, Dick AJ, et al. Endocardial versus epicardial electrical synchrony during LV free-wall pacing. Am J Physiol Heart Circ Physiol 2003;285:H1864–70.

84. Ellenbogen KA, Gold MR, Meyer TE, et al. Primary results from the SmartDelay determined AV optimization: a comparison to other AV delay methods used in cardiac resynchronization therapy (SMART-AV) trial: a randomized trial comparing empirical, echocardiography-guided, and algorithmic atrioventricular delay programming in cardiac resynchronization therapy. Circulation 2010; 122:2660–8.

85. Ryu K, D'Avila A, Heist EK, et al. Simultaneous electrical and mechanical mapping using 3D cardiac mapping system: novel approach for optimal cardiac resynchronization therapy. J Cardiovasc Electrophysiol 2010;21:219–22.

86. Rinaldi CA, Burri H, Thibault B, et al. A review of multisite pacing to achieve cardiac resynchronization therapy. Europace 2015;17(1):7–17.

87. Yoshida K, Seo Y, Yamasaki H, et al. Effect of triangle ventricular pacing on haemodynamics and dyssynchrony in patients with advanced heart failure: a comparison study with conventional bi-ventricular pacing therapy. Eur Heart J 2007;28:2610–9.

88. Pappone C, Calovic Z, Vicedomini G, et al. Multipoint left ventricular pacing improves acute

hemodynamic response assessed with pressure-volume loops in cardiac resynchronization therapy patients. Heart Rhythm 2014;11:394–401.

89. Leclercq C, Gadler F, Kranig W, et al. A randomized comparison of triple-site versus dual-site ventricular stimulation in patients with congestive heart failure. J Am Coll Cardiol 2008;51:1455–62.

90. Pappone C, Calovic Z, Vicedomini G, et al. Multipoint left ventricular pacing in a single coronary sinus branch improves mid-term echocardiographic and clinical response to cardiac resynchronization therapy. J Cardiovasc Electrophysiol 2015;26:58–63.

91. MultiPoint Pacing IDE Study (MPP IDE). Available at: http://clinicaltrials.gov/show/NCT01786993. Accessed October 6, 2014.

92. More Response on Cardiac Resynchronization Therapy with MultiPoint Pacing (MORE-CRT MPP). Available at: http://clinicaltrials.gov/show/NCT02006069. Accessed October 6, 2014.

93. Kamath GS, Balaram S, Choi A, et al. Long-term outcome of leads and patients following robotic epicardial left ventricular lead placement for cardiac resynchronization therapy. Pacing Clin Electrophysiol 2011;34:235–40.

94. Auricchio A, Delnoy PP, Butter C, et al. Feasibility, safety, and short-term outcome of leadless ultrasound-based endocardial left ventricular resynchronization in heart failure patients: results of the Wireless Stimulation Endocardially for CRT (WiSE-CRT) study. Europace 2014;16:681–8.

95. Alternate Site Cardiac Resynchronization (AL-SYNC) study. Available at: http://clinicaltrials.gov/show/NCT01277783. Accessed October 6, 2014.

96. Auricchio A, Stellbrink C, Block M, et al. Effect of pacing chamber and atrioventricular delay on acute systolic function of paced patients with congestive heart failure. The Pacing Therapies for Congestive Heart Failure Study Group. The Guidant Congestive Heart Failure Research Group. Circulation 1999;99:2993–3001.

97. Gras D, Gupta MS, Boulogne E, et al. Optimization of AV and VV delays in the real-world CRT patient population: an international survey on current clinical practice. Pacing Clin Electrophysiol 2009;32(Suppl 1):S236–9.

98. Barold SS, Ilercil A, Herweg B. Echocardiographic optimization of the atrioventricular and interventricular intervals during cardiac resynchronization. Europace 2008;10(Suppl 3):iii88–95.

99. Kamdar R, Frain E, Warburton F, et al. A prospective comparison of echocardiography and device algorithms for atrioventricular and interventricular interval optimization in cardiac resynchronization therapy. Europace 2010;12:84–91.

100. Singh JP, Abraham WT, Chung ES, et al. Clinical response with adaptive CRT algorithm compared with CRT with echocardiography-optimized atrioventricular delay: a retrospective analysis of multicentre trials. Europace 2013;15:1622–8.

101. Boriani G, Biffi M, Muller CP, et al. A prospective randomized evaluation of VV delay optimization in CRT-D recipients: echocardiographic observations from the RHYTHM II ICD study. Pacing Clin Electrophysiol 2009;32(Suppl 1):S120–5.

102. Leon AR, Abraham WT, Brozena S, et al. Cardiac resynchronization with sequential biventricular pacing for the treatment of moderate-to-severe heart failure. J Am Coll Cardiol 2005;46:2298–304.

103. Marsan NA, Bleeker GB, Van Bommel RJ, et al. Cardiac resynchronization therapy in patients with ischemic versus non-ischemic heart failure: differential effect of optimizing interventricular pacing interval. Am Heart J 2009;158:769–76.

104. Delnoy PP, Ritter P, Naegele H, et al. Association between frequent cardiac resynchronization therapy optimization and long-term clinical response: a post hoc analysis of the Clinical Evaluation on Advanced Resynchronization (CLEAR) pilot study. Europace 2013;15:1174–81.

105. Ritter P, Delnoy PP, Padeletti L, et al. A randomized pilot study of optimization of cardiac resynchronization therapy in sinus rhythm patients using a peak endocardial acceleration sensor vs standard methods. Europace 2012;14:1324–33.

106. Martin DO, Lemke B, Birnie D, et al. Investigation of a novel algorithm for synchronized left-ventricular pacing and ambulatory optimization of cardiac resynchronization therapy: results of the adaptive CRT trial. Heart Rhythm 2012;9:1807–14.

107. Clinical Trial of the SonRtip Lead and Automatic AV-VV Optimization Algorithm in the PARADYM RF SonR CRT-D (RESPOND CRT). Available at: http://clinicaltrials.gov/show/NCT01534234. Accessed October 6, 2014.

108. Birnie D, Lemke B, Aonuma K, et al. Clinical outcomes with synchronized left ventricular pacing: analysis of the adaptive CRT trial. Heart Rhythm 2013;10:1368–74.

109. Thibault B, Ducharme A, Harel F, et al. Left ventricular versus simultaneous biventricular pacing in patients with heart failure and a QRS complex >/=120 milliseconds. Circulation 2011;124:2874–81.

110. Singh JP, Rosenthal LS, Hranitzky PM, et al. Device diagnostics and long-term clinical outcome in patients receiving cardiac resynchronization therapy. Europace 2009;11:1647–53.

111. Auricchio A, Gold MR, Brugada J, et al. Long-term effectiveness of the combined minute ventilation and patient activity sensors as predictor of heart failure events in patients treated with cardiac resynchronization therapy: results of the clinical evaluation of the physiological diagnosis function in the

PARADYM CRT device trial (CLEPSYDRA) study. Eur J Heart Fail 2014;16:663–70.

112. Vegh EM, Kandala J, Orencole M, et al. Device-measured physical activity versus six-minute walk test as a predictor of reverse remodeling and outcome after cardiac resynchronization therapy for heart failure. Am J Cardiol 2014;113:1523–8.

113. Hayes DL, Boehmer JP, Day JD, et al. Cardiac resynchronization therapy and the relationship of percent biventricular pacing to symptoms and survival. Heart Rhythm 2011;8:1469–75.

114. Lakkireddy D, Di Biase L, Ryschon K, et al. Radiofrequency ablation of premature ventricular ectopy improves the efficacy of cardiac resynchronization therapy in nonresponders. J Am Coll Cardiol 2012; 60:1531–9.

115. Altman RK, Parks KA, Schlett CL, et al. Multidisciplinary care of patients receiving cardiac resynchronization therapy is associated with improved clinical outcomes. Eur Heart J 2012;33:2181–8.

116. CRT Implant Strategy Using the Longest Electrical Delay for Non-left Bundle Branch Block Patients (ENHANCE CRT). Available at: http://clinicaltrials.gov/show/NCT01983293. Accessed October 6, 2014.

117. Kandala J, Upadhyay GA, Altman RK, et al. QRS morphology, left ventricular lead location, and clinical outcome in patients receiving cardiac resynchronization therapy. Eur Heart J 2013;34:2252–62.

118. Multicenter Automatic Defibrillator Implantation Trial - Chemotherapy-Induced Cardiomyopathy (MADIT-CHIC). Available at: http://clinicaltrials.gov/show/NCT02164721. Accessed October 6, 2014.

119. Manfredi JA, Al-Khatib SM, Shaw LK, et al. Association between left ventricular ejection fraction post-cardiac resynchronization treatment and subsequent implantable cardioverter defibrillator therapy for sustained ventricular tachyarrhythmias. Circ Arrhythm Electrophysiol 2013;6:257–64.

120. Russo AM, Stainback RF, Bailey SR, et al. ACCF/HRS/AHA/ASE/HFSA/SCAI/SCCT/SCMR 2013 appropriate use criteria for implantable cardioverter-defibrillators and cardiac resynchronization therapy: a report of the American College of Cardiology Foundation appropriate use criteria task force, Heart Rhythm Society, American Heart Association, American Society of Echocardiography, Heart Failure Society of America, Society for Cardiovascular Angiography and Interventions, Society of Cardiovascular Computed Tomography, and Society for Cardiovascular Magnetic Resonance. J Am Coll Cardiol 2013;61:1318–68.

121. Kini V, Soufi MK, Deo R, et al. Appropriateness of primary prevention implantable cardioverter-defibrillators at the time of generator replacement: are indications still met? J Am Coll Cardiol 2014; 63:2388–94.

122. Kantharia BK. Deterioration from improved heart failure status in a recipient of a cardiac resynchronization therapy-defibrillator (CRT-D) following a single inappropriate shock. Int J Cardiol 2012; 161:e55–7.

123. Maggioni AP, Anker SD, Dahlstrom U, et al. Are hospitalized or ambulatory patients with heart failure treated in accordance with European Society of Cardiology guidelines? Evidence from 12,440 patients of the ESC Heart Failure Long-Term Registry. Eur J Heart Fail 2013;15:1173–84.

Ablation of Atrial Arrhythmias in Heart Failure

 CrossMark

Philip Aagaard, MD, PhD[a], Luigi Di Biase, MD, PhD, FACC, FHRS[a,b,d],
Andrea Natale, MD, FACC, FHRS, FESC[b,c,e,f,g,h],*

KEYWORDS

- Atrial arrhythmia • Atrial fibrillation • Atrial fibrillation ablation • Heart failure • Antiarrhythmic drugs
- Rate control • Rhythm control

KEY POINTS

- Atrial fibrillation (AF) may adversely affect outcome in heart failure (HF) patients. Restoration of sinus rhythm (SR) improves cardiac function.
- In HF patients, as in the general AF population, the choice of a rhythm or rate control strategy is controversial.
- The efficacy of antiarrhythmic drugs (AADs) is generally poor, and the benefits of maintaining SR may be outweighed by their adverse effects.
- AF ablation offers the opportunity to maintain SR while avoiding the adverse effects of AADs.
- AF ablation is superior to AADs in HF patients to improve prognostic markers including left ventricular ejection fraction, exercise tolerance, and quality of life.
- Ablation also of non-pulmonary vein triggers appear important in order to achieve long-term freedom from arrhythmia in patients with concomitant AF and HF.

INTRODUCTION

The incidence of both heart failure (HF) and atrial fibrillation (AF) are on the rise, and they often coexist. Pharmacologic rhythm control has not been shown to improve outcomes compared with pharmacologic rate control in AF patients, possibly because of the adverse effects of antiarrhythmic drugs (AADs). Catheter ablation offers an opportunity to achieve SR without the downside of AADs. Several studies have shown that AF ablation improves prognostic markers, including ventricular function, exercise tolerance, and quality of life in HF patients with AF. Large randomized controlled trials comparing AF ablation with pharmacologic therapy are ongoing.

ATRIAL ARRHYTHMIAS

AF is by far the most common form of atrial arrhythmia in HF patients. Other forms include typical atrial flutter, atypical atrial flutter, and atrial tachycardia. Catheter ablation is the treatment of choice for typical atrial flutter and has a high

Disclosures: Dr P. Aagaard reports that he has no conflicts of interest. Dr L. Di Biase is a consultant for Biosense Webster, Hansen Medical, and St Jude Medical, and has received speaker honoraria/travel from AtriCure, EpiEP, and Biotronik. Dr A. Natale is a consultant for Biosense Webster and St Jude Medical and has received speaker honoraria/travel from Medtronic, Boston Scientific, Biotronik and Janssen.
[a] Albert Einstein College of Medicine, Montefiore Hospital, Bronx, NY, USA; [b] Texas Cardiac Arrhythmia Institute, St David's Medical Center, 3000 North I-35, Austin, TX 78705, USA; [c] Department of Biomedical Engineering, University of Texas, Austin, TX, USA; [d] Department of Cardiology, University of Foggia, Foggia, Italy; [e] Division of Cardiology, Stanford University, Stanford, CA, USA; [f] Case Western Reserve University, Cleveland, OH, USA; [g] EP Services, California Pacific Medical Center, San Francisco, CA, USA; [h] Interventional Electrophysiology, Scripps Clinic, San Diego, CA, USA
* Corresponding author. Texas Cardiac Arrhythmia Institute, St David's Medical Center, 3000 North I-35, Suite 720, Austin, TX 78705.
E-mail address: dr.natale@gmail.com

Heart Failure Clin 11 (2015) 305–317
http://dx.doi.org/10.1016/j.hfc.2014.12.008
1551-7136/15/$ – see front matter © 2015 Elsevier Inc. All rights reserved.

success rate and low complication rate. For the other atrial arrhythmias, various medical therapy strategies or ablation can be considered. This article focuses on ablation of AF.

EPIDEMIOLOGY

AF and HF are considered the 2 current epidemics of cardiovascular disease.[1] AF is the most common arrhythmia in clinical practice, and both its incidence and prevalence are expected to rise due to the aging population.[2] HF is the most common hospital discharge diagnosis in the United States, and it consumes more health care dollars than any other disease.[3] Despite therapeutic advances, the prognosis in HF remains poor, with an estimated 5-year survival of 25% to 38%.[4]

Importantly, the 2 conditions often coexist. The prevalence of AF in HF patients ranges from 13% to 27%,[4–8] and increases with HF severity, from 5% in patients with mild HF to more than 50% in patients with severe disease.[9] Coexistence of HF and AF is associated with an increased risk for hospitalization, stroke, and mortality.[10–12]

PATHOPHYSIOLOGY

The pathophysiological relationship between AF and HF is incompletely understood. Some of the coexistence can be attributed to shared risk factors including age, diabetes, hypertension, obesity, sleep apnea, valvular disease, coronary artery disease, and structural heart disease (**Fig. 1**).[13] However, a vicious cycle, where AF begets HF, and HF begets AF also plays an important role (**Fig. 2**).[14–16]

AF may facilitate the development and progression of HF through several mechanisms:

- Heart rate (HR) elevation in AF may cause myocardial ischemia, energy depletion, and calcium handling abnormalities that eventually lead to tachycardia-induced cardiomyopathy.[17–20] This mechanism is thought to contribute to left ventricular dysfunction in up to 50% of patients with concomitant HF and AF.
- The decreased ventricular filling during short cardiac cycles in AF cannot be fully compensated for during longer cycles, which leads to a decrease in total cardiac output.[21]
- The loss of atrial contraction and atrioventricular synchrony in AF further reduces cardiac output.
- Antiarrhythmic drug (AAD) therapy used to maintain sinus rhythm (SR) may worsen HF through negative inotropic and proarrhythmic effects.[17]

Conversely, there are also several ways through which HF can facilitate the development and progression of AF:

- Elevated left ventricular filling pressure, functional valvular regurgitation, and renin-angiotensin-aldosterone (RAAS) mediated volume retention in HF induce left atrial dilation.

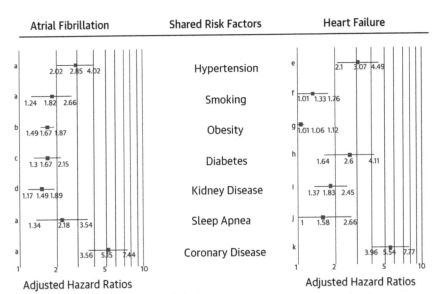

Fig. 1. Hazard ratio of incident AF and HF according to shared risk factors. Adjusted hazard ratios (95% confidence limits) of AF and HF according to 7 shared risk factors. These data were gathered through the studies of various cohorts. If overall cohort data were unavailable or not reported, results from white and/or male patients (both the largest subgroups) were reported. (*From* Trulock KM, Narayan SM, Piccini JP. Rhythm control in heart failure patients with atrial fibrillation: contemporary challenges including the role of ablation. J Am Coll Cardiol 2014;64(7):712; with permission.)

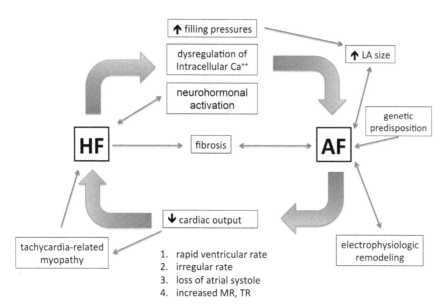

Fig. 2. AF and HF: a vicious pathophysiological cycle. AF, atrial fibrillation; HF, heart failure; LA, left atrial; MR, mitral regurgitation; TR, tricuspid regurgitation. (*Adapted from* Anter E, Jessup M, Callans DJ. Atrial fibrillation and heart failure: treatment considerations for a dual epidemic. Circulation 2009;119(18):2517; with permission.)

- The resultant myocardial stretching promotes ectopy from the pulmonary veins (PVs), the most common AF foci.[22]
- Atrial dilation also activates stretch-activated ion channels, increasing atrial dispersion of refractoriness and altering atrial conduction properties.[23]
- HF-induced fibrosis, altered myocardial calcium handling, and neurohormonal activation also contribute to alter atrial conduction properties.

Together, these mechanisms create a milieu for induction and maintenance of AF.

PROGNOSTIC SIGNIFICANCE

The prognostic significance of AF in HF is controversial owing to conflicting study results (**Table 1**). It is not clear weather AF is an independent risk factor for adverse outcomes in HF or merely represents a more advanced stage of disease, although the former opinion is generally favored.[24]

Early HF trials, such as the V-HeFT (The Vasodilator-Heart Failure) and COMET (Comparison of carvedilol and metoprolol on clinical outcomes in patients with chronic heart failure in the Carvedilol Or Metoprolol European Trial), found no independent association between the presence of AF

Table 1
The prognostic significance of atrial fibrillation in heart failure patients

Study, Year	n	% Atrial Fibrillation	Follow-up (y)	Predictor	P
Middlekauff et al,[7] 1991	390	19	1.5	Yes	.001
V-HeFT I,[4] 1993	632	15	2.5	No	.86
V-HeFT II,[4] 1993	795	13	2.0	No	.68
SOLVD,[10] 1998	6517	6	2.8	Yes	<.001
Middlekauff et al,[7] 1998	359	20	2.0	Yes	.002
Middlekauff et al,[7] 1998	391	24	2.0	No	.09
Mahoney et al,[6] 1999	234	27	1.1	No	.21
DIG,[94] 2000	7788	11	3.0	Yes	<.001
PRIME II,[45] 2000	409	84	3.4	No	n.s.
COMET,[25] 2005	3029	20	5.0	No	n.s.
VALIANT,[95] 2006	14,703	15	3.0	Yes	<.001

Adapted from Anter E, Jessup M, Callans DJ. Atrial fibrillation and heart failure: treatment considerations for a dual epidemic. Circulation 2009;119(18):2518; with permission.

and outcomes in HF patients.[4,25] However, in the more recent SOLVD (Studies of Left Ventricular Dysfunction) and Valsartan in Acute myocardial Infarction Trial (VALIANT), AF was independently associated with increased mortality.[10,26] This association was also seen in a substudy of the TRACE (The Trandolapril Cardiac Evaluation) trial, which furthermore found that the negative prognostic significance of AF was inversely related to HF severity.[27] It has since been suggested that AF may adversely affect mortality, mainly in mild-to-moderate HF but not in very advanced HF, where survival is already limited.[28]

Interestingly, new-onset AF appears to portend a particularly dismal prognosis compared with no AF or chronic AF in HF patients. In a subanalysis from the COMET study, new-onset, but not baseline, AF remained an independent predictor of all-cause mortality after multivariate analysis.[25] This finding is also supported by Framingham data.[11] A couple of explanations have been proposed:

- New-onset may AF lead to an increased metabolic demand that puts the failing heart at particularly high risk until adequate rate control is achieved, or until intrinsic compensatory mechanisms have had time to develop.
- The adverse effects of antiarrhythmic drugs (AADs) tend to cluster in the initiation phase, contributing to the particularly poor prognosis with new-onset AF.[24]

The significance of AF in patients with HF with preserved ejection fraction (HFpEF) has been understudied. However, results from the Candesartan in Heart failure-Assessment of Reduction in Mortality and morbidity (CHARM) trial suggest that the attributable risk of AF may be even higher in HFpEF patients.[29]

THERAPEUTIC OPTIONS

Although the prognostic significance of AF in HF patients is contested, it is evident that both rate control and restoration of SR improves cardiac function.[30] Rate control can be achieved either pharmacologically, or through atrioventricular node ablation and pacemaker implantation. Conversely, rhythm control can be achieved pharmacologically, or by AF ablation. In HF patients, as in the general AF population, there is controversy over which strategy represents the best treatment approach.[24,28]

RATE CONTROL

The goal of optimal rate control in AF has been considered to fall in the 60 to 80 beats per minute

range at rest, and in the 90 to 115 beats per minute range during moderate exertion.[31] However, findings from the RACE-II (Rate Control versus Electrical Cardioversion) trial failed to show a difference between strict (<80 beats per minute at rest and <110 beats per minute with moderate exertion) and more lenient rate control (<110 beats per minute at rest and with moderate exertion).[32] Importantly, most studies on rate control in AF, including the RACE-II trial, included a general AF population. It is therefore unclear if these findings can be extrapolated to HF patients, who may be more adversely affected by higher HRs. Beta-blockers are the drugs of choice for rate control in patients with concomitant HF and AF because of their known benefits in HF. However, several studies have failed to demonstrate a benefit of beta-blockade in HF patients who also have AF.[33,34] It has been speculated that a treatment-induced fall in blood pressure, particularly if greater than 10 mm Hg, may detrimentally affect cardiac function in HF patients, offsetting the benefits of rate control.[34]

When beta-blockers fail to sufficiently reduce HR, digoxin can be added as an adjunctive agent. However, its efficacy in severe HF is limited by its poor performance under high sympathetic tone conditions.[31] Nondihydropyridine calcium channel blockers have largely fallen out of favor as rate-controlling agents in HF patients because of concerns over their negative inotropic effects.[28]

In patients who fail pharmacologic rate control, atrioventricular node ablation and ventricular pacing can be attempted. Although this is an effective method to achieve rate control, there is concern that prolonged right ventricular pacing may worsen HF.[35] Therefore, atrioventricular node ablation and biventricular pacing are preferred. Although this strategy has not been compared with pharmacologic rate control in a large trial, it was inferior to AF ablation in the PABA-CHF (Pulmonary vein antrum isolation vs AV node ablation with biventricular pacing for treatment of atrial fibrillation in patients with congestive heart failure) trial.[36]

RHYTHM CONTROL

HF patients are at increased risk of adverse effects from AAD, and the agents available to maintain SR are limited in the presence of HF.[37–39] Today, amiodarone and dofetilide are the only guideline-recommended AADs for this patient population.[40] However, even their use is limited by significant drug–drug interactions and adverse effects. For example, long-term use of amiodarone is associated with significant pulmonary, hepatic, and thyroid toxicity and increases the risk for symptomatic bradycardia requiring pacemaker implantation.[41,42]

Dofetilide requires hospitalization for careful monitoring during drug initiation due to severe QT interval prolongation and torsades de points in up to 3% of patients. Furthermore, dofetilide is cleared renally and requires dose adjustment in the presence of renal dysfunction, a common HF comorbidity.[41] There are other agents that can be used in very mild HF, or when an implantable cardioverter-defibrillator (ICD) is implanted, and promising newer AAD are under investigation. However, these are topics beyond the scope of this article.[24]

RATE VERSUS RHYTHM CONTROL

Whether rhythm or rate control is the best strategy in HF failure patients with AF is controversial. The Atrial Fibrillation Follow-up Investigation of Rhythm Management (AFFIRM) and RACE trials showed no benefit of pharmacologic rhythm control over pharmacologic rate control in a general AF population.[43,44] Although these studies contained few HF patients, the results were largely mirrored in the AF-CHF trial, which randomized HF patients with AF to pharmacologic rate or rhythm control.[45] There was no difference, regardless of strategy, with respect to the end points of mortality or hospitalization for HF or stroke. However, definite conclusions should not be drawn from these trials because of substantial crossover between treatment groups. Also, only pharmacologic rhythm control therapies were evaluated, and the negative results may partly reflect the poor efficacy of AADs to maintain SR.[43–45] In fact, although not performed in an HF population, an on-treatment analysis of the AFFIRM trial showed that patients who maintained SR had better outcomes.[46] Although this may represent selection bias, it is also possible that the benefit of maintaining SR is offset by the adverse effects of the AADs. It is possible that a therapy that restores SR without the adverse effects of AADs would be superior to rate control. AF ablation may offer this opportunity.

ATRIAL FIBRILLATION ABLATION

The observation that ectopic beats originating near the pulmonary veins are responsible for the majority of paroxysmal AF episodes sparked interest in ablation as a curative therapy for AF.[47] A detailed overview of AF ablation equipment and techniques is beyond the scope of this review and can be found elsewhere.[48,49] In brief, radio

frequency catheter ablation of AF is based on percutaneous catheter insertion under fluoroscopic guidance to selectively destroy (ie, ablate) myocardial tissue regions responsible for the propagation of abnormal electrical cardiac activity in order to restore normal SR.

AF ablation by pulmonary vein isolation successfully restores SR in 60% to 80% of AF patients. The variation in procedural outcome may be explained by factors such as study heterogeneity regarding age, sex, AF types, structural heart disease, ablation methods, and operator experience.[50,51] The initial ablation success rate is comparable between the general AF population and HF patients; however, recurrence rates are higher in HF.[52–55] The latter may explain why AF ablation is not widely employed as a rhythm control strategy in HF patients. Indeed, HF patients still constitute only a small fraction of patients undergoing ablation even in experienced high-volume centers.[51]

EFFICACY OF ATRIAL FIBRILLATION ABLATION

A landmark study in 2004 showed that AF ablation resulted in significant improvements of left ventricular function, exercise tolerance, symptoms, and quality of life.[52] This improvement occurred independent of the level of preprocedural rate control, suggesting that factors other than rate (eg, loss of atrial contraction and atrioventricular dyssynchrony) also drive the deterioration of cardiac function in AF patients.

In a meta-analysis of 9 studies of AF ablation in HF patients, mean left ventricular ejection fraction (LVEF) improved 11% (95% confidence interval [CI]: 6.9–15.3, $P<.001$).[51] AF ablation also improved exercise capacity and quality of life in the majority of studies reporting on those end points. The degree of improvement was independent of the proportion of patients with paroxysmal versus persistent AF in these studies. However, the proportion of coronary artery disease patients correlated inversely with improvement in LVEF, suggesting that ischemic cardiomyopathy patients may benefit less from an AF ablation strategy. The mean procedural complication rate was 6.7%, which is comparable to the complication rates reported for AF ablation in the general population.

ATRIAL FIBRILLATION ABLATION VERSUS OTHER STRATEGIES

The PABA-CHF trial was the first trial to compare AF ablation with rate control in HF patients (**Table 2**).[36] In this study, patients with mild-to-moderate HF were randomized either to AF ablation or to atrioventricular node ablation and

Table 2
Major randomized atrial fibrillation ablation trials in heart failure patients

Study	N[a]	Ejection Fraction Before	Ejection Fraction After	P
Hsu et al,[52] 2004	116/58	35 ± 7	56 ± 13	<.001
Chen et al,[53] 2004	377/94	36 ± 7	41 ± 6	NS
Gentlesk et al,[55] 2007	366/67	42 ± 9	56 ± 8	<.001
PABA-CHF[36]	81/41	27 ± 8	35 ± 3	<.0001
MacDonald et al,[56] 2011	41/22	36 ± 12	41 ± 11	NS
ARC-CHF[57]	52/26	22 ± 8	33 ± 14	<.001
CAMTAF[58]	50/26	32 ± 8	40 ± 12	<.001
RAFT	Ongoing			
CASTLE-AF	Ongoing			
AATAC[59]	Ongoing			

[a] Total patients/randomized to ablation.
Data from Refs.[36,52,53,55–59]

biventricular pacing. The AF ablation group had superior improvements in LVEF, exercise tolerance, and quality of life during follow-up.

Several clinical trials have since compared AF ablation to pharmacologic rate control. The first of these studies demonstrated no significant differences between the groups in terms of LVEF improvement, exercise tolerance, or quality of life, although there was a trend toward improvement of LVEF in the ablation group.[56] These results should be interpreted with caution, however, as the study was small (n = 41), and only 50% of patients in the AF ablation group maintained SR, while there was a higher than anticipated percentage of patients maintaining SR in the rate control group. Moreover, this study was performed in patients with advanced HF (severely reduced LVEF) and, as discussed previously, it is possible that AF does not carry much prognostic significance in the very sickest HF patients.[28]

The results from this early study also contrast with more recent findings from the ARC-CHF (A Randomized Trial to Assess Catheter Ablation Versus Rate Control in the Management of Persistent Atrial Fibrillation in Heart Failure) and CAMTAF (A randomized controlled trial of catheter ablation versus medical treatment of atrial fibrillation in heart failure) trials, which both showed significant improvement in exercise capacity and quality of life with AF ablation compared with pharmacologic rate control.[57,58] The CAMTAF trial also showed a significant improvement of LVEF after 6 months of follow-up with AF ablation compared with pharmacologic rate control (+8.1 [95% CI: 3.0–13.1] versus -3 [95% CI: -7.7 to 0.5], $P<.001$). Similarly, the ARC-CHF trial reported a trend toward more LVEF improvement with AF ablation (mean

difference +5.6%[95% CI: −0.1 to +11.3, $P = .055$) after 12 months of follow-up. Of note, all these studies were performed in patients with HF with reduced ejection fraction (HFrEF). In fact, even in the CAMTAF trial, which had an LVEF enrollment cut-off of 50%, the actual preintervention ejection fraction was 32%. Consequently, there is a paucity of data regarding the best therapeutic approach in HFpEF patients.

The ongoing AATAC (Ablation vs Amiodarone for the Treatment of Persistent and Long Standing Persistent Atrial Fibrillation in Patients With Congestive Heart Failure), trial, a randomized trial comparing AF ablation and amiodarone for the treatment of persistent and long-standing persistent AF in HF patients recently reported preliminary results.[59] AF ablation was superior to amiodarone (75% vs 46%, lop-rank $P = .003$) in achieving freedom from AF at 10 months of follow-up. Large clinical trials, including Resynchronization—Defibrillation for Ambulatory Heart Failure Trial (RAFT)-AF (clinical trial number NCT01420393) and CASTLE-AF (Catheter ablation versus standard conventional treatment in patients with left ventricular dysfunction and atrial fibrillation) (clinical trial number NCT00643188), powered to also detect differences in mortality between AF ablation and rate control, are ongoing.

ATRIAL FIBRILLATION RECURRENCE

Even with advances in ablation techniques and equipment, AF recurs over time in 40% to 50% of patients, and repeat ablations are often necessary.[60] In a study by Gentlesk and colleagues, the initial AF ablation success rate was comparable in patients with and without heart failure

(86% vs 87%, $P =$ ns) but more repeat procedures were needed in the HF group.[55] Similarly, Chen and colleagues reported a recurrence rate of 27% in HFrEF patients compared with 13% in AF patients with normal LVEF ($P = $.003) after a single procedure, even though the groups had otherwise similar cardiovascular risk profiles.[53] Meta-analysis data also support an increased risk for recurrent AF (relative risk [RR] = 1.6, $P<$.001), as well as a need for more repeat procedures in HF patients compared with non-HF patients in order to maintain SR.[50] Evidently, a more extensive postablation follow-up detects more recurrences, which may partly explain the wide interstudy variation in recurrences.[61]

Recovery of pulmonary vein (PV) conduction and non-PV triggers are considered the 2 major causes of recurrence. The latter is thought to be a particularly important factor in HF patients and may explain their higher recurrence rate.[62] The higher repeat procedure rate in HF patients with AF increases cost and total procedural risk, and emphasizes the need for development of more effective ablation techniques in this patient population.[50]

NONPULMONARY VEIN TRIGGERS OF ATRIAL FIBRILLATION

Several studies have demonstrated that non-PV foci play an important role in initiation, maintenance, and recurrence of AF.[24,63–66] The introduction of isoprenalin (ISP) provocation has allowed more studies to address the importance of non-PV ectopic beats initiating AF.[62] High-dose ISP infusion has been shown to reveal more non-PV

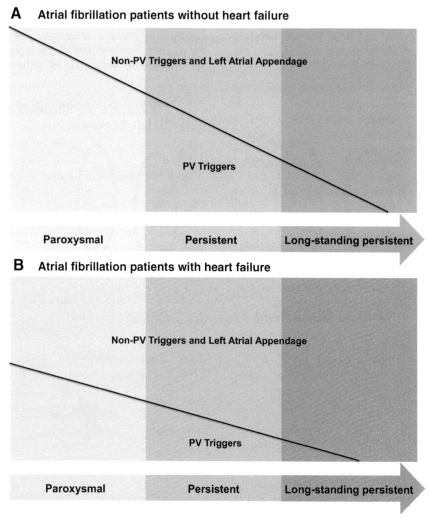

Fig. 3. Relative contribution of different ablation targets in the AF disease continuum in patients with and without heart failure. LAA, left atrial appendage; PV, pulmonary vein.

triggers than adenosine or rapid atrial pacing.[67,68] ISP may reveal non-PV foci by increasing arrhythmogenicity through vagally mediated bradycardia, while high-dose ISP may reveal non-PV foci by reducing the atrial refractory period, thereby inducing early after-depolarization and delayed after-depolarization.[69] Therefore, although PV isolation remains the cornerstone of AF ablation, the focus in recent years has expanded to also include ablation of non-PV triggers.

Non-PV triggers are particularly prevalent in patients with more long-standing AF, enlarged left atria, and underlying heart disease, including HF (**Fig. 3**).[70] Electroanatomic mapping has shown that HF patients with AF demonstrate more pronounced atrial remodeling compared with AF patients without HF. These changes include

- A more enlarged left atria[71]
- More areas of low voltage and/or electrical silence (scar), which are prone to develop into non-PV triggers[72]
- Increased atrial interstitial fibrosis, which reduces intercellular electric coupling and may predispose to ectopic firing[73]

- Intracellular calcium overload, which in animal HF models predispose to delayed after-depolarization and early after-depolarization triggered activity[74]
- Altered autonomic tone, which also increases AF susceptibility in animal models[75,76]
- Activation of atrial stretch-activated ion channels and reentry, which facilitates the development of non-PV triggers[77,78]
- Slowed atrial conduction velocities[71]
- More sinus node dysfunction[71]

It has been speculated that AF recurrence can occur either through activation of non-PV foci that were dormant during the initial procedure, or through progressive worsening of the atrial substrate causing new non-PVI foci to emerge.[79] The latter explanation is supported by evidence of progressive structural atrial remodeling in patients with AF recurrence, in contrast to the reverse atrial remodeling often seen in patients who remain free from AF.[80] Because HF is generally a progressive disease, atrial remodeling and non-PV triggers may account for the higher risk of AF recurrence after ablation in HF patients.[81]

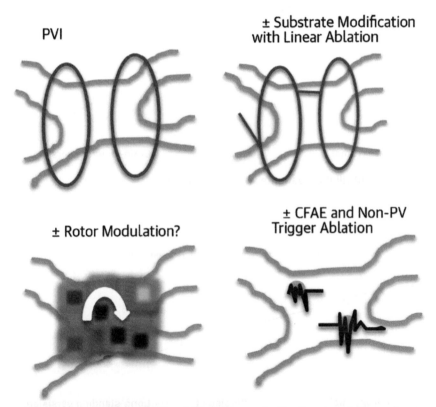

Fig. 4. Approaches to catheter ablation in HF and AF. CFAE, complex fractionated electrocardiogram; PV, pulmonary vein; PVI, pulmonary vein isolation. (*From* Trulock KM, Narayan SM, Piccini JP. Rhythm control in heart failure patients with atrial fibrillation: contemporary challenges including the role of ablation. J Am Coll Cardiol 2014;64(7):715; with permission.)

EVOLVING TECHNIQUES

The last decade has seen important development of ablation techniques and equipment. Notable examples include the invention of cryo- and laser ablation. Both these involve balloon based ablation techniques aimed at the PVs. Therefore, their applicability may be limited in patients with HF who appear to require more extensive ablation also of non-PV triggers to achieve long-term freedom from AF. Other evolving technologies include algorithms based on impedance drops, catheter stability, and contact-force sensing.[82–84]

Active areas of investigation with regards to non-PV trigger ablation include linear and focal ablation of areas with scar, or areas that demonstrate fractionation or perpetuation of rotors (**Fig. 4**). Several studies have shown that such techniques, in addition to pulmonary vein isolation, improve arrhythmia free outcomes.[85–88]

Finally, the procedural endpoint beyond PV isolation itself is a contested topic. There is an ongoing debate weather procedural AF termination improves long-term freedom from AF or not,[68,89–91] with some investigators preferring empiric lesion sets.[92] The rapid evolution of ablation equipment and techniques makes it challenging to directly compare outcomes between studies.

COST-EFFECTIVENESS

The coexistence of AF and HF increases the risk of hospitalization and significantly impacts health care cost.[93] The impact of catheter ablation to restore SR in this patient population could therefore potentially have significant implications for health care expenditure. Although there currently are no robust cost-effectiveness data regarding AF ablation in HF patients available, this issue is addressed in the ongoing RAFT-AF (NCT01420393) trial.

SUMMARY

HF and AF are on the rise and often coexist. Pharmacologic rhythm control has not been shown to improve outcomes compared with pharmacologic rate control. It is possible that the benefit in maintaining SR is offset by the adverse effects of AADs. Catheter ablation of AF offers an opportunity to achieve SR without the downside of AADs. Several studies have shown that AF ablation improves prognostic markers, including ventricular function, exercise tolerance, and perceived quality of life in HF patients. Ablation also of non-pulmonary vein triggers appear important in order to achieve long-term freedom from arrhythmia in patients with concomitant AF and HF. Studies addressing the impact of this treatment strategy on cardiovascular outcomes and cost-effectiveness are ongoing.

REFERENCES

1. Braunwald E. Shattuck lecture—cardiovascular medicine at the turn of the millennium: triumphs, concerns, and opportunities. N Engl J Med 1997; 337(19):1360–9.
2. Friberg J, Buch P, Scharling H, et al. Rising rates of hospital admissions for atrial fibrillation. Epidemiology 2003;14(6):666–72.
3. Massie BM, Shah NB. Evolving trends in the epidemiologic factors of heart failure: rationale for preventive strategies and comprehensive disease management. Am Heart J 1997;133(6):703–12.
4. Carson PE, Johnson GR, Dunkman WB, et al. The influence of atrial fibrillation on prognosis in mild to moderate heart failure. The V-HeFT studies. The V-HeFT VA Cooperative Studies Group. Circulation 1993;87(6 Suppl):VI102–10.
5. Deedwania PC, Singh BN, Ellenbogen K, et al. Spontaneous conversion and maintenance of sinus rhythm by amiodarone in patients with heart failure and atrial fibrillation: observations from the veterans affairs congestive heart failure survival trial of antiarrhythmic therapy (CHF-STAT). The Department of Veterans Affairs CHF-STAT Investigators. Circulation 1998;98(23):2574–9.
6. Mahoney P, Kimmel S, DeNofrio D, et al. Prognostic significance of atrial fibrillation in patients at a tertiary medical center referred for heart transplantation because of severe heart failure. Am J Cardiol 1999;83(11):1544–7.
7. Middlekauff HR, Stevenson WG, Stevenson LW. Prognostic significance of atrial fibrillation in advanced heart failure. A study of 390 patients. Circulation 1991;84(1):40–8.
8. Senni M, Tribouilloy CM, Rodeheffer RJ, et al. Congestive heart failure in the community: a study of all incident cases in Olmsted County, Minnesota, in 1991. Circulation 1998;98(21):2282–9.
9. Maisel WH, Stevenson LW. Atrial fibrillation in heart failure: epidemiology, pathophysiology, and rationale for therapy. Am J Cardiol 2003;91(6A): 2D–8D.
10. Dries DL, Exner DV, Gersh BJ, et al. Atrial fibrillation is associated with an increased risk for mortality and heart failure progression in patients with asymptomatic and symptomatic left ventricular systolic dysfunction: a retrospective analysis of the SOLVD trials. Studies of Left Ventricular Dysfunction. J Am Coll Cardiol 1998;32(3):695–703.
11. Wang TJ, Larson MG, Levy D, et al. Temporal relations of atrial fibrillation and congestive heart failure and their joint influence on mortality: the Framingham Heart Study. Circulation 2003;107(23):2920–5.

12. Predictors of thromboembolism in atrial fibrillation: I. Clinical features of patients at risk. The Stroke Prevention in Atrial Fibrillation Investigators. Ann Intern Med 1992;116(1):1–5.

13. Kareti KR, Chiong JR, Hsu SS, et al. Congestive heart failure and atrial fibrillation: rhythm versus rate control. J Card Fail 2005;11(3):164–72.

14. Grace AA, Narayan SM. Common threads in atrial fibrillation and heart failure. Heart Fail Clin 2013; 9(4):373–83, vii.

15. Clark DM, Plumb VJ, Epstein AE, et al. Hemodynamic effects of an irregular sequence of ventricular cycle lengths during atrial fibrillation. J Am Coll Cardiol 1997;30(4):1039–45.

16. Daoud EG, Weiss R, Bahu M, et al. Effect of an irregular ventricular rhythm on cardiac output. Am J Cardiol 1996;78(12):1433–6.

17. Shinbane JS, Wood MA, Jensen DN, et al. Tachycardia-induced cardiomyopathy: a review of animal models and clinical studies. J Am Coll Cardiol 1997;29(4):709–15.

18. Van Gelder IC, Crijns HJ, Blanksma PK, et al. Time course of hemodynamic changes and improvement of exercise tolerance after cardioversion of chronic atrial fibrillation unassociated with cardiac valve disease. Am J Cardiol 1993;72(7):560–6.

19. Wilson JR, Douglas P, Hickey WF, et al. Experimental congestive heart failure produced by rapid ventricular pacing in the dog: cardiac effects. Circulation 1987;75(4):857–67.

20. Zipes DP. Atrial fibrillation. A tachycardia-induced atrial cardiomyopathy. Circulation 1997;95(3): 562–4.

21. Gosselink AT, Blanksma PK, Crijns HJ, et al. Left ventricular beat-to-beat performance in atrial fibrillation: contribution of Frank-Starling mechanism after short rather than long RR intervals. J Am Coll Cardiol 1995;26(6):1516–21.

22. Kalifa J, Jalife J, Zaitsev AV, et al. Intra-atrial pressure increases rate and organization of waves emanating from the superior pulmonary veins during atrial fibrillation. Circulation 2003;108(6):668–71.

23. Solti F, Vecsey T, Kekesi V, et al. The effect of atrial dilatation on the genesis of atrial arrhythmias. Cardiovasc Res 1989;23(10):882–6.

24. Trulock KM, Narayan SM, Piccini JP. Rhythm control in heart failure patients with atrial fibrillation: contemporary challenges including the role of ablation. J Am Coll Cardiol 2014;64(7):710–21.

25. Swedberg K, Olsson LG, Charlesworth A, et al. Prognostic relevance of atrial fibrillation in patients with chronic heart failure on long-term treatment with beta-blockers: results from COMET. Eur Heart J 2005;26(13):1303–8.

26. Kober L, Swedberg K, McMurray JJ, et al. Previously known and newly diagnosed atrial fibrillation: a major risk indicator after a myocardial infarction complicated by heart failure or left ventricular dysfunction. Eur J Heart Fail 2006;8(6):591–8.

27. Pedersen OD, Bagger H, Kober L, et al. Impact of congestive heart failure and left ventricular systolic function on the prognostic significance of atrial fibrillation and atrial flutter following acute myocardial infarction. Int J Cardiol 2005;100(1):65–71.

28. Anter E, Jessup M, Callans DJ. Atrial fibrillation and heart failure: treatment considerations for a dual epidemic. Circulation 2009;119(18):2516–25.

29. Olsson LG, Swedberg K, Ducharme A, et al. Atrial fibrillation and risk of clinical events in chronic heart failure with and without left ventricular systolic dysfunction: results from the Candesartan in Heart failure-Assessment of Reduction in Mortality and morbidity (CHARM) program. J Am Coll Cardiol 2006;47(10):1997–2004.

30. Grogan M, Smith HC, Gersh BJ, et al. Left ventricular dysfunction due to atrial fibrillation in patients initially believed to have idiopathic dilated cardiomyopathy. Am J Cardiol 1992;69(19):1570–3.

31. Fuster V, Ryden LE, Cannom DS, et al. ACC/AHA/ESC 2006 guidelines for the management of patients with atrial fibrillation: a report of the American College of Cardiology/American Heart Association Task Force on Practice Guidelines and the European Society of Cardiology Committee for Practice Guidelines (Writing Committee to Revise the 2001 Guidelines for the Management of Patients With Atrial Fibrillation): developed in collaboration with the European Heart Rhythm Association and the Heart Rhythm Society. Circulation 2006;114(7): e257–354.

32. Van Gelder IC, Groenveld HF, Crijns HJ, et al. Lenient versus strict rate control in patients with atrial fibrillation. N Engl J Med 2010;362(15):1363–73.

33. Lechat P, Escolano S, Golmard JL, et al. Prognostic value of bisoprolol-induced hemodynamic effects in heart failure during the Cardiac Insufficiency Bisoprolol Study (CIBIS). Circulation 1997;96(7): 2197–205.

34. Lechat P, Hulot JS, Escolano S, et al. Heart rate and cardiac rhythm relationships with bisoprolol benefit in chronic heart failure in CIBIS II Trial. Circulation 2001;103(10):1428–33.

35. Doshi RN, Daoud EG, Fellows C, et al. Left ventricular-based cardiac stimulation post AV nodal ablation evaluation (the PAVE study). J Cardiovasc Electrophysiol 2005;16(11):1160–5.

36. Khan MN, Jais P, Cummings J, et al. Pulmonary-vein isolation for atrial fibrillation in patients with heart failure. N Engl J Med 2008;359(17):1778–85.

37. Coplen SE, Antman EM, Berlin JA, et al. Efficacy and safety of quinidine therapy for maintenance of sinus rhythm after cardioversion. A meta-analysis of randomized control trials. Circulation 1990;82(4):1106–16.

38. Flaker GC, Blackshear JL, McBride R, et al. Antiarrhythmic drug therapy and cardiac mortality in atrial fibrillation. The Stroke Prevention in Atrial Fibrillation Investigators. J Am Coll Cardiol 1992; 20(3):527–32.

39. Stevenson WG, Stevenson LW, Middlekauff HR, et al. Improving survival for patients with atrial fibrillation and advanced heart failure. J Am Coll Cardiol 1996;28(6):1458–63.

40. Wann LS, Curtis AB, January CT, et al. 2011 ACCF/AHA/HRS focused update on the management of patients with atrial fibrillation (updating the 2006 guideline): a report of the American College of Cardiology Foundation/American Heart Association Task Force on Practice Guidelines. J Am Coll Cardiol 2011;57(2):223–42.

41. Singla S, Karam P, Deshmukh AJ, et al. Review of contemporary antiarrhythmic drug therapy for maintenance of sinus rhythm in atrial fibrillation. J Cardiovasc Pharmacol Ther 2012;17(1):12–20.

42. Weinfeld MS, Drazner MH, Stevenson WG, et al. Early outcome of initiating amiodarone for atrial fibrillation in advanced heart failure. J Heart Lung Transplant 2000;19(7):638–43.

43. Wyse DG, Waldo AL, DiMarco JP, et al. A comparison of rate control and rhythm control in patients with atrial fibrillation. N Engl J Med 2002;347(23): 1825–33.

44. Van Gelder IC, Hagens VE, Bosker HA, et al. A comparison of rate control and rhythm control in patients with recurrent persistent atrial fibrillation. N Engl J Med 2002;347(23):1834–40.

45. Roy D, Talajic M, Nattel S, et al. Rhythm control versus rate control for atrial fibrillation and heart failure. N Engl J Med 2008;358(25):2667–77.

46. Corley SD, Epstein AE, DiMarco JP, et al. Relationships between sinus rhythm, treatment, and survival in the Atrial Fibrillation Follow-Up Investigation of Rhythm Management (AFFIRM) study. Circulation 2004;109(12):1509–13.

47. Haissaguerre M, Shah DC, Jais P, et al. Electrophysiological breakthroughs from the left atrium to the pulmonary veins. Circulation 2000;102(20):2463–5.

48. Di Biase L, Elayi CS, Fahmy TS, et al. Atrial fibrillation ablation strategies for paroxysmal patients: randomized comparison between different techniques. Circ Arrhythm Electrophysiol 2009;2(2):113–9.

49. Di Biase L, Santangeli P, Natale A. How to ablate long-standing persistent atrial fibrillation? Curr Opin Cardiol 2013;28(1):26–35.

50. Wilton SB, Fundytus A, Ghali WA, et al. Meta-analysis of the effectiveness and safety of catheter ablation of atrial fibrillation in patients with versus without left ventricular systolic dysfunction. Am J Cardiol 2010;106(9):1284–91.

51. Dagres N, Varounis C, Gaspar T, et al. Catheter ablation for atrial fibrillation in patients with left ventricular systolic dysfunction. A systematic review and meta-analysis. J Card Fail 2011;17(11): 964–70.

52. Hsu LF, Jais P, Sanders P, et al. Catheter ablation for atrial fibrillation in congestive heart failure. N Engl J Med 2004;351(23):2373–83.

53. Chen MS, Marrouche NF, Khaykin Y, et al. Pulmonary vein isolation for the treatment of atrial fibrillation in patients with impaired systolic function. J Am Coll Cardiol 2004;43(6):1004–9.

54. Tondo C, Mantica M, Russo G, et al. Pulmonary vein vestibule ablation for the control of atrial fibrillation in patients with impaired left ventricular function. Pacing Clin Electrophysiol 2006;29(9):962–70.

55. Gentlesk PJ, Sauer WH, Gerstenfeld EP, et al. Reversal of left ventricular dysfunction following ablation of atrial fibrillation. J Cardiovasc Electrophysiol 2007;18(1):9–14.

56. MacDonald MR, Connelly DT, Hawkins NM, et al. Radiofrequency ablation for persistent atrial fibrillation in patients with advanced heart failure and severe left ventricular systolic dysfunction: a randomised controlled trial. Heart 2011;97(9):740–7.

57. Jones DG, Haldar SK, Hussain W, et al. A randomized trial to assess catheter ablation versus rate control in the management of persistent atrial fibrillation in heart failure. J Am Coll Cardiol 2013;61(18): 1894–903.

58. Hunter RJ, Berriman TJ, Diab I, et al. A randomized controlled trial of catheter ablation versus medical treatment of atrial fibrillation in heart failure (the CAMTAF trial). Circ Arrhythm Electrophysiol 2014; 7(1):31–8.

59. Di Biase L, Mohanty P, Raviele A, et al. Preliminary results from AATAC: Ablation vs amiodarone for the treatment of persistent and long standing persistent atrial fibrillation in patients with congestive heart failure. Circulation 2010;122:A17358.

60. Ouyang F, Tilz R, Chun J, et al. Long-term results of catheter ablation in paroxysmal atrial fibrillation: lessons from a 5-year follow-up. Circulation 2010; 122(23):2368–77.

61. Dagres N, et al, Kottkamp H, Piorkowski C. Influence of the duration of Holter monitoring on the detection of arrhythmia recurrences after catheter ablation of atrial fibrillation: implications for patient follow-up. Int J Cardiol 2010;139(3):305–6.

62. Chen SA, Tai CT. Catheter ablation of atrial fibrillation originating from the non-pulmonary vein foci. J Cardiovasc Electrophysiol 2005;16(2):229–32.

63. Dixit S, Lin D, Frankel DS, et al. Catheter ablation for persistent atrial fibrillation: antral pulmonary vein isolation and elimination of nonpulmonary vein triggers are sufficient. Circ Arrhythm Electrophysiol 2012;5(6):1216–23 [discussion: 1223].

64. Miyazaki S, Kuwahara T, Kobori A, et al. Long-term clinical outcome of extensive pulmonary vein

isolation-based catheter ablation therapy in patients with paroxysmal and persistent atrial fibrillation. Heart 2011;97(8):668–73.

65. Mainigi SK, Sauer WH, Cooper JM, et al. Incidence and predictors of very late recurrence of atrial fibrillation after ablation. J Cardiovasc Electrophysiol 2007;18(1):69–74.

66. Roten L, Derval N, Jais P. Catheter ablation for persistent atrial fibrillation: elimination of triggers is not sufficient. Circ Arrhythm Electrophysiol 2012; 5(6):1224–32 [discussion: 1232].

67. Crawford T, Chugh A, Good E, et al. Clinical value of noninducibility by high-dose isoproterenol versus rapid atrial pacing after catheter ablation of paroxysmal atrial fibrillation. J Cardiovasc Electrophysiol 2010;21(1):13–20.

68. Elayi CS, Di Biase L, Barrett C, et al. Atrial fibrillation termination as a procedural endpoint during ablation in long-standing persistent atrial fibrillation. Heart Rhythm 2010;7(9):1216–23.

69. Chen PS, Maruyama M, Lin SF. Arrhythmogenic foci and the mechanisms of atrial fibrillation. Circ Arrhythm Electrophysiol 2010;3(1):7–9.

70. Lo LW, Chiou CW, Lin YJ, et al. Differences in the atrial electrophysiological properties between vagal and sympathetic types of atrial fibrillation. J Cardiovasc Electrophysiol 2013;24(6):609–16.

71. Sanders P, Morton JB, Davidson NC, et al. Electrical remodeling of the atria in congestive heart failure: electrophysiological and electroanatomic mapping in humans. Circulation 2003;108(12):1461–8.

72. Higa S, Tai CT, Lin YJ, et al. Focal atrial tachycardia: new insight from noncontact mapping and catheter ablation. Circulation 2004;109(1):84–91.

73. Akkaya M, Higuchi K, Koopmann M, et al. Higher degree of left atrial structural remodeling in patients with atrial fibrillation and left ventricular systolic dysfunction. J Cardiovasc Electrophysiol 2013; 24(5):485–91.

74. Stambler BS, Fenelon G, Shepard RK, et al. Characterization of sustained atrial tachycardia in dogs with rapid ventricular pacing-induced heart failure. J Cardiovasc Electrophysiol 2003;14(5):499–507.

75. Chou CC, Nguyen BL, Tan AY, et al. Intracellular calcium dynamics and acetylcholine-induced triggered activity in the pulmonary veins of dogs with pacing-induced heart failure. Heart Rhythm 2008; 5(8):1170–7.

76. Boyden PA, Tilley LP, Albala A, et al. Mechanisms for atrial arrhythmias associated with cardiomyopathy: a study of feline hearts with primary myocardial disease. Circulation 1984;69(5):1036–47.

77. Kalman JM, Sparks PB. Electrical remodeling of the atria as a consequence of atrial stretch. J Cardiovasc Electrophysiol 2001;12(1):51–5.

78. Lin YJ, Tai CT, Kao T, et al. Electrophysiological characteristics and catheter ablation in patients with

paroxysmal right atrial fibrillation. Circulation 2005; 112(12):1692–700.

79. Kurotobi T, Iwakura K, Inoue K, et al. Multiple arrhythmogenic foci associated with the development of perpetuation of atrial fibrillation. Circ Arrhythm Electrophysiol 2010;3(1):39–45.

80. Tsao HM, Wu MH, Huang BH, et al. Morphologic remodeling of pulmonary veins and left atrium after catheter ablation of atrial fibrillation: insight from long-term follow-up of three-dimensional magnetic resonance imaging. J Cardiovasc Electrophysiol 2005;16(1):7–12.

81. Yamaguchi T, Tsuchiya T, Miyamoto K, et al. Characterization of non-pulmonary vein foci with an EnSite array in patients with paroxysmal atrial fibrillation. Europace 2010;12(12):1698–706.

82. Anter E, Tschabrunn CM, Contreras-Valdes FM, et al. Radiofrequency ablation annotation algorithm reduces the incidence of linear gaps and reconnection after pulmonary vein isolation. Heart Rhythm 2014;11(5):783–90.

83. Metzner A, Reissmann B, Rausch P, et al. One-year clinical outcome after pulmonary vein isolation using the second-generation 28-mm cryoballoon. Circ Arrhythm Electrophysiol 2014;7(2):288–92.

84. Kimura M, Sasaki S, Owada S, et al. Comparison of lesion formation between contact force-guided and non-guided circumferential pulmonary vein isolation: a prospective, randomized study. Heart Rhythm 2014;11(6):984–91.

85. Kong MH, Piccini JP, Bahnson TD. Efficacy of adjunctive ablation of complex fractionated atrial electrograms and pulmonary vein isolation for the treatment of atrial fibrillation: a meta-analysis of randomized controlled trials. Europace 2011;13(2): 193–204.

86. Shivkumar K, Ellenbogen KA, Hummel JD, et al. Acute termination of human atrial fibrillation by identification and catheter ablation of localized rotors and sources: first multicenter experience of focal impulse and rotor modulation (FIRM) ablation. J Cardiovasc Electrophysiol 2012;23(12):1277–85.

87. Calkins H. Catheter ablation to maintain sinus rhythm. Circulation 2012;125(11):1439–45.

88. Narayan SM, Krummen DE, Shivkumar K, et al. Treatment of atrial fibrillation by the ablation of localized sources: CONFIRM (Conventional Ablation for Atrial Fibrillation With or Without Focal Impulse and Rotor Modulation) trial. J Am Coll Cardiol 2012; 60(7):628–36.

89. O'Neill MD, Wright M, Knecht S, et al. Long-term follow-up of persistent atrial fibrillation ablation using termination as a procedural endpoint. Eur Heart J 2009;30(9):1105–12.

90. Park YM, Choi JI, Lim HE, et al. Is pursuit of termination of atrial fibrillation during catheter ablation of great value in patients with longstanding persistent

atrial fibrillation? J Cardiovasc Electrophysiol 2012; 23(10):1051–8.

91. Faustino M, Pizzi C, Capuzzi D, et al. Impact of atrial fibrillation termination mode during catheter ablation procedure on maintenance of sinus rhythm. Heart Rhythm 2014;11(9):1528–35.

92. Gaita F, Caponi D, Scaglione M, et al. Long-term clinical results of 2 different ablation strategies in patients with paroxysmal and persistent atrial fibrillation. Circ Arrhythm Electrophysiol 2008;1(4):269–75.

93. Bleumink GS, Knetsch AM, Sturkenboom MC, et al. Quantifying the heart failure epidemic: prevalence, incidence rate, lifetime risk and prognosis of heart failure The Rotterdam Study. Eur Heart J 2004; 25(18):1614–9.

94. Crijns HJ, Tjeerdsma G, de Kam PJ, et al. Prognostic value of the presence and development of atrial fibrillation in patients with advanced chronic heart failure. Eur Heart J 2000;21(15):1238–45.

95. McMurray J, Solomon S, Pieper K, et al. The effect of valsartan, captopril, or both on atherosclerotic events after acute myocardial infarction: an analysis of the Valsartan in Acute Myocardial Infarction Trial (VALIANT). J Am Coll Cardiol 2006;47(4):726–33.

Ablation of Ventricular Arrhythmia in Patients with Heart Failure

William W.B. Chik, MBBS, MD, PhD,
Francis E. Marchlinski, MD*

KEYWORDS

- Ablation • Ventricular arrhythmia • Heart failure • Ventricular assist device

KEY POINTS

- Radiofrequency (RF) catheter ablation for ventricular arrhythmias (VAs) is usually beneficial for patients with structural heart disease and recurrent VAs or ventricular tachycardia (VT) storm resulting in multiple implantable cardiac defibrillator (ICD) shocks.
- Recognition of arrhythmia-induced cardiomyopathy is essential as it is a reversible condition with successful RF catheter ablation.
- VAs occur in more than one-third of patients on long-term ventricular assist device (VAD) support (HeartMate II, Thoratec Corporation Laboratories, Pleasanton, CA) for advanced heart failure.
- Options for treating VAs in patients with VAD include prophylactic ablation in patients at high risk for VAs after VAD, but the risk/benefit ratio must be considered in this sick population.
- Substrate and pace mapping–based ablation approach is primarily undertaken for unstable VT that occurs in 50% to 80% of patients with structural heart disease referred for ablation.

INTRODUCTION
Ventricular Arrhythmias in Heart Failure

Ventricular arrhythmias (VAs) in patients with cardiomyopathy and advanced-symptom class heart failure (HF) are associated with significant morbidity and mortality. VAs are typically managed with antiarrhythmic drug (AAD) therapy and an implantable cardiac defibrillator (ICD). Unfortunately, AAD therapy fails to prevent arrhythmia recurrence in greater than 40% of patients with prior myocardial infarction (MI) scars.[1] Although ICDs are highly effective in reducing sudden cardiac death by termination of VAs, they do not prevent arrhythmia recurrences. Recurrent shocks are not only associated with poor quality of life but also progressive HF and increased mortality and morbidity.[2–5] Radiofrequency (RF) catheter ablation (RFCA) has emerged as an important

therapeutic option for patients with drug-refractory ventricular tachycardia (VT) to reduce or prevent ICD shocks (**Box 1**).[6–8] The primary reason for VT development in the setting of structural heart disease is the presence of scars.[9] Patients with prior MI and left ventricular (LV) systolic dysfunction are at high risk, not only for developing monomorphic VT but also VT that can degenerate to ventricular fibrillation (VF) and sudden cardiac death.[9–11] However, it has also become apparent that an arrhythmogenic scar is present in individuals with nonischemic heart disease, including idiopathic cardiomyopathy (CM) and arrhythmogenic right ventricular CM/dysplasia.[12,13] The predominant mechanism for VT is reentry in these patients. To be clear, it is not the scar per se that is arrhythmogenic but the presence of living tissue intermixed within the scar that provides the ideal milieu for reentrant circuits to initiate and propagate

Division of Cardiovascular Medicine, Department of Cardiac Electrophysiology, Hospital of the University of Pennsylvania, 3400 Spruce Street, Philadelphia, PA 19104, USA
* Corresponding author. Cardiac Electrophysiology, University of Pennsylvania Health System, Hospital of the University of Pennsylvania, 9 Founders Pavilion, 3400 Spruce Street, Philadelphia, PA 19104.
E-mail address: francis.marchlinski@uphs.upenn.edu

Heart Failure Clin 11 (2015) 319–336
http://dx.doi.org/10.1016/j.hfc.2014.12.009
1551-7136/15/$ – see front matter © 2015 Elsevier Inc. All rights reserved.

Box 1
Indications for catheter ablation of VAs

Patients with structural heart disease

Catheter ablation is recommended for

1. Symptomatic sustained MMVT, including those treated by an ICD that recurs despite AAD therapy or when AADs are not tolerated or not desired

2. Incessant MMVT or VT storm not caused by a reversible cause

3. Frequent PVC, NSVT, or VT that is presumed to be causing ventricular dysfunction

4. Bundle branch reentrant or interfascicular VTs

5. Recurrent PMVT and VF refractory to AAD when there is a suspected trigger that can be targeted for ablation

Catheter ablation should be considered for

1. Recurrent MMVT despite therapy with one or more class I or III AADs

2. Recurrent MMVT and LVEF greater than 30% to 35% caused by prior MI even if they have not failed AADs or as an alternative to long-term amiodarone therapy

Patients without structural heart disease

Catheter ablation is recommended for

1. Symptomatic MMVT

2. Drug-refractory MMVT or when AADs are not tolerated or desired

3. Recurrent sustained PMVT or VF (electrical storm) that is refractory to AADs when there is a suspected trigger that can be targeted for ablation

Contraindications to catheter ablation for ventricular arrhythmias

1. Presence of a mobile ventricular thrombus (epicardial ablation or alcohol ablation may be considered)

2. Asymptomatic PVCs and/or NSVT that are not suspected of causing or contributing to ventricular dysfunction

3. VT caused by transient reversible causes, such as acute ischemia, hyperkalemia, or drug-induced torsade de pointes

Abbreviations: LVEF, left ventricular ejection fraction; MMVT, monomorphic ventricular tachycardia; NSVT, nonsustained ventricular tachycardia; PMVT, polymorphic ventricular tachycardia; PVC, premature ventricular complexes; VF, ventricular fibrillation.

Adapted from Aliot EM, Stevenson WG, Almendral-Garrote JM, et al. EHRA/HRS expert consensus on catheter ablation of ventricular arrhythmias: developed in a partnership with the European Heart Rhythm Association (EHRA), a registered branch of the European Society of Cardiology (ESC), and the Heart Rhythm Society (HRS); in collaboration with the American College of Cardiology (ACC) and the American Heart Association (AHA). Heart Rhythm 2009;6(6):886–933; with permission.

---

areas with (1) fixed or functional unidirectional block and (2) relatively slow conduction that permits recovery of previously depolarized tissue. The evolution of ablation techniques followed pioneering studies establishing the reentrant mechanism of postinfarction scar-related VT circuits.[14,15]

An estimated 40% of individuals who have an ICD placed for an index event of sustained VT will have recurrent VT.[5] This VT often necessitates the initiation of AAD to suppress additional VT episodes and prevent recurrent shocks. Unfortunately, the long-term success of these drugs in preventing recurrent arrhythmias or sudden death

is limited[1,16–18]; long-term use is often hindered by intolerance caused by side effects or drug toxicity.[16] With catheter mapping, critical components of the VT circuit can often be identified and targeted successfully with ablation.

Catheter Ablation: Entrainment Mapping Versus Substrate-Based Ablation

Hemodynamically stable ventricular tachycardia

Hemodynamically stable, slow VT that is easily inducible and stable in response to pacing composes a small minority of reentrant VT. However, when it is present, detailed activation and entrainment mapping can be performed. The goal is to identify critical elements of the reentrant circuit that are protected by anatomic or functional boundaries (dense scar or valvular structures) and that would, therefore, be easiest to successfully target with ablation. The surface electrocardiogram (ECG) recording of VT typically represents the wave front as it exits the scarred area and begins to depolarize healthy myocardium. The exit is frequently at the end of the most critical portion (isthmus) of the circuit and is located at the border of a scar. One goal during activation mapping is to identify areas with mid-diastolic potentials or abnormal, low-amplitude signals recorded during electrical diastole. These recordings are thought to represent depolarization of the aforementioned important portions of the reentrant circuit, including the most critical (isthmus).[19–21] Isolated potentials recorded during VT have been found to be present in about half of isthmus sites and represent areas at which RF energy application may be most effective in terminating VT.[19] Identifying sites critical to the reentrant circuit can sometimes be better characterized with entrainment mapping or with pacing from a remote site to dissociate the potential from the VT. The presence of bystander sites, as well as the presence of multiple loops of reentry, can often confound analysis.

Entrainment mapping can be performed in hemodynamically tolerated VT that remains stable during pacing. Pacing slightly faster than the VT will cause continuous resetting of the reentry circuit. Sites within the circuit will have a postpacing interval (PPI), or time to return to the site of pacing, within 30 milliseconds of the tachycardia cycle length (TCL). The farther away from the circuit that entrainment is attempted, the larger the difference will be between the PPI and TCL. Additionally, the presence of antiarrhythmic medications may further decrease conduction velocities during pacing and can potentially confound analysis particularly when pacing at even modestly faster rates.[22] Even after detailed mapping is performed, it may not be possible to delineate the entire circuit, as parts of the reentry circuit may not be confined to the endocardium but may course through the mid-myocardium or epicardium.

Hemodynamically unstable ventricular tachycardia

Detailed activation and entrainment mapping cannot be performed for VT associated with hemodynamic instability, unreliable inducibility, spontaneous termination of nonsustained runs, nonuniform cycle lengths, and/or morphologies during attempts at entrainment mapping. Multiple recent trials indicate only one-third of patients have exclusively mappable VT circuits.[7] For post-infarction VT, 31% had unmappable VT and 38% had both mappable and unmappable VT.[7,23] Similarly in patients with nonischemic CM (NICM), less than 50% of induced VT was hemodynamically stable and amenable to entrainment mapping. When entrainment mapping is not feasible, an alternative strategy to identify the sinus rhythm or pace mapping footprints of the VT circuit is necessary.

SINUS RHYTHM VOLTAGE MAP

The authors described the concept of *substrate mapping* in sinus rhythm to target the footprints of VT within the scar defined by voltage mapping.[24] Electroanatomic mapping used magnetic field–based or electrical impedance–based triangulation of a catheter's location in 3-dimensional space to create color-coded voltage maps in sinus rhythm as the catheter roves and records electrical signals within a cardiac chamber. A detailed substrate and voltage map should target areas of known infarction or scar based on prior imaging. The endocardial extent of the anatomic abnormality has been well characterized using bipolar voltage criteria of 1.5 to 2.0 mV for identifying normal signal amplitude recorded from the LV endocardium using a commercially available electroanatomic mapping system with a 4-mm electrode tip mapping catheter.[25,26] Low-voltage areas of endocardium typically identify arrhythmia substrate for most patients with sustained VT. Thus, a color range corresponding to endocardial bipolar voltages of 0.5 to 1.5 mV will highlight areas of densely scarred myocardium or aneurysm (<0.5 mV), border zone of scar (0.5–<1.5 mV), and healthy myocardium (>1.5 mV) (**Figs. 1** and **2**). Regions of scar identified on either MRI or computed tomography (CT) have shown good correlation with low-voltage areas on electroanatomic mapping, and integrated systems may provide incremental utility in VT mapping and ablation.[27,28]

Most isthmus regions of the VT circuit in patients with post-MI VT are located in the dense scar (<0.5 mV), whereas exit sites from the VT circuit are situated in the border zone as the VT circuit leaves the scar and engages normal myocardium. Once the myocardial scar has been accurately identified, ablation targets within the scar are chosen based on identification of (1) channels, (2) sites of good pace maps associated with long stem-QRS times, and (3) locations of abnormal electrogram morphologies (fractionated electrograms or

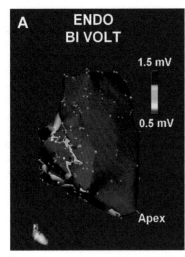
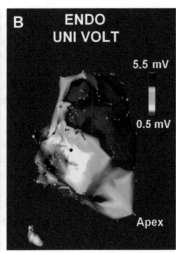
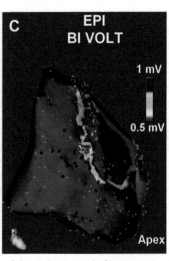

Fig. 1. Right anterior oblique (RAO) projection of sinus rhythm voltage maps of the right ventricle from a patient with arrhythmogenic right ventricular CM. Violet represented areas of preserved bipolar voltage (BI VOLT) (>1.5 mV in panel [A] and >1 mV in panel [C]) and unipolar voltage (UNI VOLT) (>5.5 mV in panel [B]), respectively. Red represented dense electroanatomic scars (<0.5 mV in [A] and [C] and <3.5 mV in [B]). Rainbow colors depicted the border zone. Panel (A) A basal area of abnormal endocardium. Endocardial unipolar voltage map in panel (B) suggested a much greater area of abnormal epicardium (EPI) extending up to the pulmonic valve and anteriorly to the apical region, which was subsequently confirmed during epicardial voltage mapping panel (C).

more importantly electrograms with late components inscribed to sinus QRS). Pace mapping in sinus rhythm attempts to replicate the 12-lead surface QRS morphology of the VT by delivering threshold-pacing stimulus from various pacing sites. Sites of good 12-lead pace map morphology match in a scar-related reentrant circuit with short stimulus to QRS interval identifying VT exit sites from scar (see **Fig. 2**).[29]

EPICARDIAL VENTRICULAR TACHYCARDIA MAPPING

Features that may indicate the need for epicardial mapping and ablation can be apparent on the surface 12-lead ECG recorded during VT.[30–32] These features include the presence of a particularly wide QRS VT with a slurred initial aspect of the QRS complex. A Q wave in lead I is a particularly sensitive characteristic for identifying an epicardial VT site of origin in patients with NICM. If it is present, and there is an absence of Q waves in the inferior leads, a basal and superior lateral epicardial focus is suggested.

Premature Ventricular Contractions and Ventricular Arrhythmia-Induced Cardiomyopathy

Idiopathic VTs, commonly manifesting as premature ventricular contractions (PVCs), can lead to CM in the absence of structural heart disease.[33–38] PVCs can also exacerbate CM in patients with

known structural disease.[33–38] Typical sites of origins include the right and LV outflow tracts, though PVCs arising from nonoutflow tract sites can also produce or potentiate a CM.[33,35,39] The incidence of arrhythmia-induced CM (AIC) in patients with repetitive monomorphic PVCs and/or nonsustained VT is estimated between 9% and 34%.[33,40,41]

Mechanisms by which PVCs precipitate CM are not completely understood, and identification of predictors for AIC in patients with frequent PVCs has been the subject of extensive research. Mechanical dyssynchrony with left bundle branch block (LBBB) and disadvantageous myocardial kinetics with PVCs have been considered as possible mechanisms; however, the development of a myopathy with atrial premature depolarizations and the absence of a convincing site-specific association with the myopathy suggest that it may not be a simple matter of LV dyssynchrony. The causal relationship between PVCs and CM has been firmly established based on the reversal of the CM with elimination of PVCs using medications or, more commonly, catheter ablative therapy.[42,43]

Numerous studies have revealed several PVC characteristics associated with the development of ventricular dysfunction in patients with frequent PVCs.[33,41,44–46] A critical consideration is the frequency of PVCs over a 24-hour time period (PVC burden). A significant PVC burden has been retrospectively defined variably as greater than 10,000 to 25,000 PVCs per day and/or alternatively as

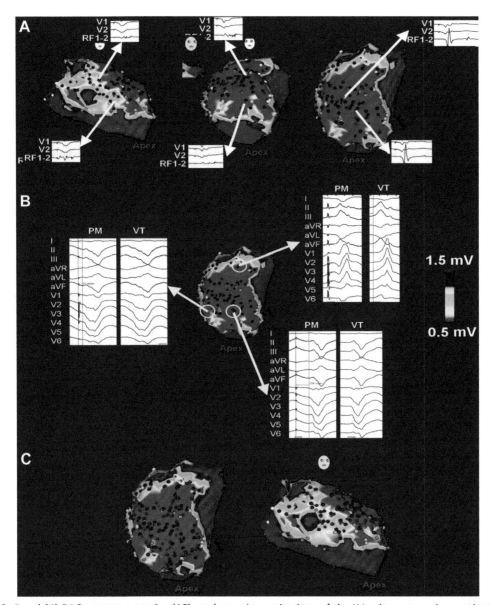

Fig. 2. Panel (*A*) RAO, antero-posterior (AP), and superior projections of the LV voltage maps in a patient with anteroseptal MI and apical aneurysm. A large area of scar involving the anterolateral wall and the interventricular septum was present. Clusters of fractionated electrograms (EGMs) and late potentials were noted. Panel (*B*) Different VTs were induced and mapped to the apical, septal, and basal aspects of the scar. The paced QRS (PM) and QRS during VT were compared at the 3 locations. Purple corresponded to areas of normal voltage (>1.5 mV) or healthy myocardium and red indicated dense scar (<0.5 mV). The border zone was depicted in rainbow colors. Panel (*C*) The final lesion set with ablations (*brown dots*) targeted the exit sites of the VT and abnormal EGMs.

greater than 12% to 24% of total heart beats per day.[46–48] Despite the absence of a definitive cutoff, the risk of developing AIC seems to be greater with a higher PVC burden with a threshold of approximately 10,000 to produce AIC.[46] Other factors, including male sex, increased body mass index, asymptomatic nature of PVCs, shorter PVC coupling interval (≤600 milliseconds), wider PVC QRS duration, an epicardial origin, interpolated PVCs, and the presence of retrograde p waves, have also been suggested to confer an increased risk of developing CM.[33,45,49–51] One study indicated that patients with PVCs of right ventricular origin (manifesting LBBB QRS morphology) have a higher propensity to develop CM.[36] Furthermore, patients developing PVC-mediated CM were more likely to be asymptomatic or had prolonged palpitations (>60 months).[36,49]

Reversibility of Cardiomyopathy with Ablation of Ventricular Arrhythmias

Recently, the authors identified a wider PVC QRS duration (>150 milliseconds) as an important independent risk factor in patients with a high PVC burden (>10,000).[52] The authors suggested that the QRS duration might be a marker for underlying myocardial fiber disruption that might predispose to frequent PVC stress-induced CM. The additional stress of frequent PVCs on top of the baseline abnormality may predispose to AIC. Carballeira Pol and colleagues[53] undertook a follow-up longitudinal study in patients with a high PVC burden but initial normal LV function. A wider QRS at the initial evaluation was documented in the cohort who subsequently developed LV dysfunction versus the cohort who maintained normal LV function. A cutoff of 150 milliseconds for PVC QRS duration was again identified to indicate increased clinical risk.[53] Additionally, a predisposition to pacing-induced CM has been suggested with a wider paced QRS complex observed in patients who later developed a CM in this setting. Of note, gross anatomic changes are not typically identified on MRI studies in patients who develop a PVC-induced CM. Subtle degrees of myocardial fiber disruption may be suggested by a minor increase in LV endocardial unipolar electrogram recordings that have been noted; but, importantly, pathologic confirmation is lacking.[54] Fortunately, most of the patients with frequent PVCs will not result in CM.[48] Although there is currently no specific risk profile that defines a group of patients that require prophylactic PVC elimination to prevent the development of the AIC, this remains an important goal of future research.

For patients with frequent PVCs or nonsustained VT and LV dysfunction, the goals of therapy should be targeted at suppressing or eliminating the PVCs. Therapeutic options include antiarrhythmic therapy and/or catheter ablation. Amiodarone or dofetilide, in conjunction with a beta-blocker, are the best choices for AAD therapy in patients with HF. Beta-blockade and non-dihydropyridine calcium channel blockade are low-risk therapies; however, they have limited efficacy. Beta-blocker therapy is frequently used if the PVC burden is high even in the absence of depressed function because of the benign nature of the treatment. Membrane-active AAD therapy including dofetilide, flecainide, mexiletine, propafenone, sotalol, or amiodarone may be more effective but at the expense of a greater side-effect profile and proarrhythmic risk. Particular caution should be exercised with the class 1 C agents in the presence of LV dysfunction. Efforts to exclude primary structural abnormalities or active ischemia are essential before initiating such treatment. In the authors' practice, treatment with membrane-active drugs is frequently reserved for patients who failed or are reluctant to undergo catheter ablation therapy.

RFCA has emerged as the definitive therapy for PVC-mediated AIC with success rates ranging from 70% to 90%.[35] Successful RFCA has been shown to improve LV ejection function (LVEF), ventricular dimensions, mitral regurgitation, and functional status (**Fig. 3**). Ablation has recently been shown to have superior efficacy than antiarrhythmic therapy in PVC reduction and improvement in LVEF in an observational series.[55]

In nonresponders of cardiac resynchronization therapy (CRT), successful catheter ablation of frequent PVCs has also been shown to improve the clinical efficacy of CRT.[56] Penela and colleagues[57] reported results from a prospective multicenter study of 80 patients with a mean PVC burden of $22 \pm 13\%$ (34% with structural heart disease). Patients undergoing successful catheter ablation without recurrence experienced significant improvements in HF parameters, including LVEF, brain natriuretic peptide levels, and New York Heart Association (NYHA) class. High baseline PVC burden ($\geq 13\%$) and persistence of ablation success were keys in predicting improvement in HF status.[57] This finding highlights the persistence of cellular and extracellular ultrastructural changes following recovery of ventricular function, which can contribute to a rapid decline in cardiac function with tachycardia recurrence. However, elimination of high-burden PVCs in patients with impaired LV function can be associated with significant improvement of LV function even when significant structural abnormalities are present.[42,43] Conversely, an epicardial origin and the presence of greater than 1 PVC morphology were factors associated with ablation failure and less improvement. In patients without structural heart disease, 5.7% had delayed gadolinium hyperenhancement suggestive of fibrosis/scar on cardiac MRI. However, no significant difference in the echocardiographic response rate was observed between patients with and without hyperenhancement on cardiac MRI.[57]

AIC caused by persistent tachyarrhythmias and frequent PVCs is an important and often underrecognized nonischemic but potentially reversible cause of CM and HF. Early recognition of the culprit VA and successful elimination of the tachyarrhythmia with targeted catheter ablation

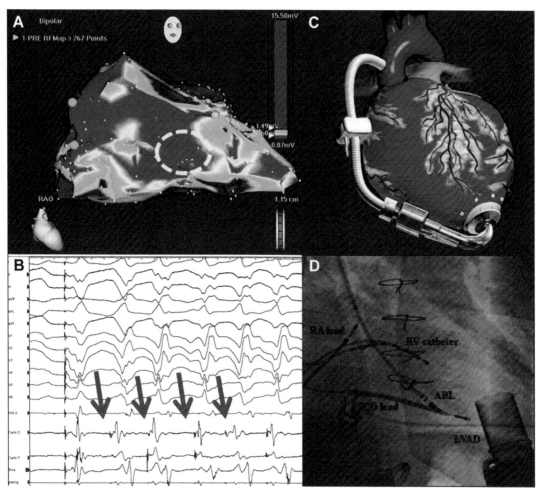

Fig. 3. This image shows a 49-year-old man with an ischemic CM and severe LV systolic dysfunction following a large anterior MI 1 month before presentation. An LV assist device (LVAD) was implanted as a bridge to heart transplantation. Panel (*A*) shows a large anteroseptal scar (represented by *red color*) corresponding to an abnormally low endocardial bipolar voltage of less than 0.5 mV (normal >2.0 mV) on 3-dimensional electroanatomical mapping. Catheter mapping was performed in the region of the endocardial anteroseptal scar and the scar border zone (outlined by the *yellow dotted lines*). (*B*) Highlights Purkinje fiber firings (*bold red arrows*) identified on the distal tip of the ablation catheter displayed as intracardiac electrograms on Prucka (labeled CARTO D) during mapping at the edge of the infarcted zone as indicated in (*A*). Radiofrequency ablation (RFA) energy at this location resulted in immediate elimination of recurrent VF for this patient. Panel (*C*) shows a graphical illustration of the LVAD (HeartMate II), and panel (*D*) demonstrates the fluoroscopic appearance of the LVAD and its anatomic proximity to the ablation catheter positioned at the site of successful RFA. EF, ejection fraction.

represents a potential therapeutic option to reverse a vicious cycle of worsening HF and deteriorating LV function.

Ventricular Assist Devices in Heart Failure

Implantable ventricular assist devices (VAD), such as HeartMate II (Thoratec Laboratories Corporation, Pleasanton, CA) have been increasingly used to extend the survival of patients with advanced HF as a bridge to cardiac transplantation, recovery, and destination therapy producing

improved quality of life.[58–61] VAs are common during left VAD (LVAD) support, with an average incidence of 33% and a range of 22% to 53% of patients.[62] The highest VA rates were observed early within the first 2 weeks after VAD implantation.[63–65] First-generation pulsatile-flow VAD devices had a reported VA incidence of 30% in the early postoperative period.[64] The Interagency Registry for Mechanically Assisted Circulatory Support reported a 10-fold increased risk for VA onset during the first month after implantation with the smaller second-generation continuous-flow VAD devices.[66,67] A history of VA before VAD implant at least doubles the risk for VA during VAD support.[64,68] Other risk factors for VA include early increases in QT interval,[69] electrolyte disturbances,[64] absence of beta-blockade therapy,[70] and atrial fibrillation before VAD support.[68] VAs in VAD-supported patients are associated with increased mortality[68] and morbidity.[65]

Mechanisms of VA in VAD-supported patients include suction events secondary to intravascular volume reduction, increased VAD flow rates, and elevated pulmonary resistance, which create negative pressure at the VAD inflow LV apical cannula site and resultant mechanical irritation triggering persistent VA.[64,71] Myocardial fibrosis–(scarring or localized injury from LVAD cannula insertion) related alteration in myocyte excitability, conduction slowing, and increased ectopic activity can lead to increased arrhythmogenicity.[72,73] Altered ventricular repolarization and prolonged QTc interval has been associated with LVAD-induced chamber decompression and implicated in the perioperative occurrence of recurrent VA.[63,69] On a cellular level, downregulation in connexin-43 expression leading to reduced conduction velocity[74,75] and upregulation of sodium-calcium exchanger affecting calcium handling and delayed after-depolarizations[76,77] have also been postulated as mechanisms for VA and mechanical dysfunction in patients with HF.

Recurrent sustained VA can cause a precipitous decrease in LVAD output (mean decrease 1.4 ± 0.6 L/min),[78] increased LVAD thrombotic risk, reduced survival to cardiac transplantation, predisposition to right HF, and death.[68,79] Myocardial scar from apical insertion of the LVAD inflow cannula creates a new substrate that promotes macroreentrant monomorphic VT (MMVT), which may be frequent, incessant, and resistant to multiple medication therapies.[64] Conversely, triggers for polymorphic VT (PMVT)/VF, including myocardial ischemia, poor hemodynamic state, and elevated intravenous inotropic requirements, are potentially alleviated by the hemodynamic support derived from LVAD.

Management of Ventricular Arrhythmias in Ventricular Assist Device–Supported Patients

Identification and reversal of treatable VA causes should be addressed, such as device malfunction, electrolyte disturbances, suboptimal LVAD continuous flow speeds, excessive diuresis or pressor use, and right HF. The optimization of durable LVAD can be used to provide additional hemodynamic support and ventricular unloading to potentially reduce recurrent or intractable VAs for both ischemic and NICM. Although AADs are routinely used in VAD-supported patients, preemptive initiation of amiodarone after VAD has not been shown to reduce VA incidence in studies.[70,80] Amiodarone instigation after recurrence of VA may reduce subsequent VA recurrence.[65] However, for patients with recurrent VAs on VAD support, the addition of another AAD (including sotalol, lidocaine, mexiletine and procainamide) has not been shown to decrease VA recurrence.[65]

The optimal management strategy for patients undergoing LVAD implantation with a history of VAs continues to be debated. The risk of developing VAs after LVAD is significantly lower in the absence of VA before LVAD implantation (4% vs 46%).[81] Patients at high risk of VA recurrence after LVAD implantation may be candidates for catheter mapping and ablation before LVAD implant provided the VA is not associated with hemodynamic decompensation in otherwise clinically stable patients. However, careful consideration of the benefits in this very sick population must be weighed against the potential risks for periprocedural complications. Alternatively, patients with refractory MMVT not stable enough to undergo catheter ablation may be candidates for pre-LVAD mapping of the arrhythmia origin or imaging studies of scar (cardiac MRI, CT) to delineate the anticipated area of interest before intraoperative cryoablation at the time of LVAD implantation to minimize cross-clamp and perfusion time.[82] Mulloy and colleagues[83] created cryoablation linear lesions connecting identified scar to fixed anatomic barriers at surgery and demonstrated reduced VA recurrence with decreased reintubation rates and duration of hospitalization. The third option is to perform RFCA for recurrent VA in the setting of LVAD-supported patients.

Catheter Ablation and Outcomes in Ventricular Assist Device–Supported Patients

Catheter ablation therapy is indicated and effective for drug-refractory VAs with recurrent ICD shocks for VAD-supported patients. An advantage in this setting is the more detailed activation and entrainment mapping that may be better tolerated because of the hemodynamic stability afforded by the VAD device, leading to improved ablation efficacy.[84] Herweg and colleagues[85] concluded that RFCA is safe and feasible in a small case series of 8 catheter ablation procedures in 6 LVAD-supported patients with refractory VT, including 5 with VT storm. Four patients had no further VT, and 2 benefited from significant reduction in VA burden.

Cantillon and colleagues[78] reported on 611 recipients of VAD, 21 were referred for 32 ablation procedures, including 52% with ICD therapies. Of the 44 inducible VTs (mean cycle length 339 ± 59 milliseconds), 91% were monomorphic macroreentrant VT. The dominant substrate harboring the reentrant circuit was composed of intrinsic myocardial scar (75%) instead of the previously proposed apical inflow cannulation site (14%). Other mechanisms of VT-induced included focal/microreentry VT (7%) or bundle-branch reentry (3.5%). PMVT/VF was identified in only 8%. RFCA succeeded acutely in 18 out of 21 (86%) of the patients with noninducibility as an endpoint, with 14 (67%) patients subsequently undergoing transplantation. VT recurrence occurred in 7 out of 21 patients (33%) at a mean of 133 ±98 days, but only 1 patient had recurrence of previously ablated arrhythmia. Six patients (29%) required repeat procedures, with subsequent recurrences observed in 4 out of 21 patients (19%).[78]

Catheter ablation of PVC-triggered VF/PMVT arising from the outflow tracts,[86] Purkinje network,[87] papillary muscle,[88] or moderator band[89] may also represent unique opportunities to provide hemodynamic support during RFCA despite the severity of the arrhythmia (**Fig. 4**).

However, several unique technical challenges pertain specifically to catheter ablation in the VAD-supported population. Firstly, catheter manipulation within the LV may be severely limited by the significantly reduced LV volumes following LVAD unloading. Secondly, the ablation catheter may rarely become entrapped within the LVAD or causes damage to the inflow cannula secondary to suction effects. This event is fortunately a very rare. Thirdly, vascular access may be difficult in continuous-flow LVAD because of the loss of systemic pulsatile flow. The absence of pulsatile flow mandates the reliance on invasive arterial monitoring given the unreliable readings from an automatic sphygmomanometer. Fourthly, crossing the aortic valve in the case of retrograde aortic access may be particularly challenging because of the absence of aortic valve opening. This crossing may be facilitated by transiently reducing LVAD flow rates. For transseptal access, a steerable sheath may be especially helpful. Finally, right

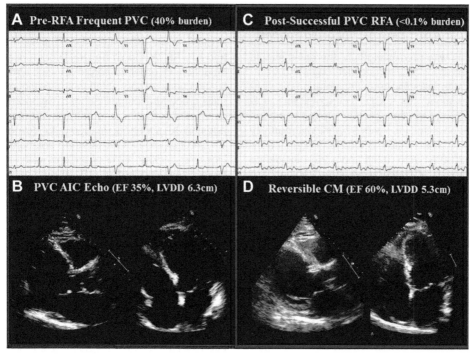

Fig. 4. This figure highlights the importance of early recognition and treatment by RF ablation (RFA) of premature ventricular complexes (PVC)–induced dilated CM (or AIC). This Fig. shows a 68-year-old gentleman with frequent symptomatic PVC (burden 40% on Holter monitoring) and progressive decline in LVEF (baseline 60%–35%) referred for RFA. Panel (*A*) shows the preablation 12-lead ECG documenting the electrocardiographic characteristics of the clinical PVCs. Panel (*B*) illustrates the preablation transthoracic echocardiographic images (parasternal and 4-chamber views, respectively). LVEF was reported as 60%, and LV end-diastolic dimension (LVDD) measured 6.3 cm. Panel (*C*) diagrams the ECG following successful RFA of 2 PVCs originating from the LV septum and the left coronary cusp. Panel (*D*) confirms recovery of the LV systolic function and reversal of CM after ablation.

ventricular (RV) decompensation may not be well tolerated for prolonged periods of mapping and ablation time during periods of VT. Indeed for cases of known severe RV dysfunction with hemodynamically significant VT, biventricular VAD implantation should be considered.

VAD provides additional hemodynamic stability for RFCA procedures allowing them to be successfully and safely performed by experienced operators and centers.[62,78,90] Ablation may be undertaken for VAD-supported patients with drug-resistant recurrent VAs, multiple ICD shocks, and/or side effects from AADs to improve the quality of life among patients with a bridge to transplant or destination therapy. In such cases, the option of percutaneous RF ablation should be considered if there is a good likelihood of procedural efficacy and survival based on substrate and relevant clinical features. A multidisciplinary approach in the decision-making process should at least involve the HF physician, electrophysiologist, and implanting surgeon for the periprocedural discussion with patients and their families.

Implantable Cardioverter Defibrillators in Ventricular Assist Device–Supported Patients

In patients with preexisting ICD, therapies should be activated for appropriate detection and treatment of VAs following VAD implantation. For patients without an ICD, concomitant ICD implantation at the time of VAD implant has been shown to be associated with a significant mortality reduction (hazard ratio 0.55 [95% confidence interval 0.32–0.94, $P = .028$]) and a 25% incidence of appropriate ICD therapies after implant.[91] A 2-fold increase in post-VAD survival has been similarly reported by adopting a de novo ICD strategy.[92] Oswald and colleagues[93] observed 34% of appropriate ICD therapies in LVAD-supported patients within the first 12 months. Patients with a prior history of VAs and a secondary prophylactic ICD indication have a 2-fold increased risk for any ICD intervention, supporting the argument for ongoing ICD use in this subgroup of patients. ICD therapies are effective with rare reports of arrhythmia undersensing or VA refractory to defibrillation. Antitachycardia pacing has been successful in terminating 25% to 50% of VT.[80,91] A high-energy ICD device may be preferred given the higher defibrillation threshold that has been observed in patients with end-stage CM on VAD and potential electrical interference of conducting artifacts inside the thorax.[93] Inappropriate therapies are relatively uncommon (6.5%) in continuous-flow VAD-supported patients.[68]

Electromagnetic interference from the LVAD (HeartMate II) causing telemetry inhibition between certain ICD models (Atlas V-193, V-240, V-243, St Jude Medical [SJM], Saint Paul, MN; Paradym CRT 8750, Sorin Group, Milan, Italy) and their programmer has been reported.[94–96] Repositioning of the programmer head (Paradym) and metal plate shielding (SJM V-243) may be effective in reestablishing telemetry; but Boudghene-Stambouli and colleagues[94] reported that 2 patients required replacement of ICDs to devices that communicated at a different frequency. Nonclinical RV lead parameter changes (reduction in sensing and impedance) were also observed after LVAD. Neither LVAD-induced RV lead interferences were associated with inappropriate therapies. Although VAD may interact with ICD resulting in loss of telemetry function necessitating reprogramming or replacement,[66] the benefits of VA detection and treatment offered by ICDs should be used in most long-term VAD-supported patients.

Catheter Ablation of Ventricular Tachycardia in Percutaneously Left Ventricular Assist Device–Supported Patients

In patients with advanced structural heart disease and HF, RFCA should be ideally composed of VT induction in order to target clinical arrhythmias limiting unnecessary ablation and potentially minimize procedural complications. This approach necessitates activation and entrainment mapping in addition to substrate mapping to delineate the VT circuitry isthmus for targeted ablation (**Fig. 5**). However, 50% to 80% of patients with structural heart disease undergoing VT ablation have hemodynamically unstable VT that is poorly tolerated during activation and entrainment mapping.[97,98] In such patients, mapping is limited to substrate and pace mapping often leading to extensive ablation for substrate modification that may worsen cardiac dysfunction if ablation is given outside scar. For patients with unstable VTs or VT storm who are acutely decompensated, external hemodynamic support devices, including intra-aortic balloon pump (IABP) and the superior percutaneous LVAD (pLVAD) devices, have been successfully used to provide hemodynamic support during mapping of induced VT episodes and removed following catheter ablation.[99–101]

The 2 pLVADs currently in clinical use are TandemHeart (CardiacAssist, Inc, Pittsburgh, PA) and Impella (Abiomed, Danvers, MA). The TandemHeart uses a left atrial-to-femoral artery bypass system and microprocessor-based pump to provide hemodynamic support at rates up to

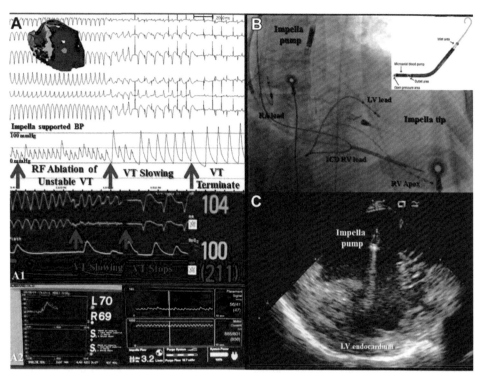

Fig. 5. An 81-year-old man with a past history significant for multivessel coronary artery disease, ischemic CM (LVEF 30%), and biventricular (BiV)-ICD implanted presented with recurrent ICD shocks for VT. He had failed medical management of his VT with amiodarone, mexiletine, and propafenone. In the electrophysiology laboratory, the surface ECG leads and the invasive arterial blood pressure (BP) tracing (0 mm Hg–100 mm Hg) were displayed as in panel (*A*). The percutaneous LVAD (pLVAD) was used to allow detailed activation and entrainment mapping during VT. The distal input port of the Impella (3.5 L/min) device was positioned in the LV cavity while the output port remained in the proximal aorta, confirmed on the fluoroscopic image in panel (*B*). The insert of panel (*B*) illustrates the standard Impella device deployed for hemodynamic support. LV, left ventricle; RA, right atrium; RV, right ventricle. Panel (*C*) shows the position of the Impella deployed in the LV cavity on intracardiac echocardiography (ICE). Panel (*A1*) depicts the left- and right-sided cerebral oximetry, respectively. Panel (*A2*) displays the corresponding BP (56/41, mean arterial pressure 47 mm Hg) recorded by the Impella device pumping at a flow rate of 3.2 L/min. During one of the multiple VT morphologies induced, RF ablation energy was successfully delivered while the patient was in VT, panel (*A*), resulting in slowing of VT cycle length before VT termination. Panel (*A1*) illustrates the impact of his rapid VT on the corresponding arterial BP despite Impella support. RF ablation could be continued while the patient remained in VT because of an acceptable level of cerebral oximetry saturation (panel [*A2*]; an acceptable cerebral oximetry threshold greater than 55%[103] was maintained throughout the ablation). Recovery of his arterial BP was noted (*A*) immediately on slowing and subsequent termination of his rapid VT during ablation.

5 L/min. The Impella device is a catheter-mounted continuous-flow motor-driven microaxial rotary pump, which removes oxygenated blood from the LV then injects into the ascending aorta at up to 5 L/min. It is percutaneously inserted at the femoral artery and advanced retrograde across the aortic valve into the left ventricle.

The first case of VT ablation with a pLVAD was reported by Friedman and colleagues[100] using a TandemHeart to perform successful endocardial and epicardial mapping and ablation of an unstable VT. The Impella pLVAD was first described by Abuissa and colleagues[101] for successfully ablating multiple unstable VTs in 3 patients by providing hemodynamic support and allowed

combined substrate, activation, and entrainment mapping resulting in termination of VT during ablation in one patient. Carbucicchio and colleagues[102] reported on using pLVAD for ablation in 19 patients with severe CM and recurrent unstable VT or VT storm causing acute cardiac decompensation. They abolished 45 out of 56 (80%) unstable VTs guided by activation mapping, and all clinical VTs were suppressed in 10 out of 19 (53%) patients without any complications, demonstrating pLVAD-supported catheter ablation for unstable VT in an emergent setting was safe and efficacious.

Miller and colleagues[99] described a retrospective observational study of 23 procedures in patients with structural heart disease and hemodynamically unstable VT performed with either pLVAD support (Impella = 10 patients) or no pLVAD support (IABP = 6; no support = 7). Patients on Impella were able to safely maintain end-organ perfusion despite spending significantly longer in hemodynamically unstable VT to permit activation/entrainment mapping and required fewer rescue shocks than the non-Impella–supported patients. Impella also permitted more VT termination during ablation than those without. This finding provided the platform for the subsequent prospective Percutaneous Hemodynamic Support With Impella 2.5 During Scar-related Ventricular Tachycardia Ablation study.[103] In this study, a cerebral oximetry threshold of greater than 55% was identified as the complementary monitoring modality for early detection of cerebral desaturations caused by end-organ hypoperfusion independent of mean arterial pressure. This hemodynamic support translated to a 40% increase in activation/entrainment mapping time during periods of hemodynamically significant VT. The pLVAD-supported ablation was associated with a more favorable hemodynamic profile and reduced cerebral desaturations than pharmacologic agents alone during fast VT.

Electromagnetic interference (EMI) between the magnetic-based electroanatomical mapping system (CARTO) and the magnetic motor of the pLVAD was nonprohibitive for continuation of the procedure but interfered with acquisition of mapping points, distortion of the catheter position, and integration of respiratory compensation algorithms.[104] Electrical impedance–based mapping systems are less likely to be affected by EMI, and accurate endocardial/epicardial maps could be obtained without titration of the microaxial flow rate.[104,105] The pLVAD functionality was not adversely impacted by EMI.

This finding was consistent with results reported by Bunch and colleagues[106] who compared 13 patients in a retrospective observational study with TandemHeart-assisted unstable VT ablation against 18-matched patients undergoing conventional substrate-based VT ablation without pLVAD support. The number of inducible MMVT intraprocedurally was greater, and procedure times were longer for the pLVAD group; however, there was no difference in acute complications and no short- and long-term outcomes between pLVAD-assisted activation/entrainment-guided ablations and substrate-based ablations without pLVAD support.[106]

Reddy and colleagues[107] recently confirmed the lack of superiority of activation/entrainment mapping over substrate mapping in their multicenter prospective observational study of 66 consecutive patients undergoing VT ablations with pLVAD. They showed that the hemodynamic support afforded by the use of TandemHeart or Impella permitted (1) a greater number of activation/entrainment mapping of VTs, (2) more unstable VTs ablated, (3) more VTs terminated during ablation, and (4) fewer rescue shocks required to terminate VTs compared with IABP.[107] However, despite more entrainment, better delineation of the critical isthmus, and targeting of VTs, these did not translate to improved short-term success or greater long-term freedom from VT.

Aryana and colleagues[108] recently published the largest retrospective nonrandomized evaluation of 68 consecutive patients with unstable, scar-mediated endocardial and/or epicardial VT with 34 (50%) patients undergoing mapping and ablation with and 34 without pLVAD, respectively. Consistent with prior studies, VT was sustained longer with a pLVAD than without a pLVAD (27.4 ±18.7 vs 5.3 ±3.6 minutes, P<.001); more VTs terminated during ablation for pLVAD-supported patients (1.2 ± 0.9 vs 0.4 ± 0.6/procedure, P<.001). Total RF ablation time was less for the pLVAD group (53 ± 30 vs 68 ± 33 minutes, P = .022), but again no difference in acute success (71% for both groups; P = 1.0). Of note, although pLVAD did not reduce VT recurrence at 19 ± 12 months' follow-up (pLVAD 26% vs control 41%, P = .31), the composite end point of 30-day rehospitalization, redo-VT ablation, recurrent ICD therapies, and 3-month mortality was lower in the pLVAD group (12% vs 35%, P = .043).

Considering the additional time and potential risks for complications to implant/explant the LVAD and the additional costs added to the procedure, it raises the question of whether a combined approach of pLVAD-assisted activation/entrainment mapping followed by substrate modification is overall superior to a conventional substrate-based ablation strategy. This question sets the foundation for a large prospective randomized study to identify patients who are most likely to benefit from the use of pLVAD for VT ablation in the advanced HF population. In the meantime, use of the device has been primarily restricted to patients who failed substrate-based ablation and have recurrence of rapid VTs. Additional consideration is given in patients with very poor LV function to help them better tolerate long ablation procedures.

Predictors of Poor Outcome and Poor Survival

The only independent predictor of in-hospital mortality identified by Reddy and colleagues[107] was a low LVEF of 15% or less. In their study of pLVAD-assisted scar VT ablation, in-hospital deaths occurred in 11 out of 66 (17%) patients. Of those who died, 9 out of 66 (14%) patients had an LVEF of 15% or less. Indeed, in-hospital mortality was significantly more likely in patients with an LVEF of 15% or less compared with those with an LVEF of 15% or more (53% vs 4%, P<.001). There were no significant differences between the pLVAD-assisted versus IABP group in terms of acute procedural success, duration of hospital stay, discharge on antiarrhythmic, or major complications (32% vs 14%, P = .143). In terms of long-term outcomes, 45% patients had VT recurrence at 12 ± 5 months and 21% underwent a repeat ablation. Unfortunately, 30% of patients died during follow-up; but there was no difference between the two study groups. The presence of CRT (odds ratio [OR] 13, P = .03) and intensive-care-unit status at the time of VT ablation (OR 21, P = .02) were the only independent predictors of long-term mortality on multivariate analysis.[107]

The authors' group recently assessed the incidence, predictors, and impact on mortality of periprocedural acute hemodynamic decompensation (AHD) during RF ablation of scar-related VT.[109] The authors identified univariate predictors of periprocedural AHD in 193 consecutive patients undergoing RF ablation of scar-related VT. ADH occurring in 22 (11%) patients was associated with a significantly higher risk of mortality over follow-up. Patients with the following clinical predictors were identified at a significantly higher risk for AHD and poor prognosis: advanced age (68.5 ± 10.7 vs 61.6 ± 15.0 years, P = .037), ischemic cardiomyopathy (86% vs 52%, P = .002), more advanced HF status (NYHA class III/IV: 55% vs 15%, P<.001; LVEF: 26 ± 10% vs 36 ± 16%, P = .003), diabetes (36% vs 18%, P = .045), chronic obstructive pulmonary disease (41% vs 13%, P = .001), presentation with VT storm (77% vs 43%, P = .002), and administration of periprocedural general anesthesia (59% vs 29%, P = .004). Importantly, the mortality rate was higher in the AHD group compared with the control group (50% vs 11%, log-rank P<.001) at 21 ± 7 months' follow-up.[109]

Furthermore, the authors previously evaluated 76 consecutive patients with LV NICM undergoing VT ablation at the University of Pennsylvania.[110] Thirty-two (42%) patients with apical VTs were identified with a significantly larger endocardial (14.9% vs 8.1%, P = .01) and epicardial (15.5% vs 5.5%, P = .03) voltage abnormality (defined as endocardial bipolar voltage <1.5 mV, endocardial unipolar voltage <8.3 mV, and epicardial bipolar voltage <1.0 mV) extending further from the base toward the apex. Apical VT is a poor prognostic predictor conferring a higher likelihood of death, heart transplantation, or LVAD for end-stage HF. More than 25% of patients at less than 1 year of follow-up had died or needed transplant/LVAD. Advanced HF optimization is, therefore, essential in this group with a poor long-term prognosis. Additionally, the endocardial bipolar scar percentage and LVEF were independent complementary predictors for adverse outcomes on multivariate analysis.[110]

SUMMARY

VAs are an important cause of morbidity and mortality in patients with advanced HF. RFCA for VAs is indicated and potentially beneficial for patients with structural heart disease and drug-refractory recurrent VAs or VT storm resulting in ICD shocks. RFCA efficacy depends on the underlying substrate (ischemic and nonischemic), location, and extent of scar distribution and accessibility of scar areas for catheter ablation. HF is a major predictor of mortality following VT ablation, and optimization of HF management is critical for the best long-term outcomes. Recognition of AIC is essential as it is a reversible condition with RFCA. VAs after VAD implant are common and associated with increased mortality and morbidity. Options include prophylactic ablation in patients at high risk for VA, cryoablation at the time of VAD implantation, and RFCA for recurrent VAs in VAD-supported patients. The benefits of percutaneous LVAD (Impella, TandemHeart) on acute and long-term outcomes are unclear as detailed activation/entrainment mapping during unstable VT has not been definitely shown to be superior to conventional substrate-based ablation. A thorough clinical evaluation for poor prognostic predictors is important for patient selection and preprocedural planning to minimize periprocedural morbidity and mortality for catheter ablation of VT. A multidisciplinary approach to the management of advanced HF, consideration, and timing for prophylactic mechanical support devices and preprocedure ablation planning for high-risk patients can improve success and optimize the safety of catheter ablation for recurrent VAs in this sick population.

REFERENCES

1. Mason JW. A comparison of seven antiarrhythmic drugs in patients with ventricular tachyarrhythmias. Electrophysiologic study versus electrocardiographic monitoring investigators. N Engl J Med 1993;329:452–8.
2. Powell BD, Saxon LA, Boehmer JP, et al. Survival after shock therapy in implantable cardioverter-defibrillator and cardiac resynchronization therapy-

defibrillator recipients according to rhythm shocked. The altitude survival by rhythm study. J Am Coll Cardiol 2013;62:1674–9.

3. Kamphuis HC, de Leeuw JR, Derksen R, et al. Implantable cardioverter defibrillator recipients: quality of life in recipients with and without ICD shock delivery: a prospective study. Europace 2003;5:381–9.

4. Poole JE, Johnson GW, Hellkamp AS, et al. Prognostic importance of defibrillator shocks in patients with heart failure. N Engl J Med 2008;359:1009–17.

5. Moss AJ, Greenberg H, Case RB, et al. Long-term clinical course of patients after termination of ventricular tachyarrhythmia by an implanted defibrillator. Circulation 2004;110:3760–5.

6. Aliot EM, Stevenson WG, Almendral-Garrote JM, et al. EHRA/HRS expert consensus on catheter ablation of ventricular arrhythmias: developed in a partnership with the European Heart Rhythm Association (EHRA), a registered branch of the European Society of Cardiology (ESC), and the Heart Rhythm Society (HRS); in collaboration with the American College of Cardiology (ACC) and the American Heart Association (AHA). Heart Rhythm 2009;6:886–933.

7. Stevenson WG, Wilber DJ, Natale A, et al. Irrigated radiofrequency catheter ablation guided by electroanatomic mapping for recurrent ventricular tachycardia after myocardial infarction: the multicenter thermocool ventricular tachycardia ablation trial. Circulation 2008;118:2773–82.

8. Reddy VY, Reynolds MR, Neuzil P, et al. Prophylactic catheter ablation for the prevention of defibrillator therapy. N Engl J Med 2007;357:2657–65.

9. Zipes D, Camm A, Borggrefe M, et al. ACC/AHA/ESC 2006 guidelines for management of patients with ventricular arrhythmias and the prevention of sudden cardiac death: a report of the American College of Cardiology/American Heart Association Task Force and the European Society of Cardiology Committee for Practice Guidelines (writing committee to develop guidelines for management of patients with ventricular arrhythmias and the prevention of sudden cardiac death). J Am Coll Cardiol 2006;48:e247–346.

10. Henkel DM, Witt BJ, Gersh BJ, et al. Ventricular arrhythmias after acute myocardial infarction: a 20-year community study. Am J Cardiol 2006;151:806–12.

11. Kempf FC Jr, Josephson ME. Cardiac arrest recorded on ambulatory electrocardiograms. Am J Cardiol 1984;53:1577–82.

12. Hsia HH, Callans DJ, Marchlinski FE. Characterization of endocardial electrophysiological substrate in patients with nonischemic cardiomyopathy and monomorphic ventricular tachycardia. Circulation 2003;108:704–10.

13. Marchlinski FE, Zado E, Dixit S, et al. Electroanatomic substrate and outcome of catheter ablative therapy for ventricular tachycardia in setting of right ventricular cardiomyopathy. Circulation 2004;110:2293–8.

14. Josephson ME, Harken AH, Horowitz LN. Endocardial excision: a new surgical technique for the treatment of recurrent ventricular tachycardia. Circulation 1979;60:1430–9.

15. Stevenson WG, Khan H, Sager P, et al. Identification of reentry circuit sites during catheter mapping and radiofrequency ablation of ventricular tachycardia late after myocardial infarction. Circulation 1993;88:1647–70.

16. Randomized antiarrhythmic drug therapy in survivors of cardiac arrest (the cascade study). CASCADE Investigators. Am J Cardiol 1993;72:280–7.

17. Connolly SJ, Hallstrom AP, Cappato R, et al. Meta-analysis of the implantable cardioverter defibrillator secondary prevention trials. AVID, CASH and CIDS studies. Antiarrhythmics vs implantable defibrillator study. Cardiac arrest study Hamburg. Canadian implantable defibrillator study. Eur Heart J 2000;21:2071–8.

18. Connolly SJ, Dorian P, Roberts RS, et al. Comparison of beta-blockers, amiodarone plus beta-blockers, or sotalol for prevention of shocks from implantable cardioverter defibrillators: the optic study: a randomized trial. JAMA 2006;295:165–71.

19. Kocovic DZ, Harada T, Friedman PL, et al. Characteristics of electrograms recorded at reentry circuit sites and bystanders during ventricular tachycardia after myocardial infarction. J Am Coll Cardiol 1999;34:381–8.

20. El-Shalakany A, Hadjis T, Papageorgiou P, et al. Entrainment/mapping criteria for the prediction of termination of ventricular tachycardia by single radiofrequency lesion in patients with coronary artery disease. Circulation 1999;99:2283–9.

21. Soejima K, Delacretaz E, Suzuki M, et al. Saline-cooled versus standard radiofrequency catheter ablation for infarct-related ventricular tachycardias. Circulation 2001;103:1858–62.

22. Stevenson WG, Friedman PL, Ganz LI. Radiofrequency catheter ablation of ventricular tachycardia late after myocardial infarction. J Cardiovasc Electrophysiol 1997;8:1309–19.

23. Callans DJ, Zado E, Sarter BH, et al. Efficacy of radiofrequency catheter ablation for ventricular tachycardia in healed myocardial infarction. Am J Cardiol 1998;82:429–32.

24. Marchlinski FE, Callans DJ, Gottlieb CD, et al. Linear ablation lesions for control of unmappable ventricular tachycardia in patients with ischemic and nonischemic cardiomyopathy. Circulation 2000;101:1288–96.

25. Cassidy DM, Vassallo JA, Buxton AE, et al. The value of catheter mapping during sinus rhythm to localize site of origin of ventricular tachycardia. Circulation 1984;69:1103–10.

26. Marchlinski FE, Garcia F, Siadatan A, et al. Ventricular tachycardia/ventricular fibrillation in the setting of ischemic heart disease. J Cardiovasc Electrophysiol 2005;16(Suppl 1):S59–70.

27. Tian J, Jeudy J, Smith MF, et al. Three-dimensional contrast-enhanced multidetector CT for anatomic, dynamic, and perfusion characterization of abnormal myocardium to guide ventricular tachycardia ablations. Circ Arrhythm Electrophysiol 2010;3:496–504.

28. Wijnmaalen AP, Schalij MJ, von der Thusen JH, et al. Early reperfusion during acute myocardial infarction affects ventricular tachycardia characteristics and the chronic electroanatomic and histological substrate. Circulation 2010;121:1887–95.

29. Josephson ME, Waxman HL, Cain ME, et al. Ventricular activation during ventricular endocardial pacing. Ii. Role of pace-mapping to localize origin of ventricular tachycardia. Am J Cardiol 1982;50:11–22.

30. Bazan V, Gerstenfeld EP, Garcia F, et al. Site-specific twelve-lead ECG features to identify an epicardial origin for left ventricular tachycardia in the absence of myocardial infarction. Heart Rhythm 2007;4:1403–10.

31. Bazan V, Bala R, Garcia F, et al. Twelve-lead ECG features to identify ventricular tachycardia arising from the epicardial right ventricle. Heart Rhythm 2006;3:1132–9.

32. Garcia F, Bazan V, Zado ES, et al. Epicardial substrate and outcome with epicardial ablation of ventricular tachycardia in arrhythmogenic right ventricular cardiomyopathy/dysplasia. Circulation 2009;120:366–75.

33. Kawamura M, Badhwar N, Vedantham V, et al. Coupling interval dispersion and body mass index are independent predictors of idiopathic premature ventricular complex-induced cardiomyopathy. J Cardiovasc Electrophysiol 2014;25:756–62.

34. Chugh SS, Shen WK, Luria DM, et al. First evidence of premature ventricular complex-induced cardiomyopathy: a potentially reversible cause of heart failure. J Cardiovasc Electrophysiol 2000;11:328–9.

35. Bogun F, Crawford T, Reich S, et al. Radiofrequency ablation of frequent, idiopathic premature ventricular complexes: comparison with a control group without intervention. Heart Rhythm 2007;4:863–7.

36. Del Carpio Munoz F, Syed FF, Noheria A, et al. Characteristics of premature ventricular complexes as correlates of reduced left ventricular systolic function: study of the burden, duration, coupling interval, morphology and site of origin of PVCS. J Cardiovasc Electrophysiol 2011;22:791–8.

37. Taieb JM, Maury P, Shah D, et al. Reversal of dilated cardiomyopathy by the elimination of frequent left or right premature ventricular contractions. J Interv Card Electrophysiol 2007;20:9–13.

38. Efremidis M, Letsas KP, Sideris A, et al. Reversal of premature ventricular complex-induced cardiomyopathy following successful radiofrequency catheter ablation. Europace 2008;10:769–70.

39. Grimm W, Menz V, Hoffmann J, et al. Reversal of tachycardia induced cardiomyopathy following ablation of repetitive monomorphic right ventricular outflow tract tachycardia. Pacing Clin Electrophysiol 2001;24:166–71.

40. Hasdemir C, Yuksel A, Camli D, et al. Late gadolinium enhancement CMR in patients with tachycardia-induced cardiomyopathy caused by idiopathic ventricular arrhythmias. Pacing Clin Electrophysiol 2012;35:465–70.

41. Yokokawa M, Good E, Crawford T, et al. Recovery from left ventricular dysfunction after ablation of frequent premature ventricular complexes. Heart Rhythm 2013;10:172–5.

42. Mountantonakis SE, Frankel DS, Gerstenfeld EP, et al. Reversal of outflow tract ventricular premature depolarization-induced cardiomyopathy with ablation: effect of residual arrhythmia burden and preexisting cardiomyopathy on outcome. Heart Rhythm 2011;8:1608–14.

43. Sarrazin JF, Labounty T, Kuhne M, et al. Impact of radiofrequency ablation of frequent postinfarction premature ventricular complexes on left ventricular ejection fraction. Heart Rhythm 2009;6:1543–9.

44. Yokokawa M, Good E, Chugh A, et al. Intramural idiopathic ventricular arrhythmias originating in the intraventricular septum: mapping and ablation. Circ Arrhythm Electrophysiol 2012;5:258–63.

45. Yokokawa M, Kim HM, Good E, et al. Impact of QRS duration of frequent premature ventricular complexes on the development of cardiomyopathy. Heart Rhythm 2012;9:1460–4.

46. Baman TS, Lange DC, Ilg KJ, et al. Relationship between burden of premature ventricular complexes and left ventricular function. Heart Rhythm 2010;7:865–9.

47. Kanei Y, Friedman M, Ogawa N, et al. Frequent premature ventricular complexes originating from the right ventricular outflow tract are associated with left ventricular dysfunction. Ann Noninvasive Electrocardiol 2008;13:81–5.

48. Niwano S, Wakisaka Y, Niwano H, et al. Prognostic significance of frequent premature ventricular contractions originating from the ventricular outflow tract in patients with normal left ventricular function. Heart 2009;95:1230–7.

49. Yokokawa M, Kim HM, Good E, et al. Relation of symptoms and symptom duration to premature

ventricular complex-induced cardiomyopathy. Heart Rhythm 2012;9:92–5.

50. Olgun H, Yokokawa M, Baman T, et al. The role of interpolation in PVC-induced cardiomyopathy. Heart Rhythm 2011;8:1046–9.

51. Ban JE, Park HC, Park JS, et al. Electrocardiographic and electrophysiological characteristics of premature ventricular complexes associated with left ventricular dysfunction in patients without structural heart disease. Europace 2013;15:735–41.

52. Deyell MW, Park KM, Han Y, et al. Predictors of recovery of left ventricular dysfunction after ablation of frequent ventricular premature depolarizations. Heart Rhythm 2012;9:1465–72.

53. Carballeira Pol L, Deyell MW, Frankel DS, et al. Ventricular premature depolarization QRS duration as a new marker of risk for the development of ventricular premature depolarization-induced cardiomyopathy. Heart Rhythm 2014;11:299–306.

54. Campos B, Jauregui ME, Park KM, et al. New unipolar electrogram criteria to identify irreversibility of nonischemic left ventricular cardiomyopathy. J Am Coll Cardiol 2012;60:2194–204.

55. Zhong L, Lee YH, Huang XM, et al. Relative efficacy of catheter ablation vs antiarrhythmic drugs in treating premature ventricular contractions: a single-center retrospective study. Heart Rhythm 2014;11:187–93.

56. Lakkireddy D, Di Biase L, Ryschon K, et al. Radiofrequency ablation of premature ventricular ectopy improves the efficacy of cardiac resynchronization therapy in nonresponders. J Am Coll Cardiol 2012; 60:1531–9.

57. Penela D, Van Huls Van Taxis C, Aguinaga L, et al. Neurohormonal, structural, and functional recovery pattern after premature ventricular complex ablation is independent of structural heart disease status in patients with depressed left ventricular ejection fraction: a prospective multicenter study. J Am Coll Cardiol 2013;62:1195–202.

58. Birks EJ, Tansley PD, Hardy J, et al. Left ventricular assist device and drug therapy for the reversal of heart failure. N Engl J Med 2006;355:1873–84.

59. Rose EA, Moskowitz AJ, Packer M, et al. The rematch trial: rationale, design, and end points. Randomized evaluation of mechanical assistance for the treatment of congestive heart failure. Ann Thorac Surg 1999;67:723–30.

60. Rose EA, Gelijns AC, Moskowitz AJ, et al. Long-term use of a left ventricular assist device for end-stage heart failure. N Engl J Med 2001;345: 1435–43.

61. Kirklin JK, Naftel DC, Kormos RL, et al. Second INTERMACS annual report: more than 1,000 primary left ventricular assist device implants. J Heart Lung Transplant 2010;29:1–10.

62. Cesario DA, Saxon LA, Cao MK, et al. Ventricular tachycardia in the era of ventricular assist devices. J Cardiovasc Electrophysiol 2011;22: 359–63.

63. Harding JD, Piacentino V 3rd, Gaughan JP, et al. Electrophysiological alterations after mechanical circulatory support in patients with advanced cardiac failure. Circulation 2001;104:1241–7.

64. Ziv O, Dizon J, Thosani A, et al. Effects of left ventricular assist device therapy on ventricular arrhythmias. J Am Coll Cardiol 2005;45:1428–34.

65. Raasch H, Jensen BC, Chang PP, et al. Epidemiology, management, and outcomes of sustained ventricular arrhythmias after continuous-flow left ventricular assist device implantation. Am Heart J 2012;164:373–8.

66. Kuhne M, Sakumura M, Reich SS, et al. Simultaneous use of implantable cardioverter-defibrillators and left ventricular assist devices in patients with severe heart failure. Am J Cardiol 2010;105:378–82.

67. Pagani FD, Miller LW, Russell SD, et al. Extended mechanical circulatory support with a continuous-flow rotary left ventricular assist device. J Am Coll Cardiol 2009;54:312–21.

68. Brenyo A, Rao M, Koneru S, et al. Risk of mortality for ventricular arrhythmia in ambulatory LVAD patients. J Cardiovasc Electrophysiol 2012;23: 515–20.

69. Harding JD, Piacentino V 3rd, Rothman S, et al. Prolonged repolarization after ventricular assist device support is associated with arrhythmias in humans with congestive heart failure. J Card Fail 2005;11:227–32.

70. Refaat M, Chemaly E, Lebeche D, et al. Ventricular arrhythmias after left ventricular assist device implantation. Pacing Clin Electrophysiol 2008;31: 1246–52.

71. Vollkron M, Voitl P, Ta J, et al. Suction events during left ventricular support and ventricular arrhythmias. J Heart Lung Transplant 2007;26:819–25.

72. Askar SF, Ramkisoensing AA, Schalij MJ, et al. Anti-proliferative treatment of myofibroblasts prevents arrhythmias in vitro by limiting myofibroblast-induced depolarization. Cardiovasc Res 2011;90: 295–304.

73. Kleber AG, Rudy Y. Basic mechanisms of cardiac impulse propagation and associated arrhythmias. Physiol Rev 2004;84:431–88.

74. Saez JC, Nairn AC, Czernik AJ, et al. Phosphorylation of connexin43 and the regulation of neonatal rat cardiac myocyte gap junctions. J Mol Cell Cardiol 1997;29:2131–45.

75. Gutstein DE, Morley GE, Fishman GI. Conditional gene targeting of connexin43: exploring the consequences of gap junction remodeling in the heart. Cell Commun Adhes 2001;8:345–8.

76. Tomaselli GF. Calcium and arrhythmias: ignore at your peril. J Cardiovasc Electrophysiol 2012;23: 1372–3.
77. Pogwizd SM, Bers DM. Calcium cycling in heart failure: the arrhythmia connection. J Cardiovasc Electrophysiol 2002;13:88–91.
78. Cantillon DJ, Bianco C, Wazni OM, et al. Electrophysiologic characteristics and catheter ablation of ventricular tachyarrhythmias among patients with heart failure on ventricular assist device support. Heart Rhythm 2012;9:859–64.
79. Shirazi JT, Lopshire JC, Gradus-Pizlo I, et al. Ventricular arrhythmias in patients with implanted ventricular assist devices: a contemporary review. Europace 2013;15:11–7.
80. Andersen M, Videbaek R, Boesgaard S, et al. Incidence of ventricular arrhythmias in patients on long-term support with a continuous-flow assist device (HeartMate II). J Heart Lung Transplant 2009; 28:733–5.
81. Garan AR, Yuzefpolskaya M, Colombo PC, et al. Ventricular arrhythmias and implantable cardioverter-defibrillator therapy in patients with continuous-flow left ventricular assist devices: need for primary prevention? J Am Coll Cardiol 2013;61:2542–50.
82. Emaminia A, Nagji AS, Ailawadi G, et al. Concomitant left ventricular assist device placement and cryoablation for treatment of ventricular tachyarrhythmias associated with heart failure. Ann Thorac Surg 2011;92:334–6.
83. Mulloy DP, Bhamidipati CM, Stone ML, et al. Cryoablation during left ventricular assist device implantation reduces postoperative ventricular tachyarrhythmias. J Thorac Cardiovasc Surg 2013;145:1207–13.
84. Osaki S, Alberte C, Murray MA, et al. Successful radiofrequency ablation therapy for intractable ventricular tachycardia with a ventricular assist device. J Heart Lung Transplant 2008;27:353–6.
85. Herweg B, Ilercil A, Kristof-Kuteyeva O, et al. Clinical observations and outcome of ventricular tachycardia ablation in patients with left ventricular assist devices. Pacing Clin Electrophysiol 2012; 35:1377–83.
86. Van Herendael H, Garcia F, Lin D, et al. Idiopathic right ventricular arrhythmias not arising from the outflow tract: prevalence, electrocardiographic characteristics, and outcome of catheter ablation. Heart Rhythm 2011;8:511–8.
87. Van Herendael H, Zado ES, Haqqani H, et al. Catheter ablation of ventricular fibrillation: importance of left ventricular outflow tract and papillary muscle triggers. Heart Rhythm 2014;11:566–73.
88. Yamada T, Doppalapudi H, McElderry HT, et al. Idiopathic ventricular arrhythmias originating from the papillary muscles in the left ventricle: prevalence, electrocardiographic and electrophysiological characteristics, and results of the radiofrequency catheter ablation. J Cardiovasc Electrophysiol 2010;21:62–9.
89. Sadek MM, Benhayon D, Sureddi R, et al. Idiopathic ventricular arrhythmias originating from the moderator band: electrocardiographic characteristics and treatment by catheter ablation. Heart Rhythm 2015;12:67–75.
90. Dandamudi G, Ghumman WS, Das MK, et al. Endocardial catheter ablation of ventricular tachycardia in patients with ventricular assist devices. Heart Rhythm 2007;4:1165–9.
91. Cantillon DJ, Tarakji KG, Kumbhani DJ, et al. Improved survival among ventricular assist device recipients with a concomitant implantable cardioverter-defibrillator. Heart Rhythm 2010;7:466–71.
92. Refaat MM, Tanaka T, Kormos RL, et al. Survival benefit of implantable cardioverter-defibrillators in left ventricular assist device-supported heart failure patients. J Card Fail 2012;18:140–5.
93. Oswald H, Schultz-Wildelau C, Gardiwal A, et al. Implantable defibrillator therapy for ventricular tachyarrhythmia in left ventricular assist device patients. Eur J Heart Fail 2010;12:593–9.
94. Boudghene-Stambouli F, Boule S, Goeminne C, et al. Clinical implications of left ventricular assist device implantation in patients with an implantable cardioverter-defibrillator. J Interv Card Electrophysiol 2014;39:177–84.
95. Matthews JC, Betley D, Morady F, et al. Adverse interaction between a left ventricular assist device and an implantable cardioverter defibrillator. J Cardiovasc Electrophysiol 2007;18:1107–8.
96. Rohit M, Charles JL, Sai-Sudhakar C, et al. A device-device interaction between a Thoratec HeartMate II left ventricular assist device and a St. Jude Atlas (v-193) implantable cardioverter defibrillator. J Cardiovasc Electrophysiol 2007;18: E27 [author reply: E28].
97. Soejima K, Suzuki M, Maisel WH, et al. Catheter ablation in patients with multiple and unstable ventricular tachycardias after myocardial infarction: short ablation lines guided by reentry circuit isthmuses and sinus rhythm mapping. Circulation 2001;104:664–9.
98. Carbucicchio C, Santamaria M, Trevisi N, et al. Catheter ablation for the treatment of electrical storm in patients with implantable cardioverter-defibrillators: short- and long-term outcomes in a prospective single-center study. Circulation 2008; 117:462–9.
99. Miller MA, Dukkipati SR, Mittnacht AJ, et al. Activation and entrainment mapping of hemodynamically unstable ventricular tachycardia using a percutaneous left ventricular assist device. J Am Coll Cardiol 2011;58:1363–71.

100. Friedman PA, Munger TM, Torres N, et al. Percutaneous endocardial and epicardial ablation of hypotensive ventricular tachycardia with percutaneous left ventricular assist in the electrophysiology laboratory. J Cardiovasc Electrophysiol 2007;18:106–9.

101. Abuissa H, Roshan J, Lim B, et al. Use of the Impella microaxial blood pump for ablation of hemodynamically unstable ventricular tachycardia. J Cardiovasc Electrophysiol 2010;21:458–61.

102. Carbucicchio C, Della Bella P, Fassini G, et al. Percutaneous cardiopulmonary support for catheter ablation of unstable ventricular arrhythmias in high-risk patients. Herz 2009;34:545–52.

103. Miller MA, Dukkipati SR, Chinitz JS, et al. Percutaneous hemodynamic support with Impella 2.5 during scar-related ventricular tachycardia ablation (PERMIT1). Circ Arrhythm Electrophysiol 2013;6: 151–9.

104. Miller MA, Dukkipati SR, Koruth JS, et al. How to perform ventricular tachycardia ablation with a percutaneous left ventricular assist device. Heart Rhythm 2012;9:1168–76.

105. Vaidya VR, Desimone CV, Madhavan M, et al. Compatibility of electroanatomical mapping systems with a concurrent percutaneous axial flow ventricular assist device. J Cardiovasc Electrophysiol 2014;25:781–6.

106. Bunch TJ, Darby A, May HT, et al. Efficacy and safety of ventricular tachycardia ablation with mechanical circulatory support compared with substrate-based ablation techniques. Europace 2012;14:709–14.

107. Reddy YM, Chinitz L, Mansour M, et al. Percutaneous left ventricular assist devices in ventricular tachycardia ablation: multicenter experience. Circ Arrhythm Electrophysiol 2014;7:244–50.

108. Aryana A, Gearoid O'Neill P, Gregory D, et al. Procedural and clinical outcomes after catheter ablation of unstable ventricular tachycardia supported by a percutaneous left ventricular assist device. Heart Rhythm 2014;11:1122–30.

109. Santangeli P, Muser D, Zado E, et al. Acute hemodynamic decompensation during catheter ablation of scar-related VT: incidence, predictors and impact on mortality. Circ Arrhythm Electrophysiol 2014. [Epub ahead of print].

110. Frankel DS, Tschabrunn CM, Cooper JM, et al. Apical ventricular tachycardia morphology in left ventricular nonischemic cardiomyopathy predicts poor transplant-free survival. Heart Rhythm 2013; 10:621–6.

Interventional and Device-Based Autonomic Modulation in Heart Failure

Mark J. Shen, MD[a], Douglas P. Zipes, MD[b],*

KEYWORDS

- Heart failure • Autonomic nervous system • Spinal cord stimulation • Vagus nerve stimulation
- Baroreflex activation therapy • Renal sympathetic nerve denervation

KEY POINTS

- Heart failure is a disease categorized by sympathetic hyperactivity, parasympathetic withdrawal, and impaired baroreflex control of sympathetic activation.
- Several measures of autonomic modulation either by implanted devices or interventions seek to restore the autonomic balance in heart failure and improve outcomes; these measures include spinal cord stimulation, vagus nerve stimulation, baroreceptor activation therapy, and renal sympathetic nerve denervation.
- Preclinical work and most early clinical trials show the benefits of these modalities in HF; additional larger, well-designed, outcome-based clinical trials are warranted to verify the results and determine whether these evolving, innovative neuromodulation approaches can be recommended to the growing population of patients with heart failure.

INTRODUCTION

Congestive heart failure (HF), a disease with high mortality and increasing prevalence,[1] is characterized by autonomic imbalance, including decreased parasympathetic tone,[2,3] hyperactive sympathetic tone,[4,5] and impaired baroreflex control of sympathetic activity.[6,7] Pharmacotherapy attempting to restore the autonomic imbalance with drugs such as β-blockers, angiotensin-converting enzyme inhibitors/angiotensin II receptor blockers, and aldosterone receptor antagonists are found to improve survival among HF patients and are recommended for HF patients with reduced ejection fraction.[1] However, the daunting prospect of HF burden and lack of recent breakthroughs in pharmacotherapy have led to the investigations of nonpharmacologic approaches that can favorably modulate the autonomic tone.[8–11] This article discusses the latest avenues of research and clinical trials regarding the application of interventional or device-based approaches in treating HF through modulating autonomic activity—specifically, spinal cord stimulation (SCS), vagus nerve stimulation (VNS), baroreflex activation therapy (BAT) and renal sympathetic nerve denervation (RSDN).

SPINAL CORD STIMULATION

Technical Aspects

SCS has been used clinically for chronic pain (approved by the US Food and Drug Administration), peripheral vascular disease, and refractory angina (in Europe). The procedure involves the subcutaneous placement of an epidural stimulation lead with distal poles at the level of T_2 to T_4, which is connected to an implanted pulse generator in the para-spinal lumbar region (**Fig. 1**).

Conflicts of Interest: The authors have nothing to disclose.
[a] Krannert Institute of Cardiology, Department of Medicine, Indiana University School of Medicine, 1800 North Capitol Avenue, Room E371, Indianapolis, IN 46202, USA; [b] Krannert Institute of Cardiology, Department of Medicine, Indiana University School of Medicine, 1800 North Capitol Avenue, Indianapolis, IN 46202, USA
* Corresponding author.
E-mail address: dzipes@iu.edu

Heart Failure Clin 11 (2015) 337–348
http://dx.doi.org/10.1016/j.hfc.2014.12.010
1551-7136/15/$ – see front matter © 2015 Elsevier Inc. All rights reserved.

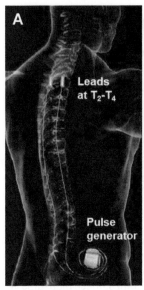 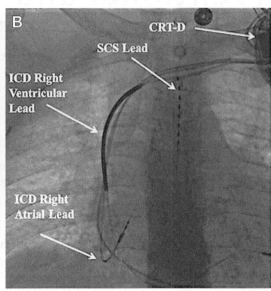

Fig. 1. (A) Schematic representation of SCS system. (B) X-ray image shows the placement of the SCS lead with concurrent cardiac resynchronization therapy-defibrillator (CRT-D) device and leads. ICD, Implantable cardioverter defibrillator. (*From* Torre-Amione G, Alo K, Estep JD, et al. Spinal cord stimulation is safe and feasible in patients with advanced heart failure: early clinical experience. Eur J Heart Fail 2014;16(7):788–95; with permission.)

SCS can be applied at 90% of the motor threshold at a frequency of 50 Hz and a pulse width of 200 ms for 2 hours at a time, 3 times a day. It can also be applied for longer intervals.

Preclinical Research

Olgin and colleagues[12] found that SCS at the level of T_1 to T_2 increased the sinus cycle length and prolonged atrioventricular nodal conduction. These effects were abolished after transection of bilateral cervical vagus nerves but not transection of ansa subclavia (sympathectomy), suggesting the effect of SCS is vagally mediated. In a canine model of ischemic HF, SCS during transient myocardial ischemia reduced the incidence of spontaneous ventricular tachyarrhythmias.[13] This antiarrhythmic effect was again associated with vagal effects—reduction in sinus rate, prolongation of PR interval, and lowering of blood pressure. With direct nerve recordings in ambulatory dogs, Garlie and colleagues[14] found that SCS attenuated augmented sympathetic activity from the stellate ganglion following myocardial infarction and pacing-induced HF in an animal model similar to the one noted below.

The chronic cardio-protective effect of SCS in HF was best shown by a canine study[15] from the same investigator group. All canines first underwent foam embolization of the left anterior descending artery followed by ventricular tachypacing to create an ischemic HF model. Then the animals were equally randomly divided into 4 groups:

- SCS (T_4 level, 90% motor threshold, 50 Hz, 0.2-m pulse duration, 2 hours at a time, 3 times daily).
- Medical therapy (carvedilol + ramipril).
- Combined SCS and medical therapy.
- Control group.

The dogs were followed up with chronically for 10 weeks. A significant decline in serum norepinephrine and brain natriuretic peptide levels along with decrease of ischemic ventricular tachyarrhythmias were observed in dogs receiving SCS. Most interestingly, dogs receiving SCS (with or without medical therapy) had greatest improvement of left ventricular ejection fraction (LVEF) (from 17% to 52%) with reductions in ventricular volume. The improvement persisted throughout the treatment period.

Clinical Trials

Based on the preclinical work, several clinical studies sought to assess the efficacy and safety of SCS in systolic HF patients (**Table 1**).[16–19] Of those trials, the largest is Determining the Feasibility of Spinal Cord Neuromodulation for the Treatment of Chronic Heart Failure (DEFEAT-HF) with implanted PrimeAdvanced neurostimulator (Medtronic Inc, Minneapolis, MN). It is a multicenter, prospective, randomized (3:2 fashion) control trial enrolling 66 patients with LVEF ≤35%, New York Heart Association (NYHA) class III HF symptoms while on optimal medical therapy,

Table 1
Clinical trials of spinal cord stimulation in heart failure

Trial	N	Criteria	Design	Endpoint[a]	Status[b]
Neurostimulation of Spinal Nerves That Affect the Heart	9	• LVEF ≤30% • NYHA III	Randomized, double-blind, crossover	Safety, device interactions, symptoms	Results published (see text)
DEFEAT-HF	66	• LVEF ≤35% • NYHA III • Narrow QRS • Dilated LV	Randomized, single-blind, parallel	Δ in LV volume	Active, not recruiting. Preliminary result soon to be presented.
SCS HEART	20	• LVEF 20%–35% • NYHA III–IV • Dilated LV	Single-arm, open-label	Safety, Δ in LV function, exercise capacity, QoL	Recruiting
TAME-HF	20	• LVEF ≤35% • NYHA III • Narrow QRS	Single-arm, open-label	Δ in LV volume, symptoms, exercise capacity	Recruiting

Abbreviations: QoL, quality of life; QRS, QRS interval of an ECG; SCS HEART, Spinal Cord Stimulation For Heart Failure; TAME-HF, Trial of Autonomic neuroModulation for trEatment of Chronic Heart Failure.

[a] Only primary outcome measures listed.
[b] As of October 2014.

narrow QRS duration, and a dilated left ventricle (LV).[17] The preliminary data of 6 months of follow-up will soon be presented at the 2014 American Heart Association scientific sessions. The results of a smaller prospective trial that enrolled 9 patients with LVEF ≤30% and NYHA class III HF symptoms while on optimal medical therapy have been published.[16] During the 7-month period of follow-up, 5 patients had improved symptoms by at least 1 NYHA class, and 3 were unchanged, whereas no one worsened. Despite the small sample size, this study found the safety and feasibility of SCS in patients with advanced HF. In particular, SCS did not affect the functions (sensing, detection, and therapy delivery) of the implantable cardioverter defibrillator.

VAGUS NERVE STIMULATION
Technical Aspects

Chronic VNS has been used clinically for years for refractory epilepsy and depression.[20] Its use in HF has recently been studied during right cervical VNS. A cuff electrode is secured around the vagus about 3 cm below the carotid artery bifurcation. A brief stimulation that reduces heart rate by 10% is performed to ensure the correct positioning. The stimulation lead is then tunneled under the skin and over the clavicle to join the intracardiac sensing electrode (placed in the right ventricle to prevent excessive bradycardia) and the pulse generator in the subcutaneous pocket in the right subclavicular region (**Fig. 2**). The stimulation parameter then follows an up-titration protocol to achieve heart rate reduction of 5 to 10 beats per minute without eliciting adverse reactions.[21,22]

Preclinical Research

Although HF is associated with a decreased vagal activity, decreased vagal activity itself is associated with higher mortality among HF patients.[23] VNS is thus an attractive idea in treating HF. Several animal studies using rats and dogs found that chronic VNS improved LV hemodynamics[24,25] and, more importantly, improved survival in HF.[26] With an implanted device to continuously record autonomic nerve activity in ambulatory canines, Shen and colleagues[27] observed that chronic VNS led to a significant reduction in sympathetic activity from the left stellate ganglion, which may underlie the cardio-protective property of VNS. VNS also has additional benefits:

- VNS is found to attenuate systemic inflammation.[25,28]
- VNS, via the modulation of nitric oxide,[29] may reduce the slope of action potential duration restitution curve,[30] which is important in the initiation of VF.[31]
- VNS can also significantly increase the expression of connexin-43,[24] which is down-regulated in failing human hearts and thereby arrhythmogenic.[32]

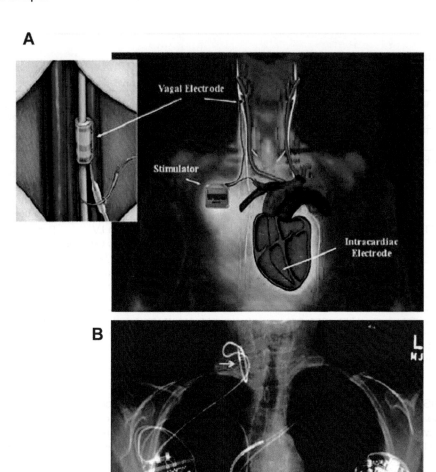

Fig. 2. (A) Schematic representation of VNS system. (B) X-ray image shows the placement of the VNS stimulator with a previously implanted implantable cardioverter defibrillator (ICD). The *arrows* show a lead attached to the vagus nerve on the right side and an additional right ventricular sensing lead connected to the vagal nerve stimulator device. (*From* [A] Schwartz PJ, De Ferrari GM, Sanzo A, et al. Long term vagal stimulation in patients with advanced heart failure: first experience in man. Eur J Heart Fail 2008;10(9):884–91; and [B] Singh JP, Kandala J, Camm AJ. Non-pharmacological modulation of the autonomic tone to treat heart failure. Eur Heart J 2014;35(2):77–85; with permission.)

- VNS is found to be associated with its prevention of mitochondrial dysfunction during ischemia-reperfusion.[33]

Clinical Trials

In a recent multicenter, single-arm, open-label pilot study enrolling 32 patients with NYHA class II to IV symptoms and LVEF $\leq$35% using Cardiofit system (BioControl Medical Ltd, Yehudi, Israel), VNS was found to be safe and tolerable and to improve quality of life and LV systolic function.[22] The positive result has prompted larger randomized trials to examine the efficacy and safety of this treatment modality in patients with severe systolic HF (**Table 2**).[34–36] The results of 2 of these

Table 2
Clinical trials of vagus nerve stimulation in heart failure

Trial	N	Criteria	Design	Endpoint[a]	Status[b]
CardioFit for the Treatment of Heart Failure	32	• LVEF ≤35% • NYHA II–IV	Single-arm, open-label	All adverse events	Results published (see text)
INOVATE-HF	650	• LVEF ≤40% • NYHA III • Dilated LV	Randomized, open-label, parallel	All-cause mortality or unplanned HF hospitalization	Recruiting
NECTAR-HF	96	• LVEF ≤35% • NYHA II–III • Dilated LV	Randomized, double-blind, crossover	Δ in LV volume, all-cause mortality	Results published (see text)
ANTHEM-HF[c]	60	• LVEF ≤40% • NYHA II–III • Dilated LV	Randomized, open-label, parallel	Δ in LV functions, adverse events	Results presented (see text)

[a] Only primary outcome measures listed.
[b] As of October 2014.
[c] Also test left-sided VNS.

trials were recently presented in the European Society of Cardiology Congress 2014 and showed conflicting findings.

- Neural Cardiac Therapy for Heart Failure Study (NECTAR-HF) is a prospective, double-blinded, randomized control study that enrolled 96 patients with NYHA class II to III symptoms and LVEF ≤35% and evaluated right-sided VNS. It failed to show an improvement in LV end-systolic diameter, the primary endpoint, in 6 months' time.[37] However, it did show that VNS was safe and able to significantly improve quality of life.
- Autonomic Neural Regulation Therapy to Enhance Myocardial Function in Heart Failure (ANTHEM-HF) is a prospective, open-label, randomized control study that enrolled 60 patients with NYHA class II to III symptoms and LVEF ≤40% and evaluated both right-sided and left-sided VNS. It showed that either right-sided or left-sided VNS was able to significantly improve LVEF and reduce LV end-systolic diameter in 6 months' time.[38]

The reason for such obvious different results is unclear. One possibility is that different types of stimulating protocols or equipment used in 2 studies may have recruited different types of fibers within the cervical vagus nerve. In fact, cervical vagus nerves invariably contain a small percentage of sympathetic nerves.[39,40] Stimulating the cervical vagus is actually stimulating a vagosympathetic trunk. Whether that reduces the beneficial effects of cervical VNS remains to be determined. Another larger trial, INcrease Of VAgal TonE in CHF (INOVATE-HF), with a plan to enroll 650 patients with similar baseline parameters (LVEF

≤40%, NYHA class III symptoms and a dilated LV) is ongoing.[34] The results of this trial may determine whether VNS is really beneficial in HF. Of note, INOVATE-HF is the only trial of VNS that chose all-cause mortality or unplanned HF hospitalization as the primary outcome measure.

BARORECEPTOR ACTIVATION THERAPY
Technical Aspects

Chronic electrical activation of the carotid baroreflex, known as BAT, has been commercially available and tested in patients with resistant hypertension.[41,42] It has since been investigated in HF. For the traditional Rheos system (CVRx Inc, Minneapolis, MN), the implantation involves surgically exposing both carotid sinuses and placing electrodes around the carotid adventitial surface bilaterally. The leads are subcutaneously tunneled and connected to an implantable stimulation device placed in the subclavian subcutaneous position on the anterior chest wall. The newer generation (Barostim neo, also from CVRx Inc) has only one carotid sinus electrode with smaller size (**Fig. 3**) that delivers less power and thus allows easier implant and fewer adverse effects.

Preclinical Research

Normally, activation of the baroreceptors within the carotid sinuses by an increase in aortic pressure or volume sends impulses to the medulla that lead to restoration of pressure homeostasis by decreasing efferent sympathetic activity while increasing efferent parasympathetic activity,[43] both desirable in HF. Furthermore, defective baroreflex control of the heart rate in the failing heart has long been recognized.[44] Therefore, BAT has the potential to

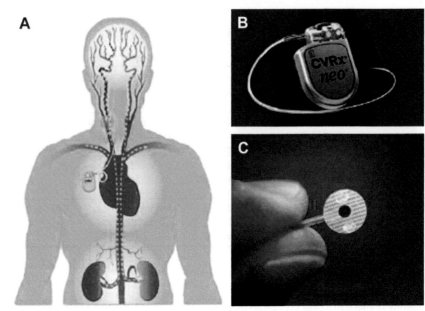

Fig. 3. (A) Schematic representation of BAT system. The new generation, Barostim neo, is shown with one carotid sinus nerve stimulator (B) that carries one electrode connected to the patch electrode (C) that will be fixed to the carotid sinus nerve. (*From* Kuck KH, Bordachar P, Borggrefe M, et al. New devices in heart failure: an A European Heart Rhythm Association report: developed by the European Heart Rhythm Association; endorsed by the Heart Failure Association. Europace 2014;16(1):109–28; with permission.)

benefit HF patients and has been studied in an experimental HF model. In a microembolization canine model of HF, chronic BAT significantly increased LV systolic function and reduced plasma norepinephrine.[45] In another study using rapid pacing model of HF, chronic BAT reduced LV filling pressure, decreased plasma norepinephrine, and doubled survival duration.[46]

Clinical Trials

A recent single-center, open-label, single-arm study enrolled 11 patients with LVEF ≤40% and NYHA class III HF symptoms while on optimal medical therapy that received BAT for 6 months.[47] Chronic BAT was associated with significant improvement in baroreflex sensitivity, LVEF, NYHA class, quality of life, and 6-minute walk distance along with significant decrease in muscle sympathetic activity. Larger clinical trials are ongoing[48–50] and summarized in **Table 3**. Of note, the Rheos Hope for Heart Failure (HOPE4HF) trial[48] is one of few trials of new treatment modalities evaluating HF with preserved ejection fraction (or diastolic HF, LVEF ≥40%) population.[51]

RENAL SYMPATHETIC NERVE DENERVATION
Technical Aspects

Catheter-based RSDN is most widely applied clinically as a treatment of resistant hypertension.[52,53] Beyond blood pressure, RSDN may prove

beneficial in other diseases associated with sympathetic hyperactivity, including HF.[54] Before the procedure, careful evaluation by imaging of the renal artery anatomy along with renal function tests is warranted to assess suitability of the intervention.[55] Via a standard femoral artery access, a flexible endovascular electrode catheter connected to a generator is placed within the renal arteries to allow delivery of radiofrequency energy. A series of lesions along each renal artery then are delivered to disrupt the renal nerves located in the adventitia of the renal arteries. For safety reasons, each lesion should be at least 5 mm apart.

Preclinical Research

RSDN ablates both efferent and afferent renal sympathetic nerves as they run together, with higher nerve density in the proximal segments and ventral region.[56] By ablating the efferent nerves, RSDN decreases the renal norepinephrine spillover by 47%[57] and attenuates the activity of renin-angiotensin-aldosterone system,[58] both important in the pathogenesis of LV remodeling in HF. More importantly, from a cardiac standpoint, afferent RSDN leads to decreased feedback activation to the central nervous system and thereby decreased sympathetic input to the heart (**Fig. 4**). In a murine model of ischemic HF, RSDN is associated with reduced LV filling pressure and improved LVEF after 4 weeks of follow-up.[59]

Table 3
Clinical trials of baroreflex activation therapy in heart failure

Trial	N	Criteria	Design	Endpoint[a]	Status[b]
The study by Gronda et al[47] from Italy	11	• LVEF ≤40% • NYHA III	Single-arm, open-label	Δ in muscle sympathetic activity	Completed. Results published (see text)
Rheos HOPE4HF	540	• LVEF ≥40% • Symptomatic • Hypertensive	Randomized, open-label, parallel	Cardiovascular death or HF event, all adverse events	Active, not recruiting
XR-1 Randomized Heart Failure study	150	• LVEF ≤35% • NYHA III	Randomized, open-label, parallel	Δ in LVEF	Active, not recruiting
Barostim HOPE4HF	60	• LVEF ≤35% • NYHA III	Randomized, open-label, parallel	Δ in HF metric, all adverse events	Active, not recruiting

[a] Only primary outcome measures listed.
[b] As of October 2014.

Among patients with resistant hypertension, RSDN leads to a reduction in heart rate and atrioventricular conduction[60] and, in another study, reduction of LV mass, reduction of LV filling pressure, shortening of isovolumetric relaxation time, and increase of LVEF.[61]

Clinical Trials

The first trial examining the safety of RSDN in HF patients is Renal Artery Denervation in Chronic Heart Failure (REACH)-Pilot trial.[62] In the 7 patients with chronic systolic HF and normotension before the procedure, there were no hypotensive or syncopal events over a 6-month follow-up period. The renal function remained stable. Although

limited in size, the pilot study found that there was a trend toward an improvement in symptoms and exercise capacity. The encouraging results call for larger randomized trials to validate the efficacy and safety of this modality in HF, despite the failure of a recent prospective, randomized, blinded study (Renal Denervation in Patients With Chronic Heart Failure and Renal Impairment Clinical Trial [SYMPLICITY HTN-3]) to show any benefit of RSDN in patients with resistant hypertension.[63] Several larger ongoing trials[64–68] are summarized in **Table 4**.

EVOLVING TECHNOLOGY

Recent preclinical work from the Cleveland Clinic found that epivascular[69] and, more excitingly,

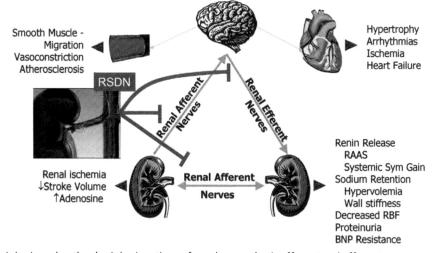

Fig. 4. Physiologic and pathophysiologic actions of renal sympathetic afferent and efferent nerves can be blocked by RSDN. RSDN, renal sympathetic denervation; RAAS, renin angiotensin aldosterone system; RBF, renal blood flow; BNP, brain natriuretic peptide. (*From* Krum H, Sobotka P, Mahfoud F, et al. Device-based antihypertensive therapy: therapeutic modulation of the autonomic nervous system. Circulation 2011;123(2):209–15; with permission.)

Table 4
Clinical trials of renal sympathetic nerve denervation in heart failure

Trial	N	Criteria	Design	Endpoint[a]	Status[b]
REACH-Pilot	7	• Chronic HF • NYHA III–IV	Single-arm, open label	Safety study	Completed. (see text)
SYMPLICITY-HF	40	• LVEF <40% • NYHA II–III • GFR 30–75	Single-arm, open label	Safety study	Recruiting
Renal Denervation in Patients With Chronic Heart Failure	100	• LVEF10%–40% • NYHA II–III • GFR >30	Randomized, open label, parallel	Safety, number of complications	Not yet recruiting
DIASTOLE	60	• HF symptoms • LVEF ≥50% • Evidence of HFpEF • HTN • GFR >30	Randomized, open label, parallel	Change in E/E′	Recruiting
RDT-PEF	40	• LVEF >40% • NYHA II–III • Evidence of HFpEF	Randomized, open label, parallel	Change in symptoms and echo findings	Recruiting
RESPECT-HF	144	• LVEF ≥50% • NYHA II–IV • Evidence of HFpEF • Episode of ADHF	Randomized, open label, parallel	Change in LA volume index	Recruiting

Abbreviations: GFR, glomerular filtration rate; HFpEF, heart failure with preserved ejection fraction; HTN = hypertension.
[a] Only primary outcome measures listed.
[b] As of October 2014.

endovascular[70] cardiac plexus stimulation can increase LV contractility without increasing heart rate. This was achieved by stimulating the cardiac plexus between the ascending aorta and right pulmonary artery. It is known that cardiac ganglionated plexi concentrated in epicardial fat pads play a cardinal role in coordinating complex interactions between the extrinsic and intrinsic cardiac autonomic nervous systems[71] and contain highly co-localized sympathetic and parasympathetic ganglion cells.[72,73] The idea that stimulating cardiac plexus endovascularly can improve LV contractility is fascinating, given that the technique is simple, requiring the placement of a stimulation catheter in the right pulmonary artery similar to that of a Swan-Ganz catheter. In addition, chronic stimulation of the cardiac plexus may help restore the impaired endogenous nerve activity from the plexus in HF.[74]

SUMMARY

HF is increasingly common and remains deadly, despite guideline-based optimal medical therapy.[1] Most currently available interventional and device-based treatment modalities for HF (defibrillator, ventricular assist device, or heart transplantation)

are often "fallbacks" instead of disease modifiers. The new modalities discussed here—SCS, VNS, BAT, and RSDN, however, have several distinct features:

• They seek to correct one of the fundamental impairments of HF—autonomic imbalance, which may underpin the survival benefits of β-blockade and inhibition of renin-angiotensin-aldosterone system. One must remember, however, that β-blockade is just blockade of β receptors. That leaves α receptors unaffected (except perhaps with carvedilol) and does not capitalize on all the other benefits of device-based neuromodulation.
• Through the same neuromodulation mechanisms, they help prevent the occurrence of ventricular tachyarrhythmias,[75] which remain a common cause of death in HF populations.
• Unlike previous device-based therapy, such as implantable cardioverter defibrillator or cardiac resynchronization therapies that focus on HF with reduced ejection fraction, some of the ongoing trials with new modalities (Rheos HOPE4HF for BAT, Denervation of the renAl sympathetic nerveS in hearT Failure With nOrmal LV Ejection Fraction [DIASTOLE],

Renal Denervation in Heart Failure With Preserved Ejection Fraction [RDT-PEF], and Renal Denervation in Heart Failure Patients With Preserved Ejection Fraction [RESPECT-HF] for RSDN) enroll patients with HF with preserved ejection fraction, a population that continues to grow and may overtake HF with reduced ejection fraction in the near future.[76]

- An attractive feature of these new modalities is that they are not new to the medical practice and have been applied to other indications for years. Their application for a new indication, therefore, should be easier and safer.

Nonetheless, caution should be exercised when examining the ongoing trials of new modalities for HF. In addition to the inherent difficulty of ensuring true double-blindness of these interventional and device-based treatment modalities, a major criticism is that most of the completed and ongoing trials have used "soft endpoints," such as changes in echocardiographic findings or periprocedural safety issues, rather than "hard endpoints," such as cardiovascular mortality or HF event that requires hospitalization. Furthermore, as the MOXonidine CONgestive Heart Failure (MOXCON) trial showed, moxonidine, an antihypertensive agent, despite reducing central sympathetic nerve activity and circulating norepinephrine concentrations, caused excessive mortality in HF patients and led to early termination of the trial.[77] This finding suggests that generalized sympathetic inhibition in HF may be harmful. In contrast, results of completed trials of the new modalities have so far been encouraging. The mechanisms of neuromodulation of these new modalities are perhaps more complex and not just antisympathetic. Altogether, autonomic modulation through interventions and devices in HF looks promising. It remains to be seen whether these new modalities can be recommended to the ever-growing population of HF patients pending results from larger randomized trials and further investigations.

REFERENCES

1. Yancy CW, Jessup M, Bozkurt B, et al. 2013 ACCF/AHA guideline for the management of heart failure: executive summary: a report of the American College of Cardiology Foundation/American Heart Association Task Force on practice guidelines. Circulation 2013;128(16):1810–52.
2. Newton GE, Parker AB, Landzberg JS, et al. Muscarinic receptor modulation of basal and beta-adrenergic stimulated function of the failing human left ventricle. J Clin Invest 1996;98(12):2756–63.
3. Porter TR, Eckberg DL, Fritsch JM, et al. Autonomic pathophysiology in heart failure patients. Sympathetic-cholinergic interrelations. J Clin Invest 1990;85(5):1362–71.
4. Cohn JN, Levine TB, Olivari MT, et al. Plasma norepinephrine as a guide to prognosis in patients with chronic congestive heart failure. N Engl J Med 1984;311:819–23.
5. Hasking GJ, Esler MD, Jennings GL, et al. Norepinephrine spillover to plasma in patients with congestive heart failure: evidence of increased overall and cardiorenal sympathetic nervous activity. Circulation 1986;73(4):615–21.
6. Grassi G, Seravalle G, Cattaneo BM, et al. Sympathetic activation and loss of reflex sympathetic control in mild congestive heart failure. Circulation 1995;92(11):3206–11.
7. Ferguson DW, Abboud FM, Mark AL. Selective impairment of baroreflex-mediated vasoconstrictor responses in patients with ventricular dysfunction. Circulation 1984;69(3):451–60.
8. Singh JP, Kandala J, Camm AJ. Non-pharmacological modulation of the autonomic tone to treat heart failure. Eur Heart J 2014;35(2):77–85.
9. Lopshire JC, Zipes DP. Device therapy to modulate the autonomic nervous system to treat heart failure. Curr Cardiol Rep 2012;14(5):593–600.
10. Florea VG, Cohn JN. The autonomic nervous system and heart failure. Circ Res 2014;114(11):1815–26.
11. Kuck KH, Bordachar P, Borggrefe M, et al. New devices in heart failure: an European Heart Rhythm Association report: developed by the European Heart Rhythm Association; endorsed by the Heart Failure Association. Europace 2014;16(1):109–28.
12. Olgin JE, Takahashi T, Wilson E, et al. Effects of thoracic spinal cord stimulation on cardiac autonomic regulation of the sinus and atrioventricular nodes. J Cardiovasc Electrophysiol 2002;13(5):475–81.
13. Issa ZF, Zhou X, Ujhelyi MR, et al. Thoracic spinal cord stimulation reduces the risk of ischemic ventricular arrhythmias in a postinfarction heart failure canine model. Circulation 2005;111(24):3217–20.
14. Garlie JB, Zhou X, Shen MJ, et al. The increased ambulatory nerve activity and ventricular tachycardia in canine post-infarction heart failure is attenuated by spinal cord stimulation [abstract]. Heart Rhythm 2012;PO3–112.
15. Lopshire JC, Zhou X, Dusa C, et al. Spinal cord stimulation improves ventricular function and reduces ventricular arrhythmias in a canine postinfarction heart failure model. Circulation 2009;120(4):286–94.
16. Torre-Amione G, Alo K, Estep JD, et al. Spinal cord stimulation is safe and feasible in patients with advanced heart failure: early clinical experience. Eur J Heart Fail 2014;16(7):788–95.
17. Determining the Feasibility of Spinal Cord Neuromodulation for the Treatment of Chronic Heart Failure

(DEFEAT-HF). Available at: http://clinicaltrials.gov/ct2/show/NCT01112579?term=NCT01112579&rank=1. Accessed August 31, 2014.

18. Spinal Cord Stimulation For Heart Failure (SCS HEART). Available at: http://www.clinicaltrials.gov/ct2/show/NCT01362725?Term=NCT01362725&rank=1. Accessed August 31, 2014.

19. Trial of Autonomic neuroModulation for trEatment of Chronic Heart Failure (TAME-HF). Available at: http://www.clinicaltrials.gov/ct2/show/NCT01820130?Term=NCT01820130&rank=1. Accessed August 31, 2014.

20. Terry R. Vagus nerve stimulation: a proven therapy for treatment of epilepsy strives to improve efficacy and expand applications. Conf Proc IEEE Eng Med Biol Soc 2009;2009:4631–4.

21. Schwartz PJ, De Ferrari GM, Sanzo A, et al. Long term vagal stimulation in patients with advanced heart failure: first experience in man. Eur J Heart Fail 2008;10(9):884–91.

22. De Ferrari GM, Crijns HJ, Borggrefe M, et al. Chronic vagus nerve stimulation: a new and promising therapeutic approach for chronic heart failure. Eur Heart J 2010;32:847–55.

23. Schwartz PJ, De Ferrari GM. Sympathetic-parasympathetic interaction in health and disease: abnormalities and relevance in heart failure. Heart Fail Rev 2011;16(2):101–7.

24. Sabbah HN, Ilsar I, Zaretsky A, et al. Vagus nerve stimulation in experimental heart failure. Heart Fail Rev 2011;16(2):171–8.

25. Zhang Y, Popovic ZB, Bibevski S, et al. Chronic vagus nerve stimulation improves autonomic control and attenuates systemic inflammation and heart failure progression in a canine high-rate pacing model. Circ Heart Fail 2009;2(6):692–9.

26. Li M, Zheng C, Sato T, et al. Vagal nerve stimulation markedly improves long-term survival after chronic heart failure in rats. Circulation 2004;109(1):120–4.

27. Shen MJ, Shinohara T, Park HW, et al. Continuous low-level vagus nerve stimulation reduces stellate ganglion nerve activity and paroxysmal atrial tachyarrhythmias in ambulatory canines. Circulation 2011;123(20):2204–12.

28. Calvillo L, Vanoli E, Andreoli E, et al. Vagal stimulation, through its nicotinic action, limits infarct size and the inflammatory response to myocardial ischemia and reperfusion. J Cardiovasc Pharmacol 2011;58(5):500–7.

29. Brack KE, Patel VH, Coote JH, et al. Nitric oxide mediates the vagal protective effect on ventricular fibrillation via effects on action potential duration restitution in the rabbit heart. J Physiol 2007;583(Pt 2):695–704.

30. Ng GA, Brack KE, Patel VH, et al. Autonomic modulation of electrical restitution, alternans and ventricular fibrillation initiation in the isolated heart. Cardiovasc Res 2007;73(4):750–60.

31. Cao JM, Qu Z, Kim YH, et al. Spatiotemporal heterogeneity in the induction of ventricular fibrillation by rapid pacing: importance of cardiac restitution properties. Circ Res 1999;84:1318–31.

32. Jongsma HJ, Wilders R. Gap junctions in cardiovascular disease. Circ Res 2000;86(12):1193–7.

33. Shinlapawittayatorn K, Chinda K, Palee S, et al. Low-amplitude, left vagus nerve stimulation significantly attenuates ventricular dysfunction and infarct size through prevention of mitochondrial dysfunction during acute ischemia-reperfusion injury. Heart Rhythm 2013;10(11):1700–7.

34. Hauptman PJ, Schwartz PJ, Gold MR, et al. Rationale and study design of the increase of vagal tone in heart failure study: INOVATE-HF. Am Heart J 2012;163(6):954–62.e1.

35. Neural Cardiac Therapy for Heart Failure Study (NECTAR-HF). Available at: https://clinicaltrials.gov/ct2/show/NCT01385176?term=NCT01385176&rank=1. Accessed August 31, 2014.

36. Dicarlo L, Libbus I, Amurthur B, et al. Autonomic regulation therapy for the improvement of left ventricular function and heart failure symptoms: the ANTHEM-HF study. J Card Fail 2013;19(9):655–60.

37. Zannad F, De Ferrari GM, Tuinenburg AE, et al. Chronic vagal stimulation for the treatment of low ejection fraction heart failure: results of the neural cardiac therapy for heart failure (NECTAR-HF) randomized controlled trial. Eur Heart J 2014. [Epub ahead of print].

38. Premchand RK, Sharma K, Mittal S, et al. Autonomic Regulation Therapy via Left or Right Cervical Vagus Nerve Stimulation in Patients with Chronic Heart Failure: Results of the ANTHEM-HF Trial. J Card Fail 2014;20(11):808–16.

39. Onkka P, Maskoun W, Rhee KS, et al. Sympathetic nerve fibers and ganglia in canine cervical vagus nerves: localization and quantitation. Heart Rhythm 2013;10(4):585–91.

40. Seki A, Green HR, Lee TD, et al. Sympathetic nerve fibers in human cervical and thoracic vagus nerves. Heart Rhythm 2014;11(8):1411–7.

41. Bakris GL, Nadim MK, Haller H, et al. Baroreflex activation therapy provides durable benefit in patients with resistant hypertension: results of long-term follow-up in the Rheos Pivotal Trial. J Am Soc Hypertens 2012;6(2):152–8.

42. Hoppe UC, Brandt MC, Wachter R, et al. Minimally invasive system for baroreflex activation therapy chronically lowers blood pressure with pacemaker-like safety profile: results from the Barostim neo trial. J Am Soc Hypertens 2012;6(4):270–6.

43. La Rovere MT, Specchia G, Mortara A, et al. Baroreflex sensitivity, clinical correlates, and cardiovascular mortality among patients with a first myocardial

infarction. A prospective study. Circulation 1988;
78(4):816–24.

44. Eckberg DL, Drabinsky M, Braunwald E. Defective
cardiac parasympathetic control in patients with
heart disease. N Engl J Med 1971;285(16):877–83.

45. Sabbah HN, Gupta RC, Imai M, et al. Chronic electrical stimulation of the carotid sinus baroreflex improves left ventricular function and promotes
reversal of ventricular remodeling in dogs with
advanced heart failure. Circ Heart Fail 2011;4(1):
65–70.

46. Zucker IH, Hackley JF, Cornish KG, et al. Chronic
baroreceptor activation enhances survival in dogs
with pacing-induced heart failure. Hypertension
2007;50(5):904–10.

47. Gronda E, Seravalle G, Brambilla G, et al. Chronic
baroreflex activation effects on sympathetic nerve
traffic, baroreflex function, and cardiac haemodynamics in heart failure: a proof-of-concept study.
Eur J Heart Fail 2014;16(9):977–83.

48. Rheos HOPE4HF Trial. Available at: http://clinical-
trials.gov/ct2/show/NCT00957073?term=NCT0095
7073&rank=1. Accessed August 31, 2014.

49. XR-1 Randomized Heart Failure study. Available at:
https://clinicaltrials.gov/ct2/show/NCT01471860?
term=NCT01471860&rank=1. Accessed August 31,
2014.

50. Barostim HOPE4HF (Hope for Heart Failure) Study.
Available at: https://clinicaltrials.gov/ct2/show/NCT0
1720160?term=NCT01720160&rank=1. Accessed
August 31, 2014.

51. Georgakopoulos D, Little WC, Abraham WT, et al.
Chronic baroreflex activation: a potential therapeutic
approach to heart failure with preserved ejection
fraction. J Card Fail 2011;17(2):167–78.

52. Krum H, Schlaich M, Whitbourn R, et al. Catheter-
based renal sympathetic denervation for resistant
hypertension: a multicentre safety and proof-of-
principle cohort study. Lancet 2009;373(9671):
1275–81.

53. Krum H, Sobotka P, Mahfoud F, et al. Device-based
antihypertensive therapy: therapeutic modulation of
the autonomic nervous system. Circulation 2011;
123(2):209–15.

54. Bohm M, Linz D, Ukena C, et al. Renal denervation
for the treatment of cardiovascular high risk-
hypertension or beyond? Circ Res 2014;115(3):
400–9.

55. Mahfoud F, Luscher TF, Andersson B, et al. Expert
consensus document from the European Society of
Cardiology on catheter-based renal denervation.
Eur Heart J 2013;34(28):2149–57.

56. Sakakura K, Ladich E, Cheng Q, et al. Anatomic
assessment of sympathetic peri-arterial renal nerves
in man. J Am Coll Cardiol 2014;64(7):635–43.

57. Esler MD, Krum H, Sobotka PA, et al. Renal sympathetic denervation in patients with treatment-

resistant hypertension (The Symplicity HTN-2 Trial):
a randomised controlled trial. Lancet 2010;
376(9756):1903–9.

58. Zhao Q, Yu S, Zou M, et al. Effect of renal sympathetic denervation on the inducibility of atrial fibrillation during rapid atrial pacing. J Interv Card
Electrophysiol 2012;35(2):119–25.

59. Nozawa T, Igawa A, Fujii N, et al. Effects of long-term
renal sympathetic denervation on heart failure after
myocardial infarction in rats. Heart Vessels 2002;
16(2):51–6.

60. Ukena C, Mahfoud F, Spies A, et al. Effects of renal
sympathetic denervation on heart rate and atrioventricular conduction in patients with resistant hypertension. Int J Cardiol 2013;167(6):2846–51.

61. Brandt MC, Mahfoud F, Reda S, et al. Renal sympathetic denervation reduces left ventricular hypertrophy and improves cardiac function in patients with
resistant hypertension. J Am Coll Cardiol 2012;
59(10):901–9.

62. Davies JE, Manisty CH, Petraco R, et al. First-in-man
safety evaluation of renal denervation for chronic systolic heart failure: primary outcome from REACH-Pilot
study. Int J Cardiol 2013;162(3):189–92.

63. Bhatt DL, Kandzari DE, O'Neill WW, et al.
A controlled trial of renal denervation for resistant hypertension. N Engl J Med 2014;370(15):1393–401.

64. Renal Denervation in Patients With Chronic Heart
Failure & Renal Impairment Clinical Trial (Sym-
plicityHF). Available at: https://clinicaltrials.gov/ct2/
show/NCT01392196?term=NCT01392196&rank=1.
Accessed August 31, 2014.

65. Renal Denervation in Patients With Chronic Heart
Failure. Available at: https://clinicaltrials.gov/ct2/
show/NCT02085668?term=NCT02085668&rank=1.
Accessed August 31, 2014.

66. Denervation of the renAl sympathetIc nerveS in
hearT Failure With nOrmal Lv Ejection Fraction
(DIASTOLE). Available at: https://clinicaltrials.gov/
ct2/show/NCT01583881?term=NCT01583881&
rank=1. Accessed August 31, 2014.

67. Renal Denervation in Heart Failure With Preserved
Ejection Fraction (RDT-PEF). Available at: https://
clinicaltrials.gov/ct2/show/NCT01840059?term=NC-
T01840059&rank=1. Accessed August 31, 2014.

68. Renal Denervation in Heart Failure Patients With Preserved Ejection Fraction (RESPECT-HF). Available
at: https://clinicaltrials.gov/ct2/show/NCT02041130?
term=NCT02041130&rank=1. Accessed August
31, 2014.

69. Kobayashi M, Sakurai S, Takaseya T, et al. Effect of
epivascular cardiac autonomic nerve stimulation on
cardiac function. Ann Thorac Surg 2012;94(4):
1150–6.

70. Kobayashi M, Sakurai S, Takaseya T, et al. Effects of
percutaneous stimulation of both sympathetic and
parasympathetic cardiac autonomic nerves on

cardiac function in dogs. Innovations (Phila) 2012; 7(4):282–9.

71. Armour JA, Murphy DA, Yuan BX, et al. Gross and microscopic anatomy of the human intrinsic cardiac nervous system. Anat Rec 1997;247(2):289–98.

72. Tan AY, Li H, Wachsmann-Hogiu S, et al. Autonomic innervation and segmental muscular disconnections at the human pulmonary vein-atrial junction: implications for catheter ablation of atrial-pulmonary vein junction. J Am Coll Cardiol 2006;48:132–43.

73. Shen MJ, Choi EK, Tan AY, et al. Neural mechanisms of atrial arrhythmias. Nat Rev Cardiol 2011;27:30–9.

74. Shinohara T, Shen MJ, Han S, et al. Heart failure decreases nerve activity in the right atrial ganglionated plexus. J Cardiovasc Electrophysiol 2012;23(4): 404–12.

75. Shen MJ, Zipes DP. Role of the autonomic nervous system in modulating cardiac arrhythmias. Circ Res 2014;114(6):1004–21.

76. Ambrosy AP, Fonarow GC, Butler J, et al. The global health and economic burden of hospitalizations for heart failure: lessons learned from hospitalized heart failure registries. J Am Coll Cardiol 2014;63(12): 1123–33.

77. Cohn JN, Pfeffer MA, Rouleau J, et al. Adverse mortality effect of central sympathetic inhibition with sustained-release moxonidine in patients with heart failure (MOXCON). Eur J Heart Fail 2003; 5(5):659–67.

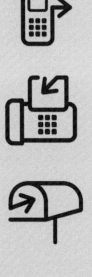

Printed and bound by CPI Group (UK) Ltd, Croydon, CR0 4YY

03/10/2024

01040375-0016